Pharmacology
for Prehospital
Emergency
Care
Second Edition

Incorporates 1992 AHA
Guidelines for Cardiopulmonary
Resuscitation and Emergency
Cardiac Care

Pharmacology
for Prehospital Emergency Care
Second Edition

Richard K. Beck, BBA, NREMT-P
Program Director
Department of Emergency Medicine
School of Primary Medical Care
University of Alabama in Huntsville
Huntsville, Alabama

Consulting Editor
James Robert Vance, PharmD
Clinical Coordinator of Pharmacy Services
Huntsville Hospital
Huntsville, Alabama
Adjunct Professor of Pharmacy
Auburn University School of Pharmacy
Auburn, Alabama

 F. A. DAVIS COMPANY • Philadelphia

F. A. Davis Company
1915 Arch Street
Philadelphia, PA 19103

Printed in the United States of America

Last digit indicates print number: 10 9 8 7 6 5 4

Acquisitions Editor: Lynn Borders Caldwell
Developmental Editor: Ralph Zickgraf
Production Editor: Rose Gabbay
Cover Design by: Steven R. Morrone

As new scientific information becomes available through basic and clinical research, recommended treatments and drug therapies undergo changes. The author(s) and publisher have done everything possible to make this book accurate, up to date, and in accord with accepted standards at the time of publication. The authors, editors, and publisher are not responsible for errors or omissions or for consequences from application of the book, and make no warranty, expressed or implied, in regard to the contents of the book. Any practice described in this book should be applied by the reader in accordance with professional standards of care used in regard to the unique circumstances that may apply in each situation. The reader is advised always to check product information (package inserts) for changes and new information regarding dose and contraindications before administering any drug. Caution is especially urged when using new or infrequently ordered drugs.

Library of Congress Cataloging-in-Publication Data

Beck, Richard K., 1947–
 Pharmacology for prehospital emergency care / Richard K. Beck ;
consulting editor, James Robert Vance.—2nd ed.
   p.   cm.
 "This edition includes the 1992 AHA recommendations for both adult
and pediatric emergency cardiac care"—Pref.
 Includes bibliographical references and index.
 ISBN 0-8036-0692-3 (softcover : alk paper) :
  1. Pharmacology. 2. Emergency medical technicians.   3. Medical
protocols.   I. Vance, James Robert.   II. American Heart
Association.   III. Title.   IV. Title: Pharmacology.
  [DNLM: 1. Drug Therapy—handbooks.   2. Emergencies—handbooks.
3. Emergency Medical Technicians.   QV 39 B393p 1994]
RM300.B38   1994
615'.1—dc20
DNLM/DLC   93-33629
for Library of Congress   CIP

This book is dedicated to my support system—my wife, Suzy, and my children, Brian and Amanda. Thank you for your love and support through what seemed to be a never-ending project.

Foreword

Each day a cry for help goes out and is answered by an EMT Paramedic, and each day an order is given by a physician to administer a therapeutic pharmacologic concoction in the hopes that a life might be saved. Day in and day out drugs are used in the prehospital setting to alleviate pain and suffering, and the EMT Paramedic is the primary administrator in most cases. The knowledge that the prehospital setting is a different environment than that of the in-house environment, coupled with the fact that physicians and nurses have their own respective pharmacology journals and manuals, makes it all too clear that the EMT Paramedic needs a manual to address the pharmacologic information that he or she will need when in the field.

This comprehensive book provides the paramedic with convenient, easy-to-understand information on the latest in prehospital emergency drug therapy. Its practicality and simplicity affords its effortless incorporation into most any paramedic curriculum, and it can also be skillfully used as a quick field reference.

Because the format and text are carefully designed without the complexities of other books and manuals, this book is very "user friendly." It uses helpful material such as ACLS algorithms, pediatric drug tables, formulas and equations, appendices, and relevant case scenarios that will be most appreciated by the reader.

Pharmacology for Prehospital Emergency Care, Second Edition, has been written with you, the paramedic, and your potential patient in mind. It should give you a better understanding of the newest techniques in administering the proper drug therapy that should give your patient the best possible chance of survival. As we all know, being in an emergency situation demands quick thinking and leaves very little margin for error. This book can help you prudently and judiciously employ the proper therapy when seconds count.

Rudy M. Veluz, MD
Diplomate of the American Board of Internal Medicine
Medical Director
    Basic Trauma Life Support, State of Alabama
Medical Director
    EMT Paramedic Program
    University of Alabama at Huntsville
    Huntsville, Alabama

Preface

Paramedics are routinely placed in positions in which quick decisions can mean the difference between life and death—especially when administering drugs. Administering drugs carries an enormous responsibility, and the knowledge the paramedic brings to the prehospital setting can make the difference in a successful patient outcome. The F. A. Davis Company agreed that there was a need for an up-to-date pharmacology textbook for paramedic students as well as a pharmacology guide for reference after graduation. This text serves both needs.

Pharmacology for Prehospital Emergency Care, Second Edition, is divided into two units. Unit One begins with an introduction to pharmacology. From there, such topics as understanding pharmacokinetics and pharmacodynamics, the autonomic nervous system, the correct methods for administering drugs, how to calculate drug dosages, and understanding fluids, electrolytes, and acid-base balance are presented. At the end of each chapter in Unit One are study questions. Correct answers and explanations as to why a particular answer is correct are presented at the end of the book.

Unit Two presents a detailed description of each drug by body system affected. This description includes the drug's generic and trade names, its therapeutic classification(s), mechanism of action, therapeutic benefits, indication(s) for prehospital use, contraindications, precautions, route and dosage, adverse reactions and side effects, any implications that the paramedic should know, and any drug interactions of which the paramedic should be aware. Chapter 7 contains the drugs that pertain to cardiovascular emergencies. On October 28, 1992, **JAMA, The Journal of the American Medical Association,** published the American Heart Association's (AHA) new recommendations of the 1992 National Conference concerning the guidelines for cardiopulmonary resuscitation and emergency cardiac care. In keeping with these recent advancements, this edition includes the 1992 AHA recommendations for both adult and pediatric emergency cardiac care.

At the end of each chapter in Unit Two, there are short case studies that illustrate how drugs can be used in various emergency situations and an extended case study.

Following Unit Two there are three appendices. Appendix A lists common medications that the paramedic may encounter, Appendix B explains the proper procedure for endotracheal intubation, and Appendix C presents a pediatric drug-dose chart.

Finally, a glossary defines terms that pertain to each chapter in this book.

I hope that *Pharmacology for Prehospital Emergency Care, Second Edition,* will be of value in the classroom and an aid for practicing paramedics.

Richard K. Beck

Acknowledgments

It has taken a lot of people to produce this text. My name is on the cover, but the book would not exist if it were not for many other talented people.

The folks at F. A. Davis were super. It was Don Weiss who first suggested that I call Jean-François Vilain, Senior Editor, to see if I was up to doing this project. Jean-François (who must like to gamble) said "Let's do it, my friend" and assigned me to Mark Wales (formerly of F. A. Davis). Mark got me on the right track to get this project going, and it was the expertise of Ralph Zickgraf who kept me on track once Mark left. A big THANK YOU to everyone at F. A. Davis.

I also want to thank Lindsey R. Thompson for his excellent artwork and to Bryan Turner for his expert photography.

The reviewers of a manuscript tell it like it is. Sometimes that was difficult to take, but their expertise and honest criticism helped with enormous recommendations for improvement. So, for their painstaking, professional manuscript review I wish to thank R. Allen Dulaney, NREMT-P, North Eastern Regional EMS, Kearneysville, West Virginia; Gary Ferguson, PhD, Northeast Louisiana University, Monroe, Louisiana; Jim Holbrook, Crafton Hills College, San Bernardino, California; Eugene Iannuzzi, RN, CEN, EMT-P; Dr. Sheldon Jacobson, Hospital of the University of Pennsylvania, Philadelphia; Peter W. Josimovich, NREMT-P; James L. Paturas, Bridgeport Hospital, Bridgeport, Connecticut; and William Toon, NREMT-P, Nyack Hospital, Nyack, New York.

I would also like to thank my students who sat patiently in class while I experimented on them with the manuscript. They too were honest and made valuable suggestions.

And finally, I want to thank my wife Suzy. She read the manuscript and also made enormous recommendations on how to make improvements. This book would not be a reality without her support.

Contents

Unit One

INTRODUCTION TO UNIT ONE

Pharmacology for Prehospital Emergency Care was written to fulfill the educational needs of paramedic students. It will also be useful as an easy-to-read reference text after graduation.

Unit One attempts to construct a foundation on which you can build. For example, Chapter 1 introduces you to pharmacology in general. It explains essential drug information about each drug presented. Also explained are such topics as drug origins, drug preparation, drug testing, and legislation governing drugs manufactured in the United States. Chapter 2 explains how drugs move through the body once they are administered and the mechanism of action a drug produces once it reaches its target receptor.

Many drugs given in prehospital emergency medicine affect the autonomic nervous system. Chapter 3 gives an overview of the autonomic nervous system and explains how selected drugs interact with its functions.

Chapter 4 explains the various routes through which drugs can be administered and gives step-by-step instruction on the procedures for correct drug administration.

Some drugs are administered according to body weight, some are given by a predetermined dosage, and some must be added to intravenous solutions before they are administered. Chapter 5 explains basic mathematics and illustrates how to calculate drug dosages.

Finally, the conditions of the body's pH, fluids, and electrolytes affect the therapeutic effects of drugs. Chapter 6 reviews fluids, electrolytes, and acid-base balance in an attempt to explain the importance of maintaining these factors within normal limits to enable drugs to produce their therapeutic effects.

The chapters in Unit One are organized to help you build your foundation. Each chapter opens with an introduction and ends with a conclusion and study questions with explanations for the correct answers. This format is designed to help you study and understand each chapter's content more fully.

Chapter 1

Introduction to Pharmacology

A **drug** is any substance that, when taken into the body, changes one or more of the body's functions. Drugs are most commonly used in medicine to treat or prevent disease. **Pharmacology** is the science of drugs and includes the study of their origin, ingredients, uses, and actions on the body. Branches of pharmacology include toxicology and therapeutics. **Toxicology** is the study of poisons and undesired drug reactions. **Therapeutics** is the use of drugs for the treatment of disease.

To understand how a drug works therapeutically, a basic understanding of both pharmacodynamics and pharmacokinetics is needed. **Pharmacodynamics** is the study of drug *actions* on the body, and it is the basis of drug treatment. **Pharmacokinetics** is the study of drug *movement* through the body over a period of time, including absorption, duration of action, distribution, metabolism or biotransformation, and elimination. Chapter 2 presents a detailed discussion of pharmacodynamics and pharmacokinetics. Figure 1-1 illustrates the

3

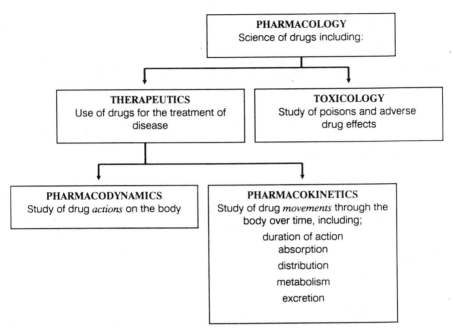

Figure 1–1. The structure of pharmacology.

relationships of therapeutics, toxicology, pharmacodynamics, and pharmaco-kinetics to the science of pharmacology.

ESSENTIAL DRUG INFORMATION

Administering drugs in the prehospital setting carries an enormous responsibility. Without question, you are placed in a position that may save many lives through proper drug administration. Drugs produce a variety of physiologic responses, including raising or lowering blood pressure, increasing or decreasing heart rate, and sedating or activating the patient. If the wrong drug or the incorrect dose of the appropriate drug is given, the results could be fatal.

For example, Mrs. Clark, age 76, presented with symptomatic chest pain and premature ventricular contractions (PVCs). Normally, the first drug Mrs. Clark should receive is oxygen. Oxygen may prevent further injury to the heart or may eliminate some of the PVCs. The next drug Mrs. Clark should receive is lidocaine, an **antiarrhythmic** drug used to suppress PVCs. Patients over 70, however, usually have a reduced **volume of distribution.** This means that Mrs. Clark has fewer plasma proteins in her body to which the lidocaine can bind, causing more of the drug to be free (or active) than would be normal in a younger person. (See Chapter 7.) Persons over 70 should initially receive the normal bolus dose, followed by half the normal maintenance infusion. This is just one example of why it is essential that you be thoroughly familiar with the following categories of information for all the drugs you are permitted to give:

Mechanism of Action

A drug's mechanism of action describes how the drug produces its desired therapeutic effects. For example, lidocaine works by decreasing the excitability of the heart muscle and the cardiac conduction system.

Therapeutic Benefits

Therapeutic benefits describe the results expected from administering a drug. For example, the therapeutic effects expected from lidocaine include suppressing PVCs in the presence of an acute myocardial infarction (MI).

Indications for Prehospital Use

The indications for a drug's use include the most common uses for that drug in the prehospital setting. For example, common uses for lidocaine in the prehospital setting include treatment of ventricular ectopy, ventricular tachycardia, and ventricular fibrillation.

Contraindications

A drug's contraindications are the circumstances under which it should not be used or alternative drugs should be considered. For example, lidocaine may be contraindicated in a patient who is experiencing a cardiac conduction problem, because the decrease in cardiac excitability that lidocaine causes may further deteriorate the patient's condition.

Precautions

Precautions describe situations in which drug use may be dangerous to the patient or when **dosage** or administration techniques may have to be modified. For example, rapid administration of lidocaine may cause an unexpected drop in blood pressure or slowing of the heart rate.

Route and Dosage

The route of a drug describes how the drug is given and the dosage tells how much of the drug should be given. For example, the initial adult dose for lidocaine when treating ventricular tachycardia is 1 to 1.5 milligrams per kilogram of body weight given through an established intravenous line. If an intravenous line has not been established, another route in which lidocaine can be given is down an established endotracheal tube (Appendix B describes the procedure for endotracheal tube placement). You should know or have readily available references that give both the adult and pediatric dosages of each drug that may be administered.

Adverse Reactions and Side Effects

A drug's adverse reactions and side effects are any actions or effects other than those desired. Some side effects of a drug are predictable and may occur in addition to the expected therapeutic effects. Potential side effects of lidocaine include anxiety, nausea, and twitching and numbness of the extremities.

Paramedic Implications

Paramedic implications explain special information that may be helpful when giving a specific drug. For example, patients over 70 have a reduced volume of distribution, which makes it necessary to reduce the maintenance infusion dosage of lidocaine by 50 percent.

Drug Interactions

Drug interactions explain the more common drug-drug interactions and their results that may occur in the prehospital setting. For example, simultaneous use of lidocaine and **beta-blockers** may cause lidocaine toxicity.

DRUG SOURCES

Drugs originate from four main sources: plants, animals, minerals or mineral products (inorganic), and chemicals made in the laboratory (synthetic).

Plant Sources

Leaves, roots, seeds, and other plant parts may be processed for use as drugs. For example, the drug atropine, used to treat symptomatic bradycardia, is obtained from the plant called deadly nightshade (its scientific name is *Atropa belladonna*). Other examples include the drugs digitalis and morphine. Digitalis, used to treat supraventricular arrhythmias and congestive heart failure, originates from the leaves of the foxglove plant *(Digitalis purpurea)*. Morphine, used in prehospital medicine as an analgesic, originates from the opium poppy (*Papaver somniferum*).

Animal Sources

Some of the most powerful drugs are extracted from animal tissue. These drugs are often used to replace insufficient human glandular secretions. For example, insulin, which is used for the treatment of diabetes mellitus, is a hormone extracted from the pancreas of pork or beef. Another example is oxytocin, a pituitary hormone used to control postpartum hemorrhage.

Inorganic Sources

Materials such as sulfur and iodine and mineral salts are commonly used to manufacture drugs. Probably the most common prehospital drug made from mineral sources is sodium bicarbonate, used to treat metabolic acidosis. Magnesium sulfate, used to treat eclampsia, is a naturally occurring mineral commonly obtained from well and sea water.

Synthetic Sources

Synthetic drugs are man-made, produced by chemical processes. Today, most drugs are synthetic. The most commonly used synthetic prehospital drug is lidocaine.

DRUG LEGISLATION

At the beginning of the twentieth century, no federal laws controlled drug distribution. During the first 10 years of the twentieth century, the use of chemicals in medicine increased rapidly. This increase brought with it an increased use of dangerous ingredients and complex formulas. Some drug companies used poor quality control and made unproved claims for their products. This made it necessary to develop national standards and government regulations to guarantee that drugs sold to the public were accurately identified and of uniform strength and purity. For these reasons, Congress enacted several laws.

Food and Drug Act (Pure Food Act) of 1906

Congress enacted the Pure Food Act to prevent the manufacture and trafficking of mislabeled, poisonous, or harmful food and drugs. This legislation named the *United States Pharmacopeia* (USP) and the *National Formulary* (NF) as official drug standards and established the Food and Drug Administration (FDA). The Pure Food Act authorized the FDA to determine if drugs were safe and effective and to enforce these standards.

Federal Food, Drug, and Cosmetic Act of 1938

The Federal Food, Drug, and Cosmetic Act updated the Pure Food Act. This legislation required that labels list the possible habit-forming properties and side effects of drugs. It also authorized the FDA to determine the safety of drugs before marketing and required that dangerous drugs be issued only by the prescription of a physician, dentist, or veterinarian. This act was amended by the Durham-Humphrey amendment in 1952. The Durham-Humphrey amendment classified certain drugs as "legend" drugs and restricted pharmacists from distributing legend drugs without a prescription. Legend drugs are those that must be labeled "Caution: Federal Law prohibits dispensing without a prescription." In 1962, the Federal Food, Drug, and Cosmetic Act was amended again by the Kefauver-Harris amendment, which authorized the FDA to establish official names for drugs and required drug manufacturers to prove a drug's ability to produce therapeutic results.

Harrison Narcotic Act of 1914

The Harrison Narcotic Act was the first federal legislation designed to stop drug addiction or dependence. It established federal control over the importation, manufacture, and sale of the opium and coca plants and all their compounds and derivatives.

Other Drug Laws and Regulations

The Harrison Narcotic Act and all further drug abuse amendments were superseded by the Controlled Substance Act of 1970. The Controlled Substance Act classifies drugs with abuse potential into five schedules by weighing a drug's potential for abuse against its medical usefulness (Table 1–1). For exam-

Table 1–1. SCHEDULE OF CONTROLLED DRUGS

Schedule	Characteristics	Examples
I	High potential for abuse No accepted medical use Research purposes only May lead to severe dependence	Heroin, marijuana, LSD, peyote, mescaline
II	High potential for abuse Accepted medical use May lead to severe dependence (physical and/or psychologic)	Opium, morphine, codeine, methadone, amphetamine
III	Moderate potential for abuse Accepted medical use May lead to moderate to low physical and high psychologic dependence	Drugs with limited amounts of opium, codeine, and morphine
IV	Low potential for abuse Accepted medical use May lead to limited dependence (physical or psychologic)	Barbital, chloral hydrate, phenobarbital, diazepam
V	Low potential for abuse Accepted medical use Has low potential for dependence (physical or psychologic)	Drugs used for relief of coughs or diarrhea, containing limited amounts of certain narcotics

ple, a Schedule I drug has high potential for abuse and no accepted medical usefulness, whereas a Schedule V drug has little potential for abuse and a recognized medical use.

Other federal agencies involved in regulating drugs include the Drug Enforcement Administration (DEA), the Public Health Service, and the Federal Trade Commission (FTC). The DEA is empowered to enforce the Controlled Substance Act. The Public Health Service, part of the U.S. Department of Health and Human Services, regulates biologic products. The FTC regulates drug advertising. It has the power to prevent false or misleading advertising of food, drugs, and cosmetics to the general public. The FTC also regulates prescription drug advertising to the medical profession for those drugs regulated by the FDA. The FTC relies on the FDA to regulate the claims of nonprescription drug advertisements.

DRUG STANDARDS AND TESTING

All drugs sold in the United States must meet and maintain high standards for therapeutic results, patient safety, and packaging safety. To meet these standards, drugs must go through strict and accurate testing that may take several years to complete. Initial drug testing begins with animal studies to determine the drug's toxicity, **therapeutic index** (a measurement of the relative safety of the drug), and pharmacokinetics. This initial testing must be done on two species of animals.

In addition to animal studies, drugs may undergo four phases of human testing before being approved by the FDA. Phase I is the initial drug evaluation, which involves small groups of healthy subjects. The goals of phase I are to prove the drug's safety and to identify tolerable dosages. If phase I testing shows that the drug is safe to give in expected therapeutic doses, the studies continue to phase II. Phase II consists of controlled evaluations designed to test the drug's effect on the specific illness for which it was designed. Phase II testing also helps to establish dosage and other pharmacokinetic information. It is during phase II testing that drug manufacturers determine if they have a marketable product before continuing with more expensive testing involved in phase III. Phase III consists of the full-scale or extended clinical evaluations. Phase III evaluations are performed on a large number of patients to determine therapeutic effect and possible side effects and to decide if the side effects are low enough to be acceptable. Phase IV drug testing is a postmarketing evaluation designed to update safety and product results and to clarify the incidence of adverse drug reactions and long-term effects. Phases I through III are almost always required. Although phase IV is not required of all drugs, the FDA prefers that all drugs go through all four phases.

There are several sources of drug information. The Pure Food Act of 1906 established the *USP* and the *NF* as the two official drug standards in the country. A new edition of the *USP* is issued every 5 years, and supplements are issued regularly. The *NF* was originally published to describe drugs of established usefulness that contained ingredients discontinued from the *USP*. The two books are now published as one volume.

Another source for drug information is the *United States Adopted Names (USAN)* and the *USP Dictionary of Drug Names*. This dictionary includes the **generic** and **trade names** of drugs, drug code designations, and Chemical Abstracts Service registry numbers. The ***Physician's Desk Reference (PDR)*** contains such information as the drug's indications, therapeutic effects, dosages, administration, warnings, contraindications, precautions, side effects, and drug interactions. Essentially, the information in the *PDR* is the same as that provided in drug package inserts. Professional journals are another good source for drug information. Articles in these journals can help emergency medical service (EMS) professionals keep up to date on current and possible future drugs.

DRUG NOMENCLATURE

From the time a drug is initially tested in the laborabory until it is approved and marketed, it can obtain up to four names. A drug's **chemical name**

Table 1–2. DRUG NOMENCLATURE

Chemical Name	Generic Name	Trade Name*	Official Name
Common Prehospital Drugs			
2-(diethylamino)-N-(2,6-dimethylphenyl) acetamide nomohydrochloride	Lidocaine hydrochloride	Xylocaine	Lidocaine hydrochloride, USP
1,2-benzenediol, 4-(2-aminoethyl)-, hydrochloride	Dopamine hydrochloride	Intropin	Dopamine hydrochloride, USP
Common Home Prescription Drugs			
Card-20(22)-enolide,3-[(0,2,dideoxy-β-D-ribo-hexopyranosyl-(1→4)-0-2,6-dideoxy-D-ribo-hexopyranosyl) oxy]-12, 14-dihydroxy-,(3β, 5β, 12β)-	Digoxin	Lanoxin	Digoxin, USP
Benzoic acid, 5-(aminosul-fonyl)-4-chloro-2-[(2-furanylmethyl)amino]-2-propanol, 1-[(1-methylethyl)amino]-3-(1-naphthalenyloxy)-, hydrochloride	Furosemide	Lasix	Furosemide, USP
	Propranolol hydrochloride	Inderal	Propranolol hydrochloride, USP
Common Over-the-Counter Drugs			
Benzoic acid, 2-(acetyloxy)-	Aspirin	Ecotrin	Aspirin, USP
Ethanamine, 2-(diphenylmethoxy)-N,N-dimethyl-, hydrochloride	Diphenhydramine hydrochloride	Benadryl	Diphenhydramine hydrochloride, USP
Acetamide, N-(4-hydroxy-phenyl)-	Acetaminophen	Tylenol	Acetaminophen, USP

* A single drug may have several different trade names.

is an exact description of the drug's structure and composition. For example, $C_{18}H_{23}NO_3.HCL$, *1,2-benzenediol,4-[2-[[3-(4-hydroxyphenyl)-1-methylpropyl]-,hydrochloride, ( )-* is the chemical name for a drug used in treating patients with low cardiac output. This same drug's **generic** or **nonproprietary** name is dobutamine hydrochloride; this name was given by the company that first formulated it. Third, the manufacturer registers a drug using a **trade** or **proprietary** name. A trade name is often designated in print by its initial capital letter and the raised registered symbol (*R*) following the name. For example, a trade name for dobutamine hydrochloride is Dobutrex®. Finally, the *USP* and *NF* give a drug its official name after it has met specific standards for quality, strength, purity, packaging, and labeling. Drugs meeting these standards are designated by the letters USP following their name. The official name for dobutamine hydrochloride is dobutamine hydrochloride, USP. The generic and official names of a drug are usually the same. To avoid confusion, it is best to refer to a drug by its generic name. Table 1–2 illustrates examples of the chemical, generic, trade, and official names of some common prehospital drugs as well as some common over-the-counter (OTC) and prescription drugs.

THERAPEUTIC DRUG CLASSIFICATIONS

Drugs are generally classified into categories according to the body tissues they affect and their therapeutic and physiologic effects. For example, lidocaine is therapeutically classified as a ventricular antiarrhythmic. Lidocaine works by decreasing the excitability of the heart muscle and the cardiac conduction system. Therapeutically, lidocaine suppresses ventricular ectopic activity. Understanding drug classifications will help you understand why a particular drug is prescribed and how the drug affects the body.

Drugs can have more than one therapeutic classification. For example, epinephrine can be therapeutically classified as a bronchodilator, cardiac stimulator, or peripheral vasoconstrictor. You should be familiar with the following therapeutic drug classifications.

Adrenocorticoid: An adrenocorticoid is one of a group of hormones secreted by the adrenal cortex. An adrenocorticoid drug included in this text is hydrocortisone (page 206).

Analgesics: An analgesic is a drug that relieves pain. Analgesic drugs included in this text are

butorphanol, page 101
hydromorphone, page 113
meperidine, page 120
morphine, page 122

nalbuphine, page 123
nitrous oxide–oxygen mixture, page 127
pentazocine, page 130

Antianginal: An antianginal is a drug that relieves the pain of angina pectoris. Antianginal drugs included in this text are

nitroglycerin, page 125
verapamil, page 136

Antianxiety agents: An antianxiety agent is a drug that prevents or controls anxiety episodes. The antianxiety agents included in this text are

diazepam, page 230
hydroxyzine, page 232

Antiarrhythmics: Antiarrhythmics correct cardiac arrhythmias. The drug of choice depends on the cause of the arrhythmia and the condition of the patient. Antiarrhythmics included in this text are

atropine, page 97
bretylium, page 99
digoxin, page 104
edrophonium, page 108
lidocaine, page 117

phenytoin, page 131
procainamide, page 132
propranolol, page 133
verapamil, page 136

Anticonvulsants: Anticonvulsants depress abnormal neuronal discharges in the **central nervous system (CNS)** that may cause seizures. Anticonvulsants included in this text are

diazepam, page 185
phenobarbital, page 188

phenytoin, page 189

Antidiabetic agent: An antidiabetic agent is a drug that prevents or relieves diabetes. The antidiabetic agent included in this text is insulin (page 176).

Antidote: An antidote is a drug that neutralizes poisons or their effects on the body. Antidotes included in this text are

activated charcoal, page 213
atropine, page 215

physostigmine, page 219
pralidoxime, page 220

Antihistamine: An antihistamine is a drug that blocks the effects of histamine, relieving the symptoms associated with allergic reactions. An antihistamine included in this text is diphenhydramine (page 204).

Antihypertensives: Antihypertensives lower blood pressure to a normal level (or as low as is safe for the patient). Antihypertensive drugs included in this text are

diazoxide, page 103
furosemide, page 112
hydralazine, page 113
labetalol, page 116

metoprolol, page 121
nitroprusside, page 126
propranolol, page 133
verapamil, page 136

Antihypoglycemic: An antihypoglycemic is a drug that prevents or relieves **hypoglycemia.** An antihypoglycemic agent included in this text is glucagon (page 175).

Anti-inflammatory: An anti-inflammatory agent is a drug that counteracts inflammation. Anti-inflammatory agents included in this text are

dexamethasone, page 184

methylprednisolone, page 188

Antipsychotics: An antipsychotic is a drug that blocks dopamine receptors in the brain. Antipsychotics inlcuded in this text are

chlorpromazine, page 229

haloperidol, page 231

Antitussives: Antitussives are drugs that suppress coughing. An antitussive included in this text is hydromorphone (page 113).

Bronchodilators: Bronchodilators are drugs used to treat airway obstruction caused by asthma or chronic obstructive pulmonary disease (COPD). Bronchodilators included in this text are

albuterol, page 160

aminophylline, page 161

epinephrine, page 162

isoproterenol, page 114

isoetharine, page 164

metaproterenol, page 165

terbutaline, page 167

racemic epinephrine, page 163

Calcium supplements: Calcium supplements replace needed calcium in the body. Calcium supplements included in this text are

calcium chloride, page 102

calcium gluceptate, page 102

calcium gluconate, page 102

Cardiac stimulators: A cardiac stimulator stimulates the heart to increase blood pressure and cardiac output. Cardiac stimulators included in this text are

epinephrine, page 109

isoproterenol, page 114

Cholinergic agonist: A cholinergic agonist strengthens, prolongs, or prevents the breakdown of the **neurotransmitter acetylcholine.** A cholinergic agonist included in this text is edrophonium (page 108).

Coronary vasodilator: A coronary vasodilator is a drug that increases the diameter of the coronary blood vessels. The coronary vasodilator included in this text is nitroglycerin (page 125).

Cyanide poisoning adjunct: A cyanide poisoning adjunct is a drug that degrades cyanide in cases of cyanide poisoning. A cyanide poisoning adjunct included in this text is amyl nitrate (page 214).

Diuretics: Diuretics promote the elimination of electrolytes and water. Diuretics included in this text are

bumetanide, page 100

ethacrynic acid, page 111

furosemide, page 112

Emetic: An emetic is an agent that causes vomiting. An emetic included in this text is syrup of ipecac (page 222).

Hydrogen ion buffer: A hydrogen ion buffer is used to bring the hydrogen ion concentration of the blood within normal levels. The hydrogen ion buffer included in this text is sodium bicarbonate (page 134).

Hyperglycemic: A hyperglycemic is a drug used to restore circulating blood sugar levels to normal in states of hypoglycemia. A hyperglycemic included in this text is dextrose 50% in water (page 173).

Immunosuppressant: An immunosuppressant is a drug that interferes with the body's natural immune response to an **antigen.** An immunosuppressant included in this text is methylprednisolone (page 188).

Inotropics: Inotropic drugs increase cardiac output. They are used for the short-term management of congestive heart failure or poor cardiac output. Inotropics included in this text are

amrinone, page 96   dobutamine, page 105
digoxin, page 104   dopamine, page 106

Medicinal gases: The two most common uses for medicinal gases in the prehospital setting are to increase or maintain the partial pressure of oxygen (PaO_2) in the arterial blood and to cause pain relief. Medicinal gases included in this text are

nitrous oxide–oxygen mixture,   oxygen, page 129
   page 127

Narcotic antagonist: A narcotic antagonist is a drug that reverses the adverse effects of narcotics. A narcotic antagonist included in this text is naloxone (page 217).

Oxytocic: An oxytocic is a drug that stimulates uterine contractions. An oxytocic included in this text is oxytocin (page 198).

Peripheral vasoconstrictor: A peripheral vasoconstrictor is a drug that constricts the peripheral blood vessels. A peripheral vasoconstrictor included in this text is epinephrine (page 109).

Sedative/hypnotic: Sedatives are drugs used to treat various anxiety states, and hypnotics are used to treat insomnia. A drug classified as both a sedative and hypnotic included in this text is phenobarbital (page 188). A drug included in this text classified as a sedative is hydroxyzine (page 232).

Skeletal muscle relaxant: A skeletal muscle relaxant is a drug used to relax injured muscles, as in orthopedic emergencies. A skeletal muscle relaxant included in this text is diazepam (page 185).

Vasodilator: A vasodilator is a drug that relaxes the blood vessels. A vasodilator included in this text is amrinone (page 96).

Vasopressors: A vasopressor is a drug that causes contractions of the muscles of the capillaries and arteries. Vasopressors included in this text are

dopamine, page 106   norepinephrine, page 128

Vitamin: A vitamin is a substance essential for normal **metabolism,** growth, and development. Vitamins are given to treat vitamin deficiencies. A vitamin included in this text is thiamine (page 177).

DRUG PREPARATIONS

Drugs generally come in three types of preparations: solid, liquid, or gas. A drug preparation may produce either local or systemic effects.

Drugs taken orally have the advantage of being easy to take, and oral administration is generally the safest way to take medicines. The disadvantages of oral medications are (1) the drug absorption process generally takes longer,

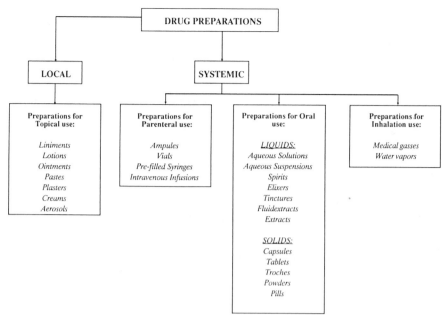

Figure 1–2. The way in which a drug is prepared determines whether it has a local or systemic effect.

and (2) the eventual concentration of the drug in the bloodstream is often unpredictable.

Drugs administered directly into the bloodstream have the advantage of bypassing the absorption process, which enables the drug to produce its desired therapeutic effect much sooner. However, this type of drug administration has the disadvantage of being more difficult and much more dangerous.

A local drug effect is confined to one specific area of the body. For example, a medicated lotion may be applied to an irritated area of the skin for the relief of a rash. A systemic effect occurs when a drug enters into the bloodstream, affecting all body tissues. Figure 1–2 categorizes types of drug preparations based on whether they produce local or systemic effects. For example, an antibiotic drug can be absorbed into the bloodstream to systemically fight off infection.

The following are common drug preparations with which you should become familiar.

Drug Preparations for Local Effects

Topical use

Liniment: A liniment is a liquid containing a medication in oil, alcohol, or water.

Lotion: A lotion is a liquid suspension for external application.

Ointment: An ointment is a semisolid preparation for external application of a drug or medicine.

Pastes: A paste is a semisolid gelatinous substance, for external application, that may contain specific active ingredients or simple materials such as oils, waxes, and starch.

Plasters: A plaster is an external medicinal preparation formed into a mass harder than an ointment and spread over muslin, linen, skin, or paper.

Cream: A cream is a smooth, thick liquid or a semisolid emulsion for external application.

Aerosol: An aerosol is a colloid or gluelike substance finely subdivided into liquid or solid particles that are dispensed in the form of a mist.

Colloid: A gluelike substance, such as a protein or starch, whose particles when dispersed in a solvent to the greatest possible degree remain uniformly distributed and fail to form a true solution.

Drug Preparations for Systemic Effects

Oral use

Liquid

Aqueous solution: An aqueous solution is a substance dissolved in water.

Aqueous suspension: An aqueous suspension consists of solid particles mixed with but not dissolved in water.

Spirits: A spirit is an alcoholic or hydroalcoholic solution of volatile substances.

Elixirs: An elixir is a sweetened hydroalcoholic liquid used alone or as a vehicle for active drugs.

Tinctures: A tincture is an alcoholic solution of vegetable or chemical material.

Fluid extracts: A fluid extract is a solution of the dissolved component part of vegetable drugs such that each milliliter equals 1.0 gram of the drug. Fluid extracts contain alcohol as a solvent or preservative or both.

Extracts: An extract is the active ingredient of a vegetable or animal drug obtained by distillation or other chemical process. There are three forms of extracts: semiliquid, solid, or powdered.

Solid

Capsule: A capsule is a gelatin container used for single-dose drug administration.

Tablet: A tablet is a small solid mass of medicinal powder. Tablets may be round, oblong, cylindrical, or triangular.

Troche or lozenge: A **troche** is a solid disk or cylindrical mass of a medicine in a flavored base.

Powder: A powder consists of fine particles of a medicine.

Pill: A pill is a medication in the form of a small solid mass or pellet.

Parenteral use

A parenteral route is defined as any route other than the alimentary canal, for example, intravenous, transtracheal, intraosseous, subcutaneous, or intramuscular.

Ampule: An ampule is a small, sealed single-dose glass container for a liquid injectable drug.

Vial: A vial is a small glass bottle that contains more than one dose of a drug.

Prefilled syringe: A prefilled syringe is usually a single-dose glass cartridge containing a liquid drug.

Intravenous infusion: An intravenous infusion is a sterile liquid preparation with or without added drugs.

Other preparations for systemic effect

Inhalants: An inhalant is a gas, a mixture of gases, or water vapors intended to be inhaled for medicinal purposes.

Suppositories: A suppository is a semisolid cylinder or cone-shaped mass that is introduced into the body by insertion into the rectum, vagina, or urethra.

PHARMACOLOGIC ABBREVIATIONS

Abbreviations are common in medicine. Using abbreviations appropriately can make you more efficient, especially in your never-ending battle with paperwork. Table 1–3 lists standard pharmacologic and other medical abbreviations with which you should be familiar.

Table 1–3. COMMON ABBREVIATIONS

Abbreviation	Meaning	Abbreviation	Meaning
$\bar{a}$	before	C	centigrade
		$\bar{c}$	with
aa	of each	CC or C/C	chief complaint
ACh	acetylcholine	cc or cm³	cubic centimeter
ACLS	Advanced Cardiac Life Support	Ca^{2+}	calcium ion
ALS	Advanced Life Support	$CaCl_2$	calcium chloride
AMA	against medical advice/American Medical Association	Caps	capsules
		CHF	congestive heart failure
		Cl^-	chloride ion
α	alpha	cm	centimeter
amp	ampule	c/o	complains of
ASA	aspirin	CO	carbon monoxide
bid	twice daily	CO_2	carbon dioxide
BLS	Basic Life Support	COPD	chronic obstructive pulmonary disease
β	beta		

Table 1–3. COMMON ABBREVIATIONS (*Continued*)

Abbreviation	Meaning	Abbreviation	Meaning
CPR	cardiopulmonary resuscitation	Ms or MSO_4	morphine sulfate
CVA	cerebrovascular accident	Na^+	sodium ion
		$NaHCO_3$	sodium bicarbonate
D/C	discontinue	Ng tube	nasogastric tube
dig.	digitalis	nitro	nitroglycerin
Dx	diagnosis	NKA	no known allergies
D_5W	dextrose 5% in water	N_2O	nitrous oxide
$D_{5\ 1/2}NS$	dextrose 5% in ½ normal saline	NPO	nothing by mouth
		NS	normal saline
$D_{50}W$	dextrose 50% in water	O_2	oxygen
ECG or EKG	electrocardiogram	OD	overdose
EGTA	esophageal gastric tube airway	oz	ounce
		p̄	after
EOA	esophageal obturator airway	p.c.	after meals
		PCO_2	carbon dioxide pressure
et	and		
ETOH	ethyl alcohol	Peds	pediatric
ETT	endotracheal tube	p.o.	by mouth
F	Fahrenheit	pH	hydrogen ion concentration
G or gm	gram		
gr	grain	PO_2	oxygen pressure or tension
gtt	drop		
gtts	drops	prn	as needed
h or hr	hour	q̄	every
Hx	history	qd	every day
IM	intramuscular	qh	every hour
IV	intravenous	qid	four times a day
K^+	potassium ion	RBC	red blood count
kg	kilogram	RL	Ringer's lactate
KO	keep open	Rx	take; treatment
KVO	keep vein open	s̄	without
L	liter	SC or SQ	subcutaneous
lb	pound	SL	sublingual
LR or RL	lactated Ringer's or Ringer's lactate	S.O.B.	shortness of breath
		ss	half
m	meter	s/s	signs/symptoms
mEq	milliequivalent	tab	tablet
mg	milligram	tid	three times a day
min	minute	TKO	to keep open
μqm/mcg	microgram	u	unit
ml	milliliter	VO	verbal order
mm	millimeter	vol	volume

Table 1–3. COMMON ABBREVIATIONS (*Continued*)

Abbreviation	Meaning	Abbreviation	Meaning
WNL	within normal limits	R	right
wt	weight	L	left
y.o.	year old	~	approximate
↑	increased	0	normal
↓	decreased	♂	male
Ø	none	♀	female

CONCLUSION

Administering drugs is a part of complete prehospital emergency care that carries an enormous responsibility. Understanding pharmacology is more than knowing which drug to administer and when to administer it. Every EMS professional who administers drugs must be familiar with the drugs used in his or her EMS system, including each drug's actions, indications, contraindications, side effects, precautions, and correct dosage; the route in which the drug should be given; and any pertinent drug interactions. Giving the correct drug appropriately can save a life—giving the same drug inappropriately can be deadly.

STUDY QUESTIONS

1. Name the four major sources of drugs, and give examples of each.

2. The primary reason for drug legislation (such as the Federal Food, Drug and Cosmetic Act) is to:
   a. Control narcotic drugs.
   b. Ensure the safety of drugs manufactured.
   c. Ensure the sterility of manufactured goods.
   d. Keep health care professionals from abusing drugs.

3. Define the following names that are given to a drug during the period from initial laboratory testing to final approval and marketing.
   a. Chemical name.
   b. Generic name.
   c. Trade name.
   d. Official name.

Chapter 2

Understanding Pharmacokinetics and Pharmacodynamics

For drugs to produce their desired therapeutic effects, they must take a complicated journey through the body. Once a drug is given, it is absorbed into the circulatory system, distributed to its site of action, and finally eliminated from the body. *Pharmacokinetics* is the study of drug absorption, distribution, **biotransformation** (or metabolism), and elimination, with emphasis on the time it takes for these processes to take place. In other words, pharmacokinetics studies *drug movement.*

Once a drug enters the circulatory system it is distributed to tissues, where certain biochemical and physiologic actions occur, producing the desired pharmacologic effects. These biochemical and physiologic actions are called the drug's *mechanism of action. Pharmacodynamics* is the study of drug actions on the body. Drug pharmacokinetics and pharmacodynamics determine the route, frequency, and dosage of drug administration.

PHARMACOKINETICS

Absorption

Absorption is the passage of a drug from the site of administration (where absorption begins) into the circulatory system. The speed at which a drug is absorbed is very important, because it determines how quickly the drug reaches its target tissue to produce its therapeutic effects.

The rate of absorption depends on several factors. First, circulatory status greatly influences drug absorption. For example, a person in shock will usually not have a positive therapeutic response from a drug administered by intramuscular injection because of poor peripheral circulation that results from shock. This poor circulation results in slow drug absorption and, therefore, inadequate therapeutic response. However, administering a drug intravenously bypasses the absorption process—the drug goes directly into the circulation, producing an adequate therapeutic response.

Another factor affecting a drug's rate of absorption is its **solubility,** that is, its ability to dissolve. The higher a drug's solubility, the faster it enters the bloodstream. Most prehospital drugs, like lidocaine and epinephrine, are already dissolved (in solution), whereas others, like nitroglycerin in tablets, are not in solution and must dissolve before they can therapeutically beneficial.

A third factor affecting drug absorption is the status of the body's **pH. Acidosis** (see Chapter 6) delays drug absorption in many cases. For example, acidosis can delay the absorption of epinephrine, thus making it inactive. That is why some patients in cardiac arrest do not respond to epinephrine—inadequate ventilations and/or chest compressions leave them acidotic. This problem is compounded by the fact that acidosis also reduces the effectiveness of electrical defibrillation in stimulating heart muscle.

Finally, drug **concentration** affects the rate of absorption (see Chapter 5). In general, the higher the percentage of drug in the preparation administered, the faster the rate of absorption.

Approximately 80 percent of drugs used in medicine are formulated to be taken orally, because taking a drug by mouth is easy and convenient for most people. The oral route, however, has two drawbacks. First, it is harder to predict and control the final concentration in the circulatory system of an orally administered drug. This unpredictability results from:

- Changes in the rate of absorption, depending on the presence or absence of food in the digestive system. Food in the stomach generally slows the absorption process.
- The destruction of some of the drug (it is hard to predict how much) by gastric enzymes.

Second, the rate of drug absorption through the digestive system is slower than the rate from subcutaneous injection and intramuscular injection. Also, because most drugs used in emergency medicine must reach their sites of action rapidly, drugs meant to be taken orally are usually not the drugs of choice in the prehospital setting.

Drugs used in prehospital emergency medicine are generally given parenterally. A **parenteral** route is any route other than the digestive system. Parenteral routes include:

- *Intravenous (IV).* The intravenous route is directly into a vein.
- *Endotracheal or Transtracheal (ET).* The endotracheal route is directly into the airway down an established ET tube.
- *Intraosseous (IO).* The intraosseous route is directly into the bone marrow. This route of drug administration is usually done only on pediatric patients under 5.
- *Intramuscular (IM).* The intramuscular route is directly into the muscle.
- *Subcutaneous (SQ or SC).* The subcutaneous route is directly into the subcutaneous fat above the muscle.
- *Sublingual (SL).* The sublingual route is into the bloodstream through absorption, when the drug is placed under the tongue.
- *Inhalation.* Some drugs are administered by inhaling the drug into the lungs, where it is absorbed into the circulation.

There are two drug routes not commonly used in prehospital emergency medicine: (1) insertion of a drug into the rectum (rectal) and (2) injection of a drug into the undersurface of the tongue **(intralingual).** The rectum is very vascular (rich in blood vessels), which allows for rapid drug absorption. However, fecal material in the rectum and the fact that patients are not always able to hold the drug in place make absorption of a therapeutic amount of a drug unpredictable. Even in the absence of fecal material, drug absorption is frequently incomplete and unpredictable. The undersurface of the tongue is also very vascular, which makes drug absorption rapid. However, improper injection of a drug under the tongue can cause severe swelling, which may lead to partial or complete airway obstruction.

Intravenous drug injection bypasses the absorption process because the drug enters directly into the circulatory system, producing desired therapeutic effects very quickly. Therefore, most emergency drugs are given intravenously.

Transtracheal drug administration allows the drug to be absorbed into the capillaries of the lungs. Most clinicians agree that transtracheal drug administration is as rapid as the intravenous route when properly performed. Transtracheal administration of five emergency drugs should be considered when an intravenous line cannot be established or if an endotracheal tube is in place before an intravenous line has been established. These five emergency drugs (for the adult patient) are: naloxone, atropine, Valium (diazepam), epinephrine, and lidocaine. Some find the acronym NAVEL helpful in remembering which drugs can be given down the endotracheal tube.

N = naloxone
A = atropine
V = Valium (trade name for diazepam)
E = epinephrine
L = lidocaine

In the pediatric patient, the drug Valium (diazepam) should not be given down the endotracheal tube if other routes are available. Valium irritates and causes inflammation in the child's bronchial tree. Therefore, it is recommended that only four emergency drugs should be administered down the endotracheal tube in the pediatric patient: lidocaine, epinephrine, atropine, and naloxone. The acronym *LEAN* may be helpful in remembering these drugs.

L = lidocaine
E = epinephrine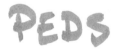
A = atropine
N = naloxone

However, endotracheal administration of Valium is justified if no other means are available.

There may be situations, such as with pediatric patients, when an intravenous line or an endotracheal tube cannot be readily established. For patients aged 5 or less, vascular access can be established and fluids and drugs given through an intraosseous line. All drugs and **crystalloid** solutions that can be given intravenously can also be given intraosseously. When fluids and drugs are administered into the bone marrow, absorption is immediate.

Table 2-1. RATES OF DRUG ABSORPTION

Route	Rate of Absorption
Intravenous	Immediate
Endotracheal/Transtracheal	Immediate
Intraosseous	Immediate
Inhalation	Rapid to immediate
Rectal	Rapid
Intramuscular	Moderate
Subcutaneous	Slow
Oral	
Sublingual	Rapid
Intralingual	Rapid
Ingestion	Slow

When drugs are administered by the intramuscular, subcutaneous, or sublingual routes, they must be absorbed through the body tissue into the capillaries and circulation and then distributed to their sites of action. For example, a drug given by intramuscular injection is injected directly into the muscle. From there, the drug must be absorbed into the capillary circulation and transported to the systemic circulation. A drug given by subcutaneous injection (SC/SQ) is injected into the subcutaneous fat above the muscle, where it too must be absorbed into the capillary circulation before it is transported to the systemic circulation. Absorption takes longer when a drug is given by subcutaneous injection because there are fewer capillaries in the subcutaneous tissue. When a drug is given by the sublingual route the drug must be absorbed through the mucosa of the undersurface of the tongue and then into the capillary circulation.

These three routes of drug administration—intramuscular, subcutaneous, and sublingual—are effective only if there is adequate circulatory status. Shock, acidosis, or peripheral vasoconstriction may delay the absorption of drugs given by one of these routes. Depending on the circulatory status of the patient, absorption by the intramuscular, subcutaneous, and sublingual routes varies from moderate to slow.

The drug used most often in emergency medicine—oxygen—is given by inhalation. Drugs administered by inhalation are absorbed into the circulation through capillaries surrounding the alveolar sacs of the lungs. The rate of absorption from inhalation is generally immediate, but the condition of the patient's lungs and circulatory status does have an effect on absorption. Table 2-1 compares the rates of absorption of different routes of drug administration.

Distribution

Once a drug is administered and absorbed into the circulatory system, it must travel to its site of action before it can be of any benefit. Once in the bloodstream the entire dose does not travel to its targeted tissues. Instead, the drug travels throughout the entire body. As Figure 2-1 illustrates, a certain amount

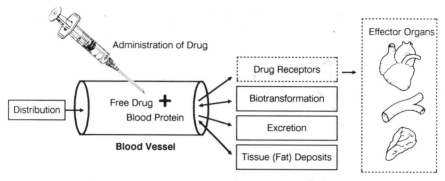

Figure 2–1. The pharmacokinetic phase of drug action.

of the drug may become bound to blood proteins (such as hemoglobin, albumen, and globulin). When this occurs, the drug is unavailable for further distribution until it is released from the blood protein. Drugs can also become stored within the body's fatty tissues. Again, until the drug is released from this fatty tissue, it is unavailable for distribution. The amount of drug that binds to blood protein or becomes stored in the body's fatty tissues is termed **bound drug.** Only the drug not bound, termed **free drug,** can be distributed for metabolism and elimination and is available targeted tissues.

Because drugs are distributed by way of the circulatory system, they generally concentrate in tissues that are well supplied with blood, such as the heart, liver, kidneys, and brain. Delivery of drugs to the brain, however, is limited by the **blood-brain barrier** and the **blood–cerebrospinal fluid barrier.** These are cell membranes that separate the circulating blood from the brain and cerebrospinal fluid. The blood-brain barrier and the blood–cerebrospinal fluid barrier restrict the movement of some damaging drugs and toxins to the brain and cerebrospinal fluid. Even drugs not completely stopped by these barriers generally enter the brain and spinal fluid at a slower rate than other tissues because of this extra barrier.

Biotransformation (Metabolism)

There are two ways in which the body eliminates a drug: biotransformation and excretion. *Biotransformation* is the chemical alteration of a drug within the body to an active or inactive water-soluble **metabolite.** *A metabolite* is any product that results from biotransformation. Changing a drug to a water-soluble metabolite makes excretion from the body easier.

Most drugs are inactivated as a result of biotransformation. Some drugs, however, become therapeutically *active* as a result of biotransformation. Two examples are the prehospital drugs diazepam and procainamide, which become therapeutically active when biotransformation begins. As biotransformation progresses, however, these drugs change back to inactive forms.

The biotransformation process of a drug to an inactive metabolite begins immediately after drug administration. The biotransformation process is actually a race against time. The drug must reach its target site of action at a sufficient therapeutic concentration in the blood before biotransformation converts the drug to an inactive state.

Biotransformation takes place primarily in the liver. Biotransformation can, however, occur in all body cells and tissues. Biotransformation that takes place in the liver is called *hepatic biotransformation.*

If the rate of drug biotransformation is slowed for any reason, **cumulative drug effects** may occur—in other words, subsequent doses have more effect. Increasing the rate of biotransformation may produce a state of apparent **tolerance,** in which the drug's effect decreases. Generally, when biotransformation is complete, a drug is no longer able to work therapeutically (unless the drug became an active metabolite), and it is excreted.

Excretion

Excretion is the elimination of waste products from the body. Drug excretion takes place through the intestines in the feces, through the kidneys in the urine, through the skin in perspiration, and through the respiratory system in exhaled air.

Volatile (easily evaporated) drugs are excreted from the body through the respiratory system in exhaled air or through the skin in perspiration. Nonvolatile, water-soluble drug metabolites are excreted in the urine. The kidney is the most important site for the excretion of drugs and drug metabolites.

Some drugs are excreted from the body through the alimentary tract. This occurs when the drug passes through the liver, is released into the bile, and is finally eliminated in the feces. When the bile enters the small intestine, however, some of the drug may be reabsorbed into the circulatory system. When this happens, the drug travels through the circulatory system until it is finally excreted in the urine. If the reabsorbed drug is in active form, this reabsorption prolongs its actions on the body.

PHARMACODYNAMICS

As we have seen, drugs enter the body by several different routes. Unless a drug enters via the intravenous, intraosseous, or endotracheal route, some time elapses before it enters the circulatory system. Once it is in the bloodstream, more time passes before the drug reaches its target site of action. The length of time from a drug's first administration until it reaches a concentration necessary to produce a therapeutic response at its target site of action is called the **onset of drug action.** Figure 2–2 compares the onset of action for a drug administered intravenously with the onset of action for the same drug given intramuscularly.

Most drugs produce their desired effects by inhibiting or increasing the action of their targeted **receptors.** A drug *receptor* is a component of a cell that combines with a drug to initiate a response. In essence, a section of the drug molecule combines with part of the molecular structure on or within a cell to produce a therapeutic effect. Once a drug reaches its site of action, it binds or unites to its receptor so it can cause the desired therapeutic response. This

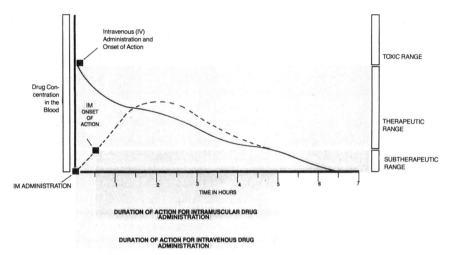

Figure 2-2. The concentration profile (how concentration changes over a period of time) of a drug administered intravenously varies significantly from that of the same drug administered intramuscularly.

action at the receptor site is also called the drug's *mechanism of action.* Chapter 3 explains how drugs and receptors interact to initiate a response.

Drug receptors are often referred to as "locks," and drugs that bind to the receptors are generally referred to as the "keys" that fit the locks. A drug's (key's) ability to fit a certain receptor (lock) enables a pharmacologic response to occur. Such a drug is called an **agonist.** In addition, some drugs bind to receptors, but their effect is to inhibit or counteract a response. These drugs are called **antagonists.**

Sometimes the terms **affinity** and **efficacy** are used to describe the nature of drug-receptor interaction. Affinity means attraction; to say that a drug has an affinity for a receptor means that it tends to combine with that receptor. Efficacy means the power to produce a desired effect. To say that a drug has efficacy means that it has the capacity to produce a pharmacologic response when it interacts with its receptor. Drugs that are agonists have both affinity and efficacy, while antagonist drugs have affinity but not efficacy.

A drug goes through four phases of activity before it produces a desired pharamacologic effect (Fig. 2-3). The *administration* phase is the introduction of a drug into the body by the appropriate route. Once administered, the drug enters the *pharmaceutical* phase. During this phase the drug dissolves so it can be made available for absorption. Drugs given by the intravenous, transtracheal, and intraosseous routes bypass the pharmaceutical phase of drug activity. Once dissolved, the drug begins the *pharmacokinetic* phase. Only free drugs capable of reaching their receptors can be said to exist in the pharmacokinetic phase. Once a drug reaches its receptors, the *pharmacodynamic* phase of drug activity occurs. It is only when the drug binds to its receptor that the pharmacologic effect occurs.

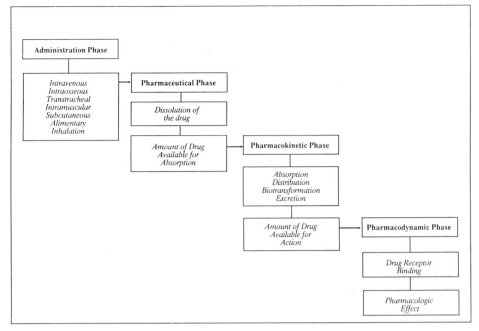

Figure 2–3. The phases of drug activity.

The minimum concentration necessary for a drug to produce the desired therapeutic response is referred to as the minimum therapeutic concentration. A drug concentration below the minimum therapeutic concentration will not produce an effective response, and drug concentrations that are too high may produce toxic effects or may even be fatal.

Most drugs have a predetermined standard dosage or the dosage is determined by body weight (see Chapter 5). Dosage guidelines are established to achieve minimum therapeutic concentrations. Any deviation from established dosage guidelines may be harmful. Remember, the goal for drug therapy is to give the minimum concentration of a drug necessary to obtain the desired therapeutic response.

PHARMACODYNAMIC TERMINOLOGY

Drug actions (pharmacodynamics) are described in a variety of ways. You should be familiar with the following descriptive terms.

Additive: An additive effect is the effect that one drug contributes to the action of another. For example, a narcotic analgesic such as morphine may have an additive effect on someone who is taking an antihistamine drug such as hydroxyzine, because both drugs cause central nervous system (CNS) depression.

Antagonistic: Antagonism is the mutual opposition in effect between two or more drugs. For example, prehospital care providers may use naloxone to oppose the effects of a morphine overdose, because naloxene and morphine are antagonists.

Cumulative: Cumulative effect is the result of repeated doses of drugs that accumulate in the body to produce symptoms of poisoning.

Depressant: A depressant is a drug that depresses a body function. For example, the drug codeine is a narcotic analgesic that produces generalized CNS depression.

Habituation: Habituation is the act of becoming accustomed. To habituate to a drug is to develop physical tolerance to and dependence on the drug.

Hypersensitiveness: Hypersensitiveness is the excessive susceptibility to the action of a drug.

Idiosyncrasy: Idiosyncrasy is an accelerated, toxic, or uncharacteristic response to the usual therapeutic dose of a drug.

Irritation: An irritation is temporary or permanent tissue inflammation caused by drug action.

Physiologic action: Physiologic action is the effect on a body function produced by a drug.

Potentiation: Potentiation is the enhanced action of two drugs, in which the total effects are greater than the sum of each drug's independent effects.

Synergism: Synergism is the joint action of two drugs producing an effect that neither drug could produce alone.

Therapeutics: Therapeutics is the production of favorable results from application of a remedy, such as a drug, in the management of disease.

Tolerance: Tolerance is the progressive decrease in the effectiveness or response of a drug.

Untoward Reaction: An untoward reaction is a harmful side effect of a drug treatment.

CONCLUSION

It is not enough for emergency medical service professionals to know when and how much of a drug to give. Understanding basic pharmacokinetics and pharmacodynamics is essential so that you know the desired therapeutic effects and can anticipate possible side effects. For each drug you administer, you should be aware of such factors as the drug's rate of absorption, minimum therapeutic concentration, and toxic levels and its possible and anticipated side effects.

STUDY QUESTIONS

1. The speed at which a drug is absorbed determines how quickly the drug reaches its target tissue to produce its therapeutic effects. The rate of drug absorption depends on what four factors?

2. When a drug tends to combine with its receptor, it is said to have:
   a. Efficacy.
   b. Tolerance.
   c. Affinity.
   d. Cumulative effects.

3. What are the four phases of activity a drug goes through before it produces a desired pharmacologic effect?

4. The goal of drug therapy is to give the minimum therapeutic concentration of a drug to obtain the effective desired therapeutic response. Explain.

Chapter 3

The Autonomic Nervous System

Many of the drugs used in prehospital emergency medicine affect tissues that receive their nerve impulses from the **autonomic nervous system.** Most of these drugs produce their effects by imitating or opposing neurotransmitters that are released by fibers that innervate (stimulate) smooth muscle, cardiac muscle, and certain glands. A **neurotransmitter** is a chemical substance located on a presynaptic neuron. When the neuron is stimulated (excited), the neurotransmitter travels across the synapse to act on the target cell to either excite or inhibit it. The specific tissues stimulated by the autonomic nervous system are called **effector organs.** The term effector simply means that when a tissue is stimulated, a specific effect should occur.

This chapter presents the general anatomy and physiology of the autonomic nervous system. Included is a discussion of how specific neurotransmitters transmit nerve impulses and how certain drugs can affect the function of these neurotransmitters. By understanding the basic functions of the autonomic nervous system, you can better predict the various effects drugs may produce on the effector organs stimulated by the autonomic nervous system.

It is not the purpose of this text to describe in detail the effects of each drug on each organ system. However, it is important to understand the basic interactions between the autonomic drugs and the autonomic nervous system since these interactions are the basis of much of the treatment in the prehospital setting.

OVERVIEW OF THE NERVOUS SYSTEM

There is only one nervous system. However, the nervous system has two major subdivisions: the **central nervous system (CNS)** and the **peripheral nervous system.** The CNS is made up of the brain and spinal cord. The peripheral nervous system is that part of the nervous system outside the CNS. Figure 3–1 illustrates the divisions and subdivisions of the nervous system.

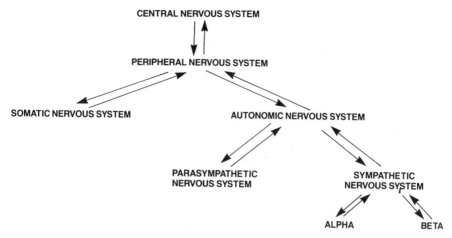

Figure 3–1. Divisions and subdivisions of the nervous system.

The *autonomic nervous system* is that portion of the peripheral nervous system that controls the body's automatic or involuntary functions. The autonomic nervous system helps to control arterial blood pressure, cardiac function, gastrointestinal functions, body temperature, bladder emptying, and many other activities. The autonomic nervous system acts on the various tissue effector organs to reduce or slow their activity or to initiate their function.

The autonomic nervous system is capable of causing rapid changes in the body's automatic functions. For example, it can double the heart rate in 3 to 5 seconds or double the arterial blood pressure within 10 to 15 seconds. Conversely, the autonomic nervous system can lower arterial blood pressure to the point of fainting within 4 to 5 seconds. In short the autonomic nervous system maintains rapid and effective control of most internal functions of the body.

The autonomic nervous system contains automatic **motoneurons.** *Motoneurons* are motor neurons that convey impulses to effector tissues from the central nervous system. In other words, they stimulate effector tissues. Automatic effector tissues include cardiac, smooth muscle, gland, and epithelial tissues.

NEUROTRANSMITTERS

The autonomic nervous system is activated mainly by centers located in the brain and spinal cord. When activated, the autonomic nervous system functions on what is termed the **reflex arc** principle. A *reflex arc* is the complete circuit of nerves involved in an involuntary movement, from the stimulus to the response: the sensory neuron ending in the spinal cord, the motoneuron from the spinal cord to the effector organ, and connecting neurons within the spinal column. The basic units of the system are its neurons and neuronal synapses (Fig. 3–2). A **synapse** is the space between two neurons, or the space between a neuron and an effector organ. An electrical signal travels along the neuron and

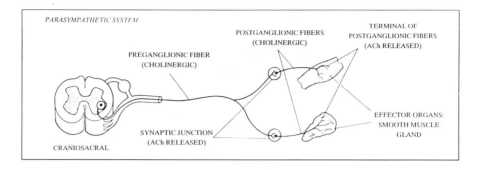

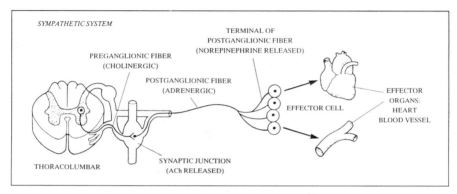

Figure 3–2. Comparison of the parasympathetic and sympathetic nervous systems. (From Hahn, AB, et al.: Mosby's Pharmacology in Nursing, ed. 16. C.V. Mosby, St. Louis, 1986, p 366, with permission.)

causes the release of a neurotransmitter (a body-produced chemical) from the *pre*synaptic neuron. The neurotransmitter moves across the synaptic space and combines with receptors on the *post*synaptic neuron. These actions cause an electrical change in the neuron's membrane ion permeability, which then starts an action impulse potential in the postsynaptic neuron of the effector organ. The result is a continuation of electrical flow causing contraction of a muscle, the secretion of a gland, the contraction of a pupil, or an alteration of heart rate. Acetylcholine (ACh), norepinephrine, and epinephrine are the primary neurotransmitters of the autonomic nervous system.

THE PARASYMPATHETIC AND SYMPATHETIC NERVOUS SYSTEMS

The autonomic nervous system is composed of two anatomically and physiologically separate divisions: the **parasympathetic** and **sympathetic nervous systems.** The *parasympathetic nervous system* is connected with the CNS through certain cranial nerves and through the middle three sacral segments of the spinal cord. The ganglia (nervous tissue) of the parasympathetic nervous system are located near the effector organs stimulated. The *sympathetic nervous system* is connected with the CNS through the thoracic and upper lumbar segments of the spinal cord. Its ganglia are located near the spinal column rather than near the effector organs stimulated (see Fig. 3–2).

Many effector organs are simultaneously stimulated by both the sympathetic and parasympathetic nervous systems. Physiologically, stimulation by the sympathetic nervous system excites a response, whereas stimulation by the parasympathetic nervous system inhibits a response. The opposition of these two systems works to produce normal automatic body functions. The neural pathways for each system frequently travel together, especially in the thorax, abdomen, and pelvis (Fig. 3–3).

Parasympathetic Nervous System

The major nerves of the parasympathetic nervous system are the two **vagus nerves.** Approximately 75 percent of all parasympathetic nerve fibers are located in the vagus nerves, which travel the entire thoracic and abdominal region of the body (Fig. 3–4).

The parasympathetic nervous system is the main regulator of many automatic effector organs including the heart, digestive tract smooth muscle, glands that secrete digestive juices, and endocrine gland cells that secrete insulin. Vagus nerve stimulation causes the following physiologic changes:

- Salivation
- Bradycardia
- A decrease in strength of cardiac contractions
- Hypotension
- Increased blood flow to the stomach and intestines
- An increase in glandular secretions of digestive juices

Vagus nerve fibers do not reach the ventricles of the heart. Therefore, vagal stimulation causes decreased heart rate by its effects on atrial muscle. These include decreased sinoatrial node firing rate, decreased contractility, and decreased conduction in the atrioventricular node. **Acetylcholine** is the neurotransmitter of the parasympathetic nervous system. Acetylcholine binds to atrial muscle receptor sites to enable vagal nerve stimulation. An example of a drug that affects the parasympathetic nervous system is atropine. Atropine is a parasympathetic blocker. It competes with acetylcholine for receptor sites, blocking its action and causing an increase in heart rate. Atropine is used in cases of severe bradycardia.

Sympathetic Nervous System

Sympathetic nerves originate in the lateral columns of the thoracic and first 3 to 4 lumbar segments of the spinal cord. Stimulation of the sympathetic nervous system prepares the body for emergencies. One of the first steps in the body's reaction to stress is a sudden increase in sympathetic activity, which

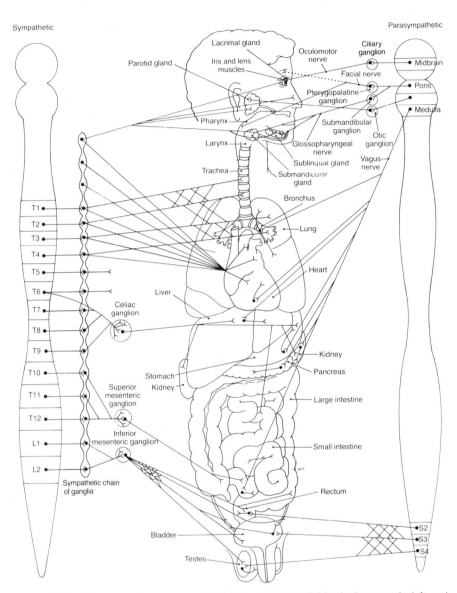

Figure 3–3. The autonomic nervous system. The sympathetic division is shown on the left, and the parasympathetic division is shown on the right. In reality, both divisions are bilateral. (From Scanlon, VC and Sanders, T: Essentials of Anatomy and Physiology. F.A. Davis, Philadelphia, 1991, p 186, with permission.)

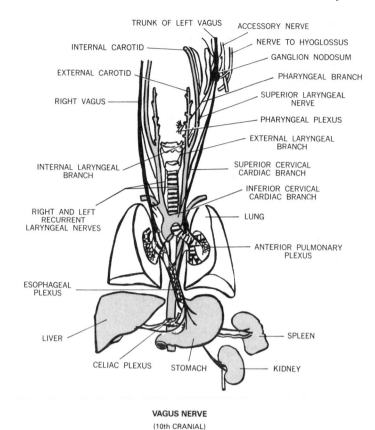

TRUNK OF LEFT VAGUS
ACCESSORY NERVE
INTERNAL CAROTID
NERVE TO HYOGLOSSUS
GANGLION NODOSUM
EXTERNAL CAROTID
PHARYNGEAL BRANCH
RIGHT VAGUS
SUPERIOR LARYNGEAL NERVE
PHARYNGEAL PLEXUS
EXTERNAL LARYNGEAL BRANCH
INTERNAL LARYNGEAL BRANCH
SUPERIOR CERVICAL CARDIAC BRANCH
INFERIOR CERVICAL CARDIAC BRANCH
RIGHT AND LEFT RECURRENT LARYNGEAL NERVES
LUNG
ANTERIOR PULMONARY PLEXUS
ESOPHAGEAL PLEXUS
LIVER
SPLEEN
CELIAC PLEXUS
STOMACH
KIDNEY

VAGUS NERVE
(10th CRANIAL)

Figure 3–4. The vagus nerve. (From Thomas, CL: Taber's Cyclopedic Medical Dictionary, ed. 15. F.A. Davis, Philadelphia, 1985, p 1832, with permission.)

makes the body ready to use maximum energy and to engage in maximum physical activity. This activity has been historically called the "fight or flight" response. Table 3–1 compares the fight or flight response of the body to sympathetic nervous system stimulation with the body's response to the parasympathetic nervous system.

Stimulation of the sympathetic nervous system causes the following physiologic changes:

- Dry mouth
- Tachycardia
- Increased strength of cardiac contractions
- Hypertension
- Dilation of pupils
- Vasoconstriction of the skin, kidneys, and digestive organs
- Vasodilation of the skeletal muscles

Table 3–1. COMPARISON OF THE BODY'S RESPONSE TO STIMULATION OF THE SYMPATHETIC NERVOUS SYSTEM WITH THAT OF STIMULATION OF THE PARASYMPATHETIC NERVOUS SYSTEM

Sympathetic (Flight or Fight)	Parasympathetic
The heart beats faster and pumps more efficiently (To aid in flight.)	The rate and strength of cardiac contractions decrease
Hypertension	Hypotension
Vasoconstriction of skin, kidneys, and digestive tract (Urination and digestion are lower priorities during flight.)	Increase in blood flow to the stomach and intestines and an increase in glandular secretions of digestive enzymes
Dry mouth (To assist in keeping the airway clear during flight.)	Salivation
Pupil dilation (For better vision during flight.)	Pupil contraction
Vasodilation of skeletal muscles (To assist in running.)	

The sympathetic nervous system has specific effects on the heart, including:

- Increased firing rate of the sinoatrial node
- Increased atrial muscle contractility and conduction velocity
- Higher conduction rate of the atrioventricular node
- Increased contractility and automaticity in the left ventricle
- Increased stroke volume

These effects caused by stimulation of the sympathetic nervous system increase cardiac output. The sympathetic nervous system stimulates all blood vessels except the capillaries. *Epinephrine* and *norepinephrine* are the main neurotransmitters of the sympathetic nervous system.

THE ADRENERGIC AND CHOLINERGIC NERVOUS SYSTEMS

The autonomic nervous system can be further described in terms of **adrenergic** (sympathetic) and **cholinergic** (parasympathetic) components. Neurons and effector organs that are activated by epinephrine are called *adrenergic.* Neurons and effector organs that are activated by acetylcholine are defined as *cholinergic.* Adrenergic drugs are drugs that imitate the action of epinephrine, and cholinergic drugs are drugs that imitate acetylcholine. Table 3–2 compares the physiologic activities of the adrenergic and cholinergic nervous systems. Drugs that oppose the action of epinephrine are called **anti**adrenergic drugs, and drugs that oppose the action of acetylcholine are called **anti**cholinergic drugs. For example, isoproterenol is classified as a beta-adrenergic agonist related to epinephrine, which is also a beta-adrenergic agonist. The drug atropine is classified as an anticholinergic agent that competes at receptor sites with acetylcholine.

Table 3–2. PHYSIOLOGIC ACTIONS OF THE ADRENERGIC AND CHOLINERGIC SYSTEMS

Effector Organ	Adrenergic Response (Sympathetic)	Cholinergic Response (Parasympathetic)
Heart		
Rate of contractions	Increase	Decrease
Force of contractions	Increase	Decrease
Blood pressure	Increase	Decrease
Blood vessels		
Skin/mucous membrane	Constriction	Dilation
Skeletal muscle	Dilation	Dilation
Coronary	Dilation; constriction	
Renal	Constriction	
Pupils	Dilation	Contraction
Bronchii	Relaxation	Contraction
Adrenal medulla	Secretion of epinephrine and norephinephrine	
Glands		
Sweat	Generalized secretion	Localized secretion
Salivary	Slight secretion	Profuse secretions
Gastrointestinal		Increased secretions
Pancreas (islets)	Inhibit insulin secretion	
Metabolic rate	Increased	

Adrenergic receptors are classified as either alpha-adrenergic receptors or beta-adrenergic receptors. Sympathetic stimulation of alpha-adrenergic receptors produces constriction of blood vessels, dilation of the pupils, and relaxation of the smooth muscles of the gastrointestinal tract. Stimulation of beta-adrenergic receptors results in an increase in the rate and force of contractions of the heart, relaxation of the smooth muscles of the bronchioles in the lungs and gastrointestinal tract, and vasodilation of blood vessels in the skeletal muscles.

Alpha-adrenergic receptors are identified according to the location of their receptors. Alpha$_1$-receptor sites are located on the **post**synaptic effector cells, and alpha$_2$-receptor sites are located on the **pre**synaptic nerve terminals. Stimulating alpha$_2$-receptors inhibits the release of additional norepinephrine. When alpha$_1$-receptors are stimulated, peripheral and coronary vasoconstriction occurs.

Beta-adrenergic receptors are also divided into two categories, beta$_1$ and beta$_2$. Most beta$_1$-adrenergic receptor sites are located in the heart. Stimulation of beta$_1$-adrenergic receptors causes increased heart rate, increased contractility, and an increase in atrioventricular conduction. Beta$_2$-adrenergic receptors are located mainly in bronchial and vascular smooth muscle. Stimulation of these receptors causes vasodilation, bronchodilation, and uterine relaxation. Blockage of these receptors opposes the effect of the neurotransmitter. Beta-

Table 3–3. ALPHA-ADRENERGIC AND BETA-ADRENERGIC RECEPTOR
SITES AND FUNCTIONS

Effector Organ	Alpha	Beta
Heart		
SA Node		Increased rate (beta$_1$)
AV Node		Increased automaticity and conduction velocity (beta$_1$)
Ventricles		Increased force of contraction and conduction velocity (beta$_1$)
Arterioles	Vasoconstriction (alpha$_1$)	Vasodilation (beta$_2$)
Veins	Vasoconstriction (alpha$_1$)	Vasodilation (beta$_2$)
Lungs		Bronchodilation (beta$_2$)
Pupils	Contraction	
Pancreas (Islets)	Decreased secretion	

blocking drugs are either selective for beta$_1$-adrenergic receptors or nonselective. Nonselective blocking drugs block both beta$_1$- and beta$_2$-receptors. Table 3–3 lists the alpha-receptor and beta-receptor sites and their functions.

Drugs that influence the sympathetic nervous system are classified according to the alpha and beta effects they produce. For example, norepinephrine activates all alpha-receptors and some beta-receptors, whereas epinephrine activates all alpha-receptors and all beta-receptors. Isoproterenol is a drug that only activates beta-receptors.

Some drugs block the effects of parasympathetic or sympathetic stimulation. These drugs occupy receptor sites, which prevents parasympathetic or sympathetic neurotransmitters from occupying the sites. For example, atropine blocks the effects of acetylcholine by attaching to the acetylcholine receptor site. Excessive parasympathetic stimulation decreases cardiac output. Atropine increases the heart rate and cardiac output by blocking the parasympathetic effects of acetylcholine on the heart.

Propranolol is a beta-adrenergic blocking drug that competes with epinephrine for beta-receptors. Propranolol is primarily used to treat angina pectoris, tachycardia, and hypertension.

CONCLUSION

The autonomic nervous system regulates automatic effectors that maintain or quickly restore the state of equilibrium of the body's automatic functions. Doubly stimulated organs receive both sympathetic and parasympathetic impulses, which influence their function in opposing ways. For example, sympathetic impulses make the heart beat faster and parasympathetic impulses slow the heart down. The relationship between the effects of the two opposing systems determines actual heart rate.

The parasympathetic or cholinergic division of the autonomic nervous system regulates the body's involuntary functions. This takes place through the vagus nerves by the release of acetylcholine. Vagal stimulation slows the heart rate, but this action can be opposed by parasympathetic blocking drugs.

The sympathetic or adrenergic division enables the body to respond to emergency, or stress. This system is regulated mainly by the release of norepinephrine and epinephrine. The sympathetic division is further subdivided into alpha-adrenergic and beta-adrenergic receptors. Stimulation of alpha-adrenergic receptors causes vasoconstriction of the blood vessels, a decrease in gastrointestinal secretion, and dilation of the pupils. Stimulation of beta-adrenergic receptors causes an increase in the rate and force of contractions of the heart, dilation of the arterioles of skeletal muscles, and dilation of the bronchiolar muscles of the lungs. Drugs that effect only alpha-adrenergic receptors have no direct effect on the heart. Their bronchoconstricting effects are minimal, but they have significant vasoconstriction action.

STUDY QUESTIONS

1. Vagus nerve stimulation causes the following physiologic changes:
   a. Bradycardia.
   b. Hypertension.
   c. Increased firing rate of the SA node.
   d. Increased stroke volume.
   e. Decreased strength of cardiac contractions.
   f. Dilation of pupils.
   (1) a and e.
   (2) b and f.
   (3) c and d.
   (4) d and a.
2. Stimulation of alpha$_1$-receptor sites causes
   a. Bronchodilation.
   b. An increase in heart rate.
   c. Peripheral and coronary vasoconstriction.
   d. Inhibition of the release of norepinephrine.

3. A neurotransmitter is
   a. An electrical impulse.
   b. A body-produced chemical.
   c. A postsynaptic neuron.
   d. A presynaptic neuron.

4. Neurons and effector organs that are activated by epinephrine are called
   a. Adrenergic.
   b. Cholinergic.
   c. Antiadrenergic.
   d. Anticholinergic.

Chapter 4

Drug Administration

Drug administration is one of the most important, demanding, and risky functions you will perform in prehospital emergency care. It will be your responsibility to interpret and carry out the drug order and to ensure its appropriateness. Drug administration requires training, a solid knowledge base, and well-developed decision-making abilities.

To have its intended therapeutic effect, a drug must reach its site of action. To do this, the drug must enter the body, be absorbed into the circulation, and then be transported to the targeted tissues. All these events vary according to the route of administration. The route of administration of a drug is determined by the amount of the drug needed, the rapidity of action desired, and the patient's condition.

Basically, there are two ways to introduce drugs into the body: by the alimentary tract and by parenteral routes. In prehospital emergency situations, drugs are most often given by parenteral routes, since these are much more rapid and generally more predictable.

ALIMENTARY TRACT ROUTES

Oral

As explained in Chapter 1, oral (PO) administration of drugs provides the most convenient, safe, and economic way to get drugs into the body. Although some orally administered drugs are absorbed from the stomach and colon, most are absorbed from the small intestines. Because they must travel through the mouth, throat, and stomach before entering the bloodstream, the onset of action of oral drugs is slower. The delay in onset sometimes means a decrease in or a lack of therapeutic effects. Therefore, when a rapid therapeutic effect is required, such as in life-threatening emergencies, parenteral drug administration is preferred.

Rectal

Rectal drug administration can have either local or systemic effects. Systemic drug absorption from rectal administration, however, can be incomplete and unpredictable, especially if the patient is unable to retain the drug long enough. On the other hand, rectal drug administration quickly results in a high concentration of the drug in the circulation, for two reasons. First, the rectum contains a rich network of capillaries. Second, because venous blood from the lower part of the rectum does not pass through the liver, drugs absorbed in the rectum are not biotransformed in the liver before reaching other body sites.

Rectal drug administration may be necessary when oral administration is unsuitable, for instance, with unconscious or nauseated patients or with small children who are unable to swallow drugs. An example of a drug administered rectally is promethazine (Phenergan), used in the treatment of motion sickness, as a sedative, and as an antiemetic.

Rectal drug administration is usually not performed in the prehospital setting.

PARENTERAL ROUTES

Parenteral drug administration includes all routes other than the alimentary tract.

Sublingual

To administer a drug sublingually (SL), place it under the patient's tongue and instruct him or her to keep it there until it is dissolved and absorbed into the capillaries. The underside of the tongue is rich in capillaries, which permits rapid absorption and therefore quick drug action. Sublingual drug administration permits the drug to enter the general circulation without passing through the liver or being affected by gastric and intestinal enzymes. This yields a higher concentration of the drug in the circulation than does oral administration.

Obviously the tongue is in the mouth, which is the beginning of the alimentary tract. However, since the drug is absorbed through the mucosa of the tongue and directly into the circulation without interference from gastric enzymes and other material found in the alimentary tract, the sublingual drug route is considered a parenteral route. An example of a prehospital drug administered sublingually is nitroglycerin, used to treat anginal attacks and for the long-term **prophylactic** management of angina pectoris. (*Prophylactics* are designed to prevent illness or disease.)

Intralingual

Intralingual (IL) drug administration is the injection of a drug into the undersurface of the patient's tongue. The tongue contains a rich supply of capillaries, which means quick drug absorption. A major disadvantage of an intralingual injection is that the tongue might swell, causing partial or complete airway obstruction. Intralingual drug administration is usually not a prehospital procedure.

Intradermal

Intradermal (ID) administration is the injection of a drug into the upper layers of the skin, with the needle almost parallel to the skin surface. These injections are usually done with a fine, short (⅝-inch by 26- to 27-gauge) needle and a small-barrel (1-milliliter) syringe. Intradermal drug administration is used to provide local drug effects for the treatment of allergies or to perform allergy skin testing. The amount of drug that can be injected intradermally is small; the rate of absorption is slow because absorption is limited to the capillaries of the dermis. Intradermal drug administration is usually not a prehospital procedure.

Subcutaneous

A subcutaneous (SQ/SC) injection is performed by inserting a small needle (½ to ⅝ inches long, with a gauge of 25 or less) into the fatty tissue above the muscle. Usually, the largest dose that can be injected by this method is 2 milliliters. Subcutaneous injection causes minimal tissue trauma and avoids damage to large blood vessels and nerves. Figure 4–1 illustrates the common subcutaneous injection sites.

Drug absorption after a subcutaneous injection largely depends on the physical condition of the patient. For example, subcutaneous injection is undesirable for patients with compromised circulatory perfusion, for instance, patients in shock or patients with peripheral vascular disease.

An example of a prehospital drug administered by subcutaneous injection is epinephrine (1:1000 solution) used in treating bronchoconstriction associated with anaphylaxis (see Chapter 12).

Intramuscular

Intramuscular (IM) injection is the most common method of administering parenteral drugs. It is not common in the prehospital setting, however. The drug is injected deep into the muscle tissue, where it is absorbed into the capillaries and enters the bloodstream. Drug doses of up to 3 milliliters can be given via the intramuscular route; it requires needles of 21 to 23 gauge and 1 to 1½ inches in length. If larger amounts of a drug are to be given, it is better to use

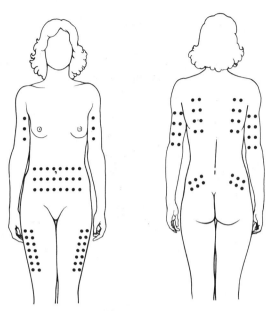

Figure 4–1. Subcutaneous injection sites. (From Deglin, JH, Vallerand, AH, and Russin, MM: Davis's Drug Guide for Nurses, ed. 2. F.A. Davis, Philadelphia, 1990, p 1219, with permission.)

two injection sites. Figure 4–2 illustrates common sites for intramuscular drug administration.

The rate of absorption of a drug administered by intramuscular injection depends on the physical condition of the patient. For example, intramuscular injection may be contraindicated for patients with decreased peripheral perfusion or inadequate muscle mass. On the other hand, intramuscular drug administration usually yields a predictable absorption rate.

In prehospital emergencies in which an intravenous line (see page 49) cannot be established, intramuscular injection is sometimes the answer. For example, prehospital emergency care providers can use intramuscular injection to administer thiamine to patients in a coma of unknown origin or a coma due to alcohol and to patients suffering delerium tremens.

Intravenous

When the situation calls for a rapid therapeutic effect, intravenous (IV) injection allows direct administration of a drug directly into the bloodstream, either as a **bolus** or as an infusion. A bolus is one dose of a drug injected into the vein all at once. Continuous infusion is the controlled introduction (at a specified rate) of a drug into the bloodstream over a period of time. Continuous infusion is a way to keep the amount of drug available to body tissues at a con-

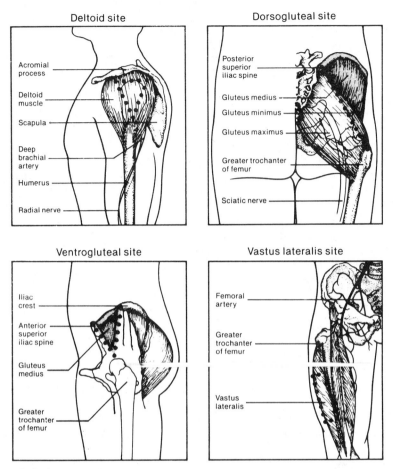

Figure 4–2. Intramuscular injection sites. (From Deglin, JH, Vallerand, AH, and Russin, MM: Davis's Drug Guide for Nurses, ed. 2. F.A. Davis, Philadelphia, 1990, p 1220, with permission.)

stant level. Most prehospital emergency drugs are administered by intravenous injection.

Drug administration by intravenous bolus yields quick, predictable therapeutic concentrations, which makes it the route of choice in most emergency situations. However, the rapidity of absorption of an intravenous bolus carries the risk of producing immediate adverse reactions and side effects.

The rate of an intravenous infusion can be set to maintain therapeutic levels of a drug. In some emergency situations, the physician or EMT-P first gives an intravenous bolus to achieve therapeutic levels quickly, then uses an intravenous infusion to maintain those established levels. For instance, lidocaine is administered in this way to treat ventricular fibrillation. The EMT-P or physician uses bolus doses of lidocaine to produce therapeutic levels as quickly as possible. Once circulation has been restored, an infusion maintains the established therapeutic level of lidocaine in the bloodstream.

Transtracheal/Endotracheal

Some emergency drugs can be administered down an endotracheal (ET) tube when an intravenous line cannot be started or cannot be established quickly enough. Drugs given down the endotracheal tube are absorbed into the capillaries of the lungs. When endotracheal administration is done correctly, the rate of absorption of the drug is just as rapid as when the drug is given by intravenous injection. For adults, drugs that can be administered down the endotracheal tube include naloxone, atropine, diazepam, epinephrine, and lidocaine. For children, drugs that can be administered down the endotracheal tube include naloxone, atropine, epinephrine, and lidocaine.

Intraosseous

Intraosseous (IO) administration is a safe, rapid, and effective way to introduce fluids and drugs into the bloodstream via the highly vascular bone marrow. The EMT-P or physician can establish an intraosseous line at the proximal tibia (the preferred site), distal femur, or distal tibia of a pediatric patient with circulatory failure or cardiac arrest. In prehospital medicine, this procedure is generally performed on patients 5 years of age or younger who are unconscious, unresponsive, and in immediate danger of dying. In most cases, the EMT-P should not try to establish a prehospital intraosseous line until at least two attempts at establishing a peripheral intravenous line have failed.

COMMON PREHOSPITAL DRUG ADMINISTRATION TECHNIQUES

Most emergency drugs are given parenterally, by the intravenous, transtracheal, intraosseous, intramuscular, or subcutaneous route. The subcutaneous and intramuscular routes are not as common as the other routes in the prehospital setting. Because of the increase in medical facilities employing paramedics as health care providers, it is becoming more important for the EMT-P to be familiar with all common drug routes and administration techniques.

Subcutaneous Injection

1. Perform a thorough patient assessment and history, confirming:
   That the medication is needed.
   That the patient does not have any allergies that contraindicate the use of the medication.
2. Receive the order.
3. Write down and confirm the order.

4. Calculate the required dosage.
5. Prepare the appropriate equipment:
   Medication
   1- to 2-milliliter syringe
   ⅝-inch by 25-gauge needle
   Antibacterial swab and alcohol prep
   4-inch x 4-inch gauze pads
   Adhesive bandage strip
6. Explain the procedure to the patient.
7. Examine the medication, reconfirming that:
   It is the correct medication.
   It has not expired.
   It is not discolored.
   There are no visible particles in the solution.
8. Gently tap the upper part of the ampule or shake the ampule down, forcing the medication to the lower portion of the ampule.* Figure 4–4 illustrates the withdrawal of a medication from an ampule.
9. Using a 4-inch x 4-inch gauze pad or alcohol prep to protect your hand, break off the top of the ampule.
10. Draw the medication into the syringe and expel any excess air from it.
11. Choose a suitable administration site. A commonly used site is the subcutaneous tissue over the triceps brachii muscle on the back of the arm.
12. Cleanse the site with an antibacterial swab.

---

* Some drugs come in a vial instead of an ampule. Figure 4–3 illustrates the procedure for withdrawing a medication from a vial. When withdrawing a drug from a vial, first clean the rubber stopper with an antibacterial swab. Insert the needle and inject a volume of air into the vial equal to the volume of drug you need to withdraw. For example, if you need 4 milliliters of a drug, inject 4 milliliters of air into the vial. Doing so makes it easier to withdraw the drug into the syringe.

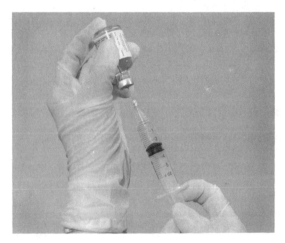

Figure 4–3. Withdrawing medication from a vial.

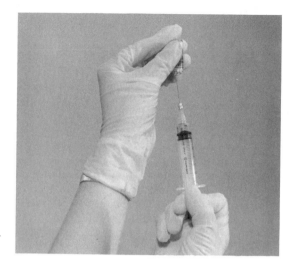

Figure 4–4. Withdrawing medication from an ampule.

13. Pinch the skin and insert the needle at a 45-degree angle (Fig. 4–5).
14. Aspirate the syringe (gently pull the plunger back to create suction) to make sure that the needle is not in a blood vessel. If blood enters the syringe, withdraw the needle and prepare another site for another attempt, *using a new needle.*

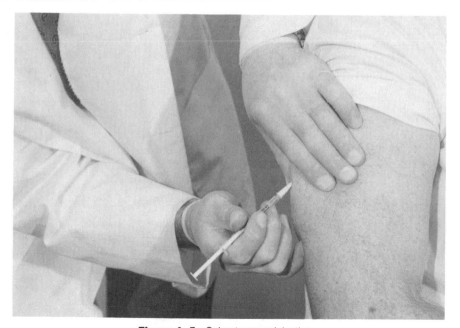

Figure 4–5. Subcutaneous injection.

15. Inject the medication slowly.
16. Remove and dispose the needle.
17. Gently massage the injection site. (This aids in drug absorption.)
18. Cover the site with an adhesive bandage strip.
19. Confirm and document administration of the medication.
20. Closely monitor the patient and report any changes.

Intramuscular Injection

In most cases, intramuscular injections should be avoided when the patient's chief complaint is chest pain. An intramuscular injection may cause a rise in the amount of certain muscle enzymes circulating within the bloodstream. The level of these enzymes can help the physician determine if a myocardial infarction (MI) is the cause of the patient's chest pain. An intramuscular injection in the prehospital setting may confuse the picture when measurements of muscle enzymes are evaluated at the hospital.

The procedure for intramuscular administration of medications is as follows:

1. Perform a thorough patient assessment and history, confirming:
   That the medication is needed.
   That the patient does not have any allergies that contraindicate the use of the medication.
2. Receive the order.
3. Write down and confirm the order.
4. Calculate the required dosage.
5. Prepare the appropriate equipment:
   Medication
   Appropriate size syringe (1- to 3-milliliter)
   1- to 1½-inch by 21- to 23-gauge needle
   Antibacterial swab and alcohol prep
   4-inch by 4-inch gauze pads
   Adhesive bandage strip
6. Explain the procedure to the patient.
7. Examine the medication, reconfirming that:
   It is the correct medication.
   It has not expired.
   It is not discolored.
   There are no visible particles in the solution.
8. Gently tap the upper part of the ampule or shake the ampule down, forcing the medication to the lower part of the ampule.
9. Using a 4-inch by 4-inch gauze pad or an alcohol prep to protect your hand, break off the top of the ampule.
10. Draw the medication into the syringe and expel any excess air from it.
11. Choose a suitable administration site. A commonly used site is the deltoid muscle of the arm.
12. Cleanse the administration site with an antibacterial swab.
13. Insert the needle into the tissue at a 90-degree angle (Fig. 4–6).

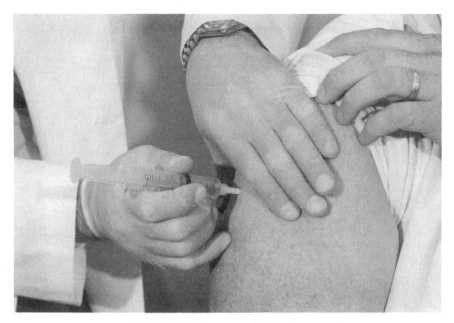

Figure 4–6. Intramuscular injection.

14. Aspirate the syringe to make sure that the needle is not in a blood vessel. If blood enters the syringe, withdraw the needle and prepare another site for another attempt, *using a new needle*.
15. Inject the medication slowly.
16. Remove and dispose the needle.
17. Gently massage the injection site. (This aids in drug absorption.)
18. Cover the site with an adhesive bandage strip.
19. Confirm and document administration of the medication.
20. Closely monitor the patient and report any changes.

Intravenous Lifeline

1. Perform a thorough patient assessment and history, confirming the need for the intravenous line.
2. Receive the order and write it down.
3. Confirm the order.
4. Prepare necessary equipment:
   Correct intravenous fluid
   Correct administration set. For example, the establishment of an intravenous lifeline requires a microdrip or minidrip set (60 drops per milliliter [60 gtt/ml]). For the replacement of fluid volume, a macrodrip set is used (10 to 15 drops per milliliter [10–15 gtt/ml]). There are other kinds of administration set for special kinds of drug administration.

Appropriate intravenous catheter. For example, volume replacement requires a large-bore (14- to 16-gauge) catheter, and a smaller bore is better for **keep-open rates.**

Extension tubing, if appropriate

Antibiotic swabs and ointment

Tourniquet

Gauze pads

Tape (½ inch and 1 inch)

5. Remove the outer wrapper from the intravenous bag and inspect the bag to make sure that:

    It contains the right fluid in the correct amount.

    The expiration date of the bag has not passed.

    The fluid is clear and free of visible particles.

6. Open, inspect, and attach the intravenous tubing to the bag.

7. Drain the fluid into the tubing, flushing out all air.

8. Stop the *venous* blood flow of the patient, using a tourniquet.

9. Identify and select a suitable vein.

10. Clean site with an antibiotic swab.

11. Using sterile technique, make a puncture, advance the catheter, and remove and dispose the needle.

12. Take a blood sample, if appropriate, and connect the tubing to the catheter.

13. Remove the tourniquet.

14. Confirm the fluid is flowing properly and adjust the rate of flow.

15. Apply antibiotic ointment and cover with sterile gauze or a bandage.

16. Tape securely.

17. Label the bag with the following information:

    The patient's name

    The date and time that the intravenous infusion was established

    Catheter size

    The name of person who established the intravenous infusion

18. Confirm and document the procedure.

19. Monitor the patient and report any changes.

Intravenous Bolus Injection

Once you have established an intravenous infusion (intravenous lifeline), you can administer a bolus injection through the intravenous line. This procedure is called an *intravenous bolus injection*. In the following description of the procedure, the bolus is packaged in a single-dose, prefilled syringe. In most prehospital emergency situations, this is the case. Sometimes, however, the necessary drug is available only in an ampule or vial, from which you must draw the proper dose.

1. Perform a thorough patient assessment and history, confirming that:

    The medication is needed.

    The patient does not have any allergies that contraindicate the use of the medication.

2. Receive the order.

3. Write down and confirm the order.
4. Prepare the appropriate equipment:
   Correct drug (prefilled syringe with needle)
   Antibacterial swab and alcohol prep
   Adhesive bandage strip
5. Explain the procedure to the patient.
6. Examine the medication, reconfirming that:
   It is the correct medication.
   It has not expired.
   It is not discolored.
   There are no visible particles in the solution.
7. Calculate the required dosage.
8. Assemble the prefilled syringe and expel excess air from it.
9. Verify the patency of the intravenous line.
10. Clean the medication port on the intravenous administration set using an antibacterial swab.
11. Recheck the medication.
12. Insert the needle into the medication port (Fig. 4-7).
13. Pinch the tubing off above the medication injection port.
14. Administer the medication at the appropriate rate. (Rates differ among different types of medication.)
15. Remove the needle and clean the administration port with an antibacterial swab; dispose of the needle and syringe.
16. Release the pinched intravenous line.

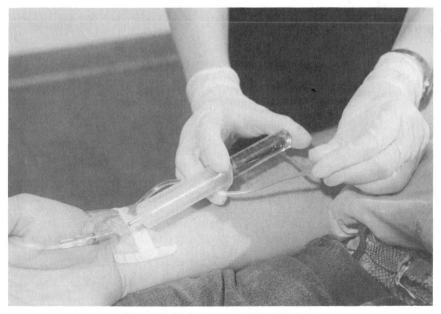

Figure 4-7. Intravenous bolus injection.

17. Flush the intravenous line by opening the line wide open for 30 seconds to 1 minute.
18. Confirm and record administration of the medication.
19. Closely monitor the patient and report any changes.

Intravenous Infusion (Piggyback)

1. Perform a thorough patient assessment and history confirming that:
   The medication is needed.
   The patient does not have any allergies that contraindicate the use of the medication.
2. Receive the order.
3. Write down and confirm the order.
4. Prepare the appropriate equipment:
   Correct drug (prefilled syringe with needle)
   Antibacterial swab and alcohol prep
   Label for the intravenous bag
5. Explain the procedure to the patient.
6. Examine the medication, reconfirming that:
   It is the correct medication.
   It has not expired.
   It is not discolored.
   There are no visible particles in the solution.
7. Recheck the medication.
8. Assemble the prefilled syringe and expel excess air from it.
9. Clean the medication port on the intravenous bag with antibacterial swab.
10. Insert the needle into the medication port of the bag and add the medication (Figure 4–8).
11. Remove the needle and cleanse the administration port with an antibacterial swab; dispose of the syringe and needle.
12. Thoroughly mix the medication in the intravenous bag.
13. Attach an intravenous line to the bag, "prime" the line, and attach a 1-inch by 18-gauge needle to the line.
14. Clean the medication port of the already-established intravenous line with an antibacterial swab, insert the needle (Fig. 4–9), and secure with tape.
15. Shut down the previously established intravenous line and begin flow of the piggyback medication line; set the flow to the necessary rate.
16. Label the piggyback intravenous bag with:
    The patient's name
    The date and time that the piggyback infusion was established
    The name and amount of the drug added to the piggyback intravenous bag
    The infusion flow rate
    The name of the person who established the piggyback infusion
17. Confirm and record the establishment of the piggyback infusion.
18. Monitor the patient and report any changes.

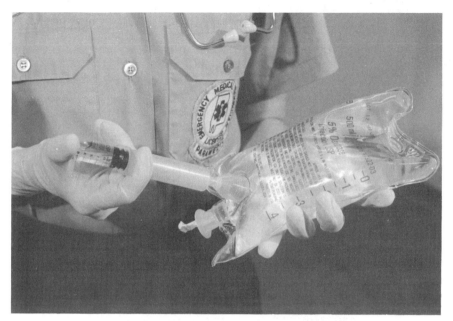

Figure 4–8. Adding medication to an intravenous bag.

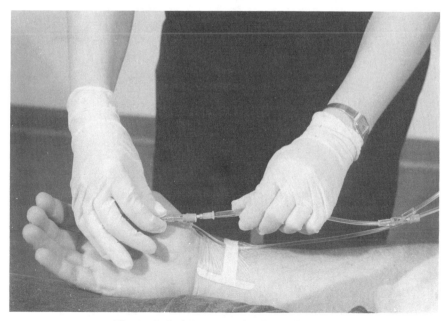

Figure 4–9. Intravenous piggyback infusion.

Transtracheal Administration

Administering drugs through an established endotracheal tube is relatively easy. When the procedure is performed properly, absorption of the drugs is as rapid as when they are administered intravenously.

1. Receive the order.
2. Write down and confirm the order.
3. Examine the medication, reconfirming that:
   It is the correct medication.
   It has not expired.
   It is not discolored.
   There are no visible particles in the solution.
4. Assemble the prefilled syringe and expel excess air from it.
5. Remove the bag-valve-mask device and inject the correct amount of medication into the endotracheal tube (Fig. 4–10). Dispose of the needle and syringe. If the medication order is for a small dose, and you must withdraw the drug from an ampule or vial, dilute the drug with 5 to 10 milliliters of sterile normal saline solution or sterile water.
6. Replace the bag-valve-mask device and hyperventilate to force drug down the tube.
7. Resume normal ventilations.
8. Confirm and record the administration of medication.
9. Monitor the patient and report any changes.

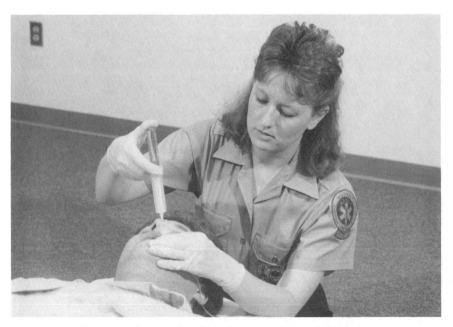

Figure 4–10. Administering a drug down an endotracheal tube.

Intraosseous Infusion

Intraosseous infusion allows rapid vascular access via the bone marrow. It is used mostly to administer fluids and drugs to children under 5 who are suffering circulatory failure or cardiac arrest. All drugs and crystalloid solutions that can be administered intravenously can be given by the intraosseous route. The procedure for establishing an intraosseous line is as follows:

1. Receive the order.
2. Write down and confirm the order.
3. Prepare the appropriate equipment:
   Intravenous solution, intravenous tubing, and a stopcock
   Spinal or bone-marrow needle with a stylet (15- to 18-gauge)
   Syringe filled with saline
   Antibacterial swab and alcohol preps

4. Examine the solution, reconfirming that:
   It is the correct solution.
   It has not expired.
   It is not discolored.
   There are no visible particles in the solution.

5. Attach a line to the bag, prime the line, and attach the needle.
6. Identify bony landmarks. For example:
   The proximal tibia: The needle will enter 1 to 3 centimeters below the tibial tuberosity just beneath the knee (Fig. 4–11). The proximal tibia is the preferred site for three reasons: (1) The prominence of the bone makes it easy to find the right injection site. (2) There is little soft tissue over the bone. (3) The flat surface of the bone makes for easier needle insertion.
   The distal femur: The needle will enter 3 centimeters above the lateral condyle just above the knee (Fig. 4–12).
   The distal tibia: The needle will enter in the flat surface of the tibia 1 to 3 centimeters above the medial malleolus at the ankle (Fig. 4–13).

7. Clean the site with antibacterial swab.
8. Insert the needle with stylet in place at a 90-degree angle to the bone or at a slight angle *away* from the joint. This is to avoid inserting the needle into the growth plate.
9. Remove the stylet.
10. Attempt to aspirate bone marrow. If no marrow enters the needle, inject a small amount of saline solution into the site. If there is resistance to the injection, or if saline solution infiltrates the soft tissue around the site, the needle is not in the bone marrow.
11. Stabilize the needle (although it should stand unsupported).
12. Connect the tubing and begin the infusion.
13. Confirm the establishment of intraosseous infusion.
14. Monitor the patient and report any changes.

Once the intraosseous infusion has been established, medications can be administered via intravenous bolus or piggyback infusion.

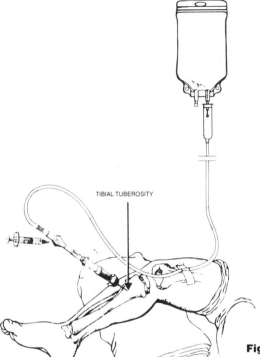

TIBIAL TUBEROSITY

Figure 4–11. Preferred site for intraosseous drug administration (proximal tibia).

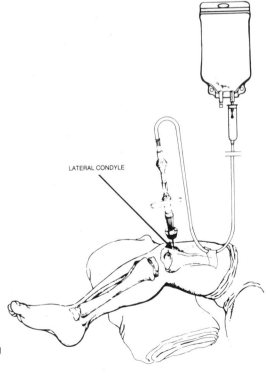

LATERAL CONDYLE

Figure 4–12. Intraosseous drug administration (distal femur).

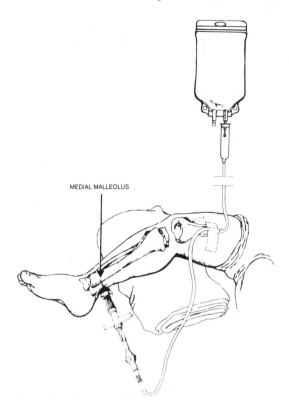

MEDIAL MALLEOLUS

Figure 4–13. Intraosseous drug
administration (distal tibia).

UNIVERSAL PRECAUTIONS

It is not possible by looking at a patient to tell if he or she is infected with
a blood-borne infection such as hepatitis or human immunodeficiency virus
(HIV), which can lead to the fatal acquired immunodeficiency syndrome
(AIDS). Therefore, the Centers for Disease Control in Atlanta, Georgia, recommends certain **universal precautions.** *Universal precautions* are infection control procedures that health care workers should apply with *all* patients, in *all*
situations.

Wear gloves whenever touching a patient. This is especially important
when you come in contact with blood or any body fluid. You should also wear
gloves when performing procedures like starting intravenous lines, drawing
blood, giving injections, or inserting an endotrachael tube. After each patient
contact, carefully remove your gloves and immediately dispose of them. If
blood or body fluids come in contact with your skin, thoroughly wash all
exposed surfaces.

If there is a chance that patient blood or body fluids may come in contact
with your face or clothing, wear protective masks and gowns. Once your contact
with the patient is completed, carefully remove mask and gown and properly
dispose of them.

Do not re-cap, bend, break, or remove needles from the syringe. Dispose of needles and disposable syringes in puncture-resistant containers immediately after use.

All of the routes for transmission of blood-borne infections have yet to be identified. Therefore, it is extremely important for you to take all appropriate precautions against coming in contact with such infections while treating your patient. All equipment used on the patient, such as a bag-valve-mask device or airway adjuncts, should be cleaned as soon after use as possible. When appropriate, use disposable equipment.

CONCLUSION

You must be knowledgeable about and competent in every drug administration procedure that you will be called on, as an emergency care provider, to perform. You must also know all the medications you are allowed to give and the routes by which they are usually given. When an emergency arises, time is precious. In an emergency, you will be required to quickly identify the drug(s) to be given, the necessary dosage, and the most appropriate route. You must be comfortable with all drugs you are responsible for administering and be able to administer them in a safe, rapid, and systematic manner.

STUDY QUESTIONS

1. You have responded to a patient in cardiac arrest. Why is an intramuscular injection not recommended for this situation?

2. The rate of action of a drug is determined by the drug concentration and the route by which the drug is administered. Of the four routes of drug administration listed below, which lists routes in order from fastest to slowest rate of drug absorption?
   a. Intramuscular, oral, subcutaneous, intravenous.
   b. Intravenous, endotracheal, oral, intramuscular.
   c. Oral, subcutaneous, intramuscular, intravenous.
   d. Intraosseous, intramuscular, subcutaneous, oral.

3. Which of the following steps is **not** appropriate when administering a drug by intravenous bolus injection?
   a. Verify the patency of the intravenous line before administering the drug.
   b. Pinch the intravenous tubing off above the medication injection port.
   c. Flush the intravenous line after drug administration.
   d. Recap the needle and save any unused drug.

Chapter 5

Fundamentals of Drug-Dosage Calculations

Administering drugs would be much easier if they all came in the same form and were packaged in the same way and in identical **concentrations.** However, drugs come in a variety of forms, packages, and concentrations (Figs. 5–1 and 5–2). Anyone with the responsibility for administering drugs must (1) be familiar with their various forms and concentrations, (2) know how to prepare the drug for administration, and (3) be able to calculate the dosage and rate of administration. The following list illustrates the bewildering variety of forms in which drugs often used in prehospital emergencies are packaged:

- *Lidocaine:* 2 grams (2 g) in solution in a 10-milliliter (10-mL) syringe. In this case, the drug concentration is 200 milligrams per milliliter (200 mg/ mL). The paramedic dilutes this in an appropriate intravenous fluid before administration. Lidocaine is also commonly available, for direct bolus intravenous injection, as 100 milligrams of a 20 milligrams-per-milliliter solution in a prefilled 5-milliliter syringe.
- *$D_{50}W$ (50% dextrose in water):* This very widely used prehospital agent is commonly available in a 50-milliliter prefilled syringe, which contains 25 grams of dextrose.
- *Furosemide:* 20 milligrams in a 2-milliliter prefilled syringe. Furosemide is also packaged in **ampules** of different sizes (e.g., 20 milligrams in a 2-milliliter ampule, 100 milligrams in a 10-milliliter ampule).
- *Nitroglycerin:* Most commonly available in tablets—$\frac{1}{150}$ grain ($\frac{1}{150}$ gr), which equals 0.4 milligram, or $\frac{1}{200}$ grain, which equals 0.3 milligram. (One grain, in **apothecaries'** measure, equals about 60 milligrams.)

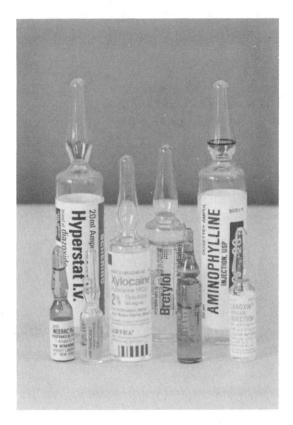

Figure 5–1. A common type of drug preparation is the liquid solution in a glass ampule.

- *Oxytocin:* Commonly packaged as 10 U.S.P. **units** in a 1-milliliter ampule. A *unit* is defined as one of anything. It is a specific amount adopted as a standard of measurement. A **U.S.P. unit** is any unit specified in the *United States Pharmacopeia.*
- *Dopamine:* One of the forms in which you may encounter this drug is as 200 milligrams in solution in a 5-milliliter prefilled syringe.
- *Sodium bicarbonate:* Sodium bicarbonate is usually packaged in prefilled 50-milliliter syringes containing either 44.4 or 50 **milliequivalents (mEq).** A *milliequivalent* is the concentration of **electrolytes** (see Chapter 6) in a certain volume of solution, usually expressed as milliequivalent per liter (mEq/L).

As the preceding list shows, drugs come in a bewildering variety of forms, concentrations, and packages. The paramedic who administers drugs must be able to use mathematical calculations to determine the right dosages.

WEIGHTS AND MEASURES

Throughout history, humans have developed various systems of weights and measures—ways of describing the size and/or amount of physical objects

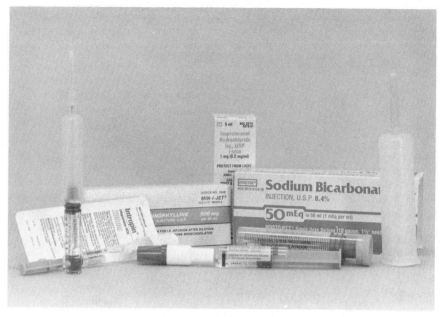

Figure 5–2. Drugs come in many forms, some of which are shown above.

or substances. Each system has units of measure for three physical characteristics:

Length: The distance between two points.

Mass: How much matter is in an object or a substance; this is commonly expressed as its weight.

Volume: How much space is occupied by an object or a substance.

Some systems use different measures for dry and liquid volume. For instance, in the system used in the United States (called the U.S. system or household system), the units of dry measure are pint, quart, peck, and bushel and the units of liquid measure include fluidounce, pint, quart, and gallon.

Because of the historic roots of pharmacology, drug dosages in the United States are expressed in any one of three systems:

1. **The metric system.** (See page 63.)
2. **The United States system.** The **United States system** is based on the traditional English system, which in England has been almost completely replaced by the metric system.
3. **The apothecaries' system.** *Apothecary* is the old name for pharmacist. The apothecaries' system has units of measure for weight (mass) and liquid weight (capacity).

Table 5–1 lists the various units of measure in each system. Table 5–2 shows the equivalents between various units in the English and metric systems.

Table 5-1. SYSTEMS OF WEIGHTS AND MEASURES

United States (English)	Metric	Apothecaries'
Mass (Weight)		
Pound (lb)	Kilogram (kg)	Pound (lb ap)
Ounce (oz)	Hectogram (hg)	Ounce (ox ap)
Dram (dr)	Dekagram (dag)	Dram (dr ap)
Grain (gr)	Gram (g)	Scruple (s)
	Decigram (dg)	Grain*
	Centigram (cg)	
	Milligram (mg)	
	Microgram (μg)	
Volume (Liquid Measure)		
Gallon (gal)	Kiloliter (kL)	Gallon (gal)
Quart (qt)	Hectoliter (hL)	Quart (qt)
Pint (pt)	Dekaliter (daL)	Pint (pt)
Gill (gi)	Liter (L)	Gill (gi)
Fluidounce (fl oz)	Deciliter (dL)	Fluidounce (fl oz)
Fluidram (fl dr)	Centiliter (cL)	Fluidram (fl dr)
Minim (min)	Milliliter (mL)	Minim (min)
	Microliter (μL)	
Length		
Mile (mi)	Kilometer (km)	
Yard (yd)	Hectometer (hm)	
Foot (ft or ')	Dekameter (dam)	
Inch (in or ")	Meter (m)	
	Decimeter (dm)	
	Centimeter (cm)	
	Millimeter (mm)	
	Micrometer (μm)	

* Although the English pound and apothecaries' pound are not equivalent, the English grain and apothecaries' grain are—each is equal to approximately 60 milligrams.

To administer drugs safely, you must be able to convert various units of measure:

- You will need to convert an amount expressed in one unit of measure into its equivalent in another unit of measure in the *same system*. For example, if a physician tells you to administer 1500 milligrams of a drug and the drug is packaged in tablets, each containing 0.5 gram of the drug, you must convert 0.5 gram to its equivalent in milligrams in order to calculate how many tablets are required. (You will learn how to do this in the "Decimal Review" section.)

Table 5–2. COMMONLY USED EQUIVALENTS

Metric-English	English-Metric
1 kilogram (k) = 2.2 pounds (lb)	1 pound (lb) = 0.454 kilograms (k)
1 gram (g) = 0.035 ounces (oz)	1 ounce (oz) = 28.35 grams (g)
1 milligram (mg) = 0.015 grains	1 grain (gr) = 0.0645 grams (gr) or 64.5 milligrams (mg)
1 liter (L) = 1.057 quarts (qt)	1 fluidounce (fl oz) = 29.57 milligrams (mg)
1 deciliter (dL) = 3.38 fluidounce (fl oz)	
1 milliliter (mL) = 0.27 fluidram	

- You must also know how to convert an amount expressed in one unit of measure into its equivalent in *another system.* For example, many drug orders are based on body weight. If the order tells you to administer 0.5 milligram per kilogram of body weight, and the patient weighs 165 pounds, you must convert pounds to kilograms. (The "U.S.-to-Metric Conversions" section shows you how.)

THE METRIC SYSTEM

The metric system is used in many countries of the world and in all scientific disciplines, including medicine and pharmacology. It is a decimal system, meaning it is based on the number 10. Every unit of length is ten times larger than the next smaller unit and ten times smaller than the next larger unit. The basic unit of length is the *meter;* the basic unit of mass (weight) is the *gram;* and the basic unit of volume is the *liter.* The names of all the other units of measure in the metric system are formed by adding prefixes to the names of the basic units. The prefix indicates how many times larger or smaller than the basic unit the new unit is. For example, a kilometer equals 1000 meters; a millimeter equals one thousandth of a meter. Table 5–3 illustrates the progression of prefixes used in the metric system.

Table 5–3. METRIC PREFIXES

Prefix	Multiple of Base
Mega-	1,000,000
Kilo-	1000
Hecto-	100
Deka-	10
Base	1
Deci-	1/10
Centi-	1/100
Milli-	1/1,000
Micro-	1/1,000,000

Review of Decimals

Converting dosages within the metric system is easy because it is a decimal system. A review of decimal arithmetic will show how simple calculating metric dosages can be.

Each amount in the metric system consists of a whole number (in many cases, the whole number is 0) and a decimal fraction separated by the decimal point (e.g., 1.5). The whole number is on the left of the decimal point, and the decimal fraction is expressed by the numbers on the right of the decimal point. The position of a number in relation to the decimal point gives that number its name and its value (Fig. 5–3). For example, the first place to the left of the decimal point is the unit place, the second is the ten place, and so on. A 2 in the second place to the left of the decimal point (e.g., 20.00) indicates that there are two tens in the ten's place. A zero in the first place to the left of the decimal point indicates that there is nothing in the units place, which means, so far, that the number is twenty. A 2 in the second place to the right of the decimal point (e.g., 0.02) indicates two one-hundredths. The number 20.02, then, means "twenty and two hundredths."

For amounts less than 1, it is a good idea to place a 0 in the unit place (the first place to the left of the decimal point); for example, the best way to express the fraction ½ in decimals is 0.5.

Adding and subtracting decimals

When adding decimal numbers, place the second number below the first number, the third below the second, and so on, just as with whole numbers—but remember to line the numbers up on the decimal point.

> **EXAMPLE**
>   Add: 3.3 + 29.75 + 4
>
> **Solution**
>   3.30
>   +29.75
>   + 4.00   [Add 0s to the right of the decimal point as needed]
>   ―――――
>   37.05

Subtracting one decimal number from another number also requires lining the two numbers up, one below the other, on the decimal point.

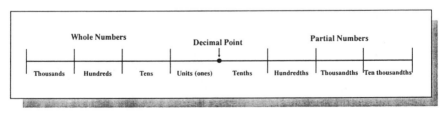

Figure 5–3. In the decimal system, the position of a number in relation to the decimal place determines the name and value of the number.

EXAMPLE
Subtract: 17.20 − 6.25

Solution

  17.20   [Add 0s to the right of the decimal point as needed]
− 6.25
  10.95

EXAMPLE
Subtract: 33.02 − 17

Solution

  33.02
−17.00   [Add 0s to the right of the decimal point as needed]
  16.02

Rounding decimals

For many decimal calculations, it is necessary or convenient to "round" the answer up or down. Round down to the nearest whole number if the decimal fraction is below 0.5 (change 6.4 to 6). If the decimal fraction is 0.5 or higher, round up to the next larger whole number (change 6.5 to 7). You can also round down or up to the next decimal place (change 6.43 to 6.4; change 6.66 to 6.7).

There are other systems for rounding numbers that you may prefer to use and that work just as well.

Multiplying decimals

First, multiply decimal numbers together as if they were whole numbers, without regard to the decimal point. Then add the number of decimal places (places to the right of the decimal point) in both of the multipliers. That total is the number of decimal places in the product of the two numbers; the decimal point goes that number of places to the left of the last number in the product.

EXAMPLE
Multiply: 12.5 × 3.7

Solution

   12.5 [1 decimal place]
× 3.7 [+1 decimal place]
   875
+375
 46.25 [2 decimal places in the product]
    21

EXAMPLE
Multiply: 25.75 × 6.05

Solution

```
        25.75  [  2 decimal places]
    ×    6.04  [+2 decimal places]
        10300
    +    0000
    +15450
       155.5300  [  4 decimal places in the product]
          4321
```
[After determining where the decimal point goes, drop any final zeros at the right of the decimal point]

Whenever you multiply by any multiple of 10, a shorter method is to move the decimal point to the right by the number of zeros in the multiple. For example, when multiplying by 10, move the decimal point one place to the right:

$15.75 \times 10 = 157.50$

When multiplying by 100, move the decimal point two places to the right:

$15.75 \times 100 = 1575.0$

When multiplying by 1000, move the decimal point three places to the right:

$15.75 \times 1000 = 15,750.0$

Dividing decimals

When dividing by a decimal number, place a caret ($\wedge$) as many places to the right of the decimal point in both the divisor and the dividend as there are places in the divisor. Then, place the decimal point in the quotient above the caret in the dividend.

EXAMPLE
Divide: $253.680 \div 10.5$

Solution

```
              2 4.16
    10.5 )253.6 80
          210
          43 6
          42 0
           1 6 8
           1 0 5
             6 3 0
             6 3 0
```

EXAMPLE
Divide: 50.2990 ÷ 0.125

Solution

```
                402.4
    0.125 ) 50.299 0
            50 0
            299
            250
             49 0
             49 0
```

There is a shorter method for dividing a decimal number by any multiple of 10. Move the decimal point in the dividend to the left by the number of zeros in the divisor. For example, when dividing by 10, move the dividend's decimal point one place to the left:

15.0 ÷ 10 = 1.5

When dividing a decimal number by a multiple of 100, move the decimal point two places to the left:

6.0 ÷ 100 = 0.06

Metric-to-Metric Conversions

Because the metric system is a decimal system, it is easy to convert from one metric unit to another. For example, to convert grams to milligrams, all you have to do is multiply by 1000. As a shortcut, move the decimal point three places to the right.

EXAMPLE
Convert 3 grams to milligrams

Solution
3.0 g × 1000 = 3000 mg [Multiply by 1000]

or simply move the decimal point three places to the right.
3.0 g = 3000 mg [Add zeros as needed to move the decimal point]
         123

EXAMPLE
Convert 5.25 grams to milligrams

Solution
5.25 g × 1000 = 5250 mg

or
5.25 g = 5250 mg

To convert milligrams to grams, divide by 1000—move the decimal point three places to the left.

EXAMPLE
Convert 4000 milligrams to grams

Solution

$$1000 \overline{)4000 \text{ mg}} \quad \frac{4 \text{ g}}{}$$

or

4000 mg = 4.000 g
           ⌣⌣⌣
           321

PROBLEM
You are a paramedic student in the emergency department. A physician orders you to administer 1500 milligrams of a drug. The drug comes in 0.5-gram tablets. You must *convert* within the metric system to find out how many milligrams are in each tablet. Then you must *calculate* to find out how many tablets are required.

Solution
To find the number of milligrams in each tablet, move the decimal point three places to the right.

Step 1 (Convert): Convert grams to milligrams.
0.5 g = 500.0 mg [Move the decimal point three places to the right]

Answer = each tablet contains 500 mg.

Step 2 (Calculate): Divide the required dosage by the amount of drug per tablet.

$$500 \overline{)1500} \quad \frac{3}{}$$

Three tablets are required for the prescribed dose.

When converting liters to milliliters (larger unit to smaller unit), you must multiply by 1000 (or just move the decimal point three places to the right). For example:

6 L = 6000 mL (6 × 1000 or 6000)
                          ⌣⌣⌣
                          123
4.5 L = 4500 mL (4.5 × 1000 or 4500)
                            ⌣⌣⌣
                            123

To convert milliliters to liters (smaller unit to larger unit), you must divide by 1000 or just move the decimal three places to the left. For example:

5000 mL = 5 L (5000 ÷ 1000 or 5,000)

$$\overline{321}$$

2500 mL = 2.5 L (2500 ÷ 1000 or 2,500)

$$\overline{321}$$

The cubic centimeter (cc) is a once-common unit of measure whose use is decreasing. Both a milliliter and a cubic centimeter are equal to one-thousandth of a liter. Even though milliliter and centimeter are equivalent expressions, milliliter is the preferred term.

U.S.-to-Metric Conversions

For many drugs administered in the prehospital setting, the drug order is expressed as a volume of drug based on body weight. For example, an order for lidocaine might call for administering 1 milligram per kilogram of body weight (1 mg/kg). Most patients do not know their body weight in kilograms, so you must be able to convert pounds (U.S.) to kilograms (metric).

If 2.2 pounds equals 1 kilogram (Table 5–2), 1 pound equals 1/2.2 kilograms.

2.2 lb = 1 kg
  1 lb = 1 ÷ 2.2 kg

To convert pounds to kilograms, simply divide the number of pounds by 2.2. For example:

100 lb = 100 ÷ 2.2 = 45 kg
150 lb = 150 ÷ 2.2 = 68 kg [68.18 is rounded down to 68]
235 lb = 235 ÷ 2.2 = 107 kg [106.82 is rounded up to 107]

THE APOTHECARIES' SYSTEM

The apothecaries' system of measurement is rarely used by physicians when ordering drugs. However, many drugs are available only in (apothecary) grains. For this reason, you should be able to use the apothecaries' system. The apothecaries' system measures solids in units of grains, drams, ounces, and pounds. It measures liquids in minims, fluidrams, fluidounces, pints, and gallons.

Converting from the metric system to the apothecaries' system is rarely necessary in the prehospital setting.

CALCULATING DRUG SOLUTIONS

Many drugs are given in solution—that is, pure drug in powder or liquid form is dissolved in a liquid. To administer a prescribed amount of a drug in solution, you must know the drug concentration of the solution. *Drug concentra-*

tion is the amount of drug per unit of volume; it is usually expressed in milligrams per milliliter. The formula for determining concentration is:

$$\text{Concentration} = \frac{\text{Amount of Drug (mg)}}{\text{Volume of Solution (mL)}}$$

For example, a common preparation of bretylium is a prefilled 10-milliliter syringe containing 500 milligrams of bretylium. In this case, the drug concentration is 50 milligrams per milliliter (50 mg/mL).

$$\text{Concentration} = \frac{500 \text{ mg [Total mg]}}{10 \text{ ml [Total mL]}} = 50 \text{ mg/mL}$$

When you know the drug concentration, you know how much drug is in one milliliter of a solution. From that, you can determine how much solution is required to deliver the amount of drug ordered. Divide the amount of drug ordered by the drug concentration:

$$\text{Required Volume of Solution (mL)} = \frac{\text{Required Drug Amount (mg)}}{\text{Drug Concentration (mg/mL)}}$$

PROBLEM

   The physician directs you to give a patient 200 milligrams of a drug. The preparation on hand is a 10-milliliter syringe containing 500 milligrams of the drug. How much of the preparation do you administer?

Solution

   First, find the drug concentration (amount of drug per milliliter of solution) in the syringe by dividing the amount of drug in the syringe by the total volume of the solution:

$$\frac{500 \text{ mg}}{10 \text{ mL}} = 50 \text{ mg/mL}$$

Next, find the volume of solution required (mL) to deliver the required drug amount (mg) by dividing the required drug amount by the drug concentration (mg/mL).

$$\frac{200 \text{ mg}}{50 \text{ mg/mL}} = 4 \text{ mL [The answer will be in mL]}$$

Give the patient 4 milliliters of the solution in the 10-milliliter syringe.

Sometimes drug concentration is expressed as a percentage. For example, a common preparation of lidocaine is a 20 percent concentration in a 10-milliliter syringe. Twenty percent means that there are 20 grams of drug in every 100 milliliters of preparation.* To find out how much lidocaine is in the syringe, multiply the percentage of drug (expressed as a decimal fraction) in solution by the total volume of the syringe.

0.20 [Concentration] $\times$ 10 mL [Volume] = 2 g

What is the concentration in milligrams per milliliter? Convert grams to milligrams and divide by the number of milliliters in the preparation.

$$2 \text{ g} \times 1000 = 2000 \text{ mg}$$

$$\frac{2000 \text{ mg}}{10 \text{ mL}} = 200 \text{ mg/mL}$$

Sometimes, as with epinephrine, the drug concentration is expressed as a ratio. For example, two often-used preparations are epinephrine in a 1:1000 solution and epinephrine in a 1:10,000 solution. The ratio of 1:1000 indicates that 1 milliliter of solution contains 1 milligram of the drug. The 1:10,000 ratio indicates that there is 1 milligram of drug in 10 milliliters of solution.

CALCULATING RATES OF INFUSION

Intravenous tubing is packaged in macrodrop or microdrop sets. Macrodrop intravenous tubing is available in both 10- and 15-drop sets. With a 10-drop intravenous set, 10 drops equals 1.0 milliliter. With a 15-drop set, 15 drops equals 1.0 milliliter. A microdrop intravenous set takes 60 drops to deliver 1.0 milliliter.

To calculate the drip rate for an intravenous infusion, you need to know three values: the volume of fluid required, the set size (10-, 15-, or 60-drop), and the total time of the infusion in minutes. For example: How many drops per minute will it take to infuse 500 milliliters of fluid using a 15-drop-per-minute (gtt/min)* macrodrop intravenous set for 45 minutes?

Infusion Rate (drops per minute)

$$= \frac{\text{Volume Required (mL)} \times \text{Set Size (drops per min)}}{\text{Infusion Time (min)}}$$

$$\text{Infusion Rate (gtt/min)} = \frac{500 \text{ mL} \times 15 \text{ gtt/mL}}{45 \text{ min}}$$

$$= \frac{7500 \text{ gtt}}{45 \text{ min}} = 167 \text{ gtt/min } [166.67 \text{ rounded to } 167]$$

---

* Remember, in the metric system the cubic centimeter, milliliter, and gram are equivalent. One cubic centimeter holds one milliliter of water, and one milliliter of water (or of most other liquids) weighs 1 gram.

* *gtt* is the abbreviation for guttae, which is Latin for drops.

EXAMPLE

How many drops per minute will it take to infuse 250 milliliters of fluid using a microdrop intravenous (60 drops per milliliter) for 1 hour?

Solution

$$\text{Infusion rate} = \frac{250 \text{ mL} \times 60 \text{ gtt/mL}}{60 \text{ min}} = \frac{15000}{60} = 250 \text{ gtt/min}$$

EXAMPLE

You are ordered to prepare a lidocaine infusion by adding 2 grams of lidocaine to 500 milliliters of dextrose 5% in water. Once the infusion is prepared, it is to run at 3 milligrams per minute, using a microdrip set. What is the concentration (milligrams per milliliter) of the lidocaine infusion, and at what rate (drops per minute) should the infusion run to deliver 3 milligrams of lidocaine per minute?

Solution

Step 1: Determine the lidocaine concentration.

$$\text{Concentration} = \frac{\text{Amount of Drug}}{\text{Volume of Solution}}$$

$$= \frac{2 \text{ g}}{500 \text{ mL}} \quad [\text{Convert g to mgs}]$$

$$= \frac{2000 \text{ mg}}{500 \text{ mL}} = 4 \text{ mg/mL}$$

Step 2: Determine the volume of solution needed to deliver 3 milligrams of lidocaine.

$$\text{Required Volume of Solution} = \frac{\text{Required Drug Amount}}{\text{Drug Concentration}}$$

$$= \frac{3 \text{ mg}}{4 \text{ mg/mL}} = 0.75 \text{ mL}$$

Step 3: Determine the infusion rate required.

$$\text{Infusion Rate} = \frac{\text{Volume of Solution Required} \times \text{Set Size}}{\text{Infusion Time}}$$

$$= \frac{0.75 \text{ mL} \times 60 \text{ gtt/mL}}{1 \text{ min}}$$

$$= 45 \text{ gtt/mL}$$

CONVERTING TEMPERATURE MEASUREMENTS

Prehospital emergency care providers must understand the Celsius system of temperature measurement as well as the metric system of weights and measures. You must be able to convert temperatures expressed in Celsius to Fahrenheit, and vice versa.

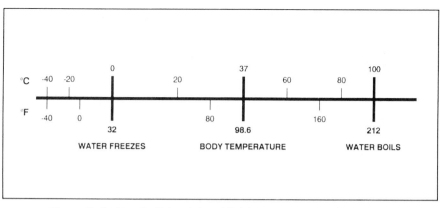

Figure 5–4. How the Fahrenheit and Celsius temperature scales compare.

Figure 5-4 compares the Fahrenheit and Celsius systems of temperature measurement. The freezing point of Celsius is 0°, and the freezing point for Fahrenheit is 32°. On the Celsius scale the boiling point of water is 100°; it is 212° on the Fahrenheit scale. Normal body temperature on the Celsius scale is 37°, and normal body temperature on the Fahrenheit scale is 98.6°.

Two formulas will help you convert between the two systems. To convert Fahrenheit to Celsius use the following formula:

Degrees Celsius = (Degrees Fahrenheit − 32) × 0.556

EXAMPLE
Convert 212°F to Celsius

Solution
C = (212 − 32) × 0.556
= 100°

To convert Celsius to Fahrenheit use this formula

Degrees Fahrenheit = Degrees Celsius × 1.8 + 32

EXAMPLE
Convert 37°C to Fahrenheit

Solution
F = 37 × 1.8 + 32
= 66.6 + 32 = 98.6°

CONCLUSION

When many of us hear the word "math" we immediately have a catecholamine release, sending our stress levels through the roof. The key to feeling comfortable with math is patience and practice.

This chapter presents basic information on which to build. As with any skill, math skill requires frequent practice to maintain acceptable proficiency levels.

PRACTICE PROBLEMS

Conversions

1. 50 kg = _____ lb

2. 180 lb = _____ kg

3. 0.2 mg = _____ μg

4. 3.0 L = _____ mL

5. 0.3 g = _____ mg

6. 10 mL = _____ cc

7. 3.0 g = _____ mg

8. 0.06 g = _____ mg

9. 200 lb = _____ kg

10. 4.0 g = _____ mg

11. 0.03 g = _____ mg

12. 8000 mg = _____ g

13. 200 mL = _____ cc

14. 2.0 mg = _____ μg

15. 0.1 L = _____ mL

PROBLEM SET A

1. A physician has ordered you to administer 1 milligram per kilogram of lidocaine to a patient in cardiac arrest. You estimate that the patient weighs 175 pounds. The lidocaine is packaged as 100 milligrams in a 5-milliliter prefilled syringe.
   a. How many milligrams of lidocaine are required?
   b. How many milliliters of solution are needed for the required dose of lidocaine?

2. You are ordered to administer 0.5 milligram of epinephrine by intravenous bolus. The epinephrine comes packaged as 1 milligram in a 10-milliliter prefilled syringe. How many milliliters will you give?

3. A physician orders you to administer an isoproterenol infusion. You are to begin the infusion at 2 micrograms per minute using a microdrip (60-drops-per-minute) infusion set. The infusion is prepared by adding 1 milligram of isoproterenol to 500 milliliters of dextrose 5% in water (D_5W).
   a. What is the concentration of isoproterenol when it is added to the D_5W (in micrograms per milliliter)?
   b. What infusion rate is needed to administer 2 micrograms per minute?

4. You are ordered to add 800 milligrams of dopamine to 500 milliliters of D₅W. What will be the resulting concentration in micrograms per milliliter?

5. You are ordered to administer 20 milligrams of furosemide. Your furosemide is packaged as 40 milligrams in a 4-milliliter prefilled syringe. How many milliliters will you administer?

6. A physician orders you to administer 5 milligrams per kilogram of bretylium. Your patient weighs 175 pounds. The bretylium is packaged as 500 milligrams in a 10-milliliter vial.
   a. How many milligrams will you administer?
   b. How many milliliters will you administer?

PROBLEM SET B

1. You have diluted 2 grams of lidocaine in 500 milliliters of D₅W.
   a. What is the resulting concentration (milligrams per milliliter)?
   b. What infusion rate is needed when using a minidrip (60-drop-per-minute) set to deliver 2 milligrams per minute?

2. You have a 20 percent solution of mannitol in 500 milliliters of fluid. The physician orders you to administer 1.5 grams per kilogram of drug to your patient over 1 hour. Your patient weighs 120 pounds. You are using a 15-drop-per-minute intravenous IV set.
   a. What is the concentration (grams per milliliter) of the mannitol solution?
   b. How many drops per minute will you administer to your patient?

3. You are ordered to administer 2 liters of lactated Ringer's over a 3-hour period. How many drops per minute will you administer if your standard intravenous set yields 10 drops per milliliter?

4. You have a patient in severe anaphylactic shock. You are ordered to administer 0.5 milligram of a 1:10,000 solution of epinephrine by intravenous bolus. The epinephrine comes packaged as 1 milligram in a 10-milliliter solution. How many milliliters will you administer?

5. After you administer the dose in question 4, you are requested to start an epinephrine infusion. The physician orders you to administer 1 microgram per minute. You add 2 milligrams of 1:1000 epinephrine to 500 milliliters of D₅W.
   a. What is your resulting concentration (micrograms per milliliter)?
   b. What infusion rate is needed with a minidrip (60-drop-per-minute) intravenous set?

6. The physician orders you to begin a norepinephrine infusion at a rate of 2 micrograms per minute. You prepare the infusion by adding 4 milligrams of norepinephrine to 500 milliliters of normal saline.
   a. What is the resulting concentration (micrograms per milliliter)?
   b. What infusion rate is needed with a minidrip (60-drop-per-minute) intravenous set?

Chapter 6

Fluids, Electrolytes, and Acid-Base Balance

BODY FLUIDS

ELECTROLYTES

FLUID TRANSPORT
Passive Transport
Filtration

Diffusion
Osmosis
Active Transport

ACID-BASE BALANCE

INTRAVENOUS THERAPY

It is important for you to be familiar with the basics of **body fluids** and **electrolytes.** Maintaining a proper balance of fluids and electrolytes within the body is necessary for life. If, for instance, you are faced with a patient who is depleted of fluids and electrolytes (such as a person with severe burns or who is a severely dehydrated patient) you must act rapidly to help restore the internal environment to increase the patient's chances.

This chapter reviews the basics of fluids, electrolytes, and **acid-base balance.** The chapter also describes some often-used intravenous fluids and their roles in the treatment of fluid and electrolyte compromise.

BODY FLUIDS

Total body fluid varies from individual to individual depending on both sex and age. However, the average adult has a total body fluid content of approximately 60 percent of body weight. This total body fluid is divided into **intracellular** and **extracellular fluid** compartments (Fig. 6–1). *Intracellular fluid* is the fluid contained inside the body's cells. It accounts for approximately 45 percent of total body weight. *Extracellular fluid* is the body fluid outside the cells. It accounts for approximately 15 percent of body weight. Extracellular fluid is further divided into two separate types: **interstitial fluid** and **intravascular fluid** or **plasma.** *Interstitial fluid* is extracellular fluid located in the spaces between the body's cells. It accounts for approximately 10.5 percent of body weight. *Intravascular fluid* is the noncellular, fluid portion of the blood. It accounts for approximately 4.5 percent of body weight.

To illustrate, a man who weighs 176 pounds (80 kilograms) has approximately 48 liters (1 liter weighs approximately 1 kg) of body fluid (80 × 0.60 = 48). This amount is broken down as follows:

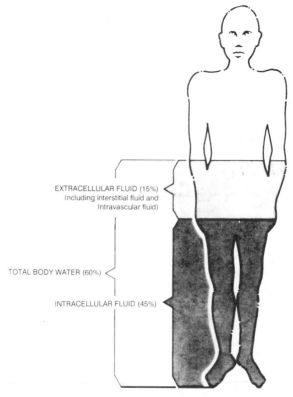

EXTRACELLULAR FLUID (15%)
Including interstitial fluid and
Intravascular fluid)

TOTAL BODY WATER (60%)

INTRACELLULAR FLUID (45%)

Figure 6–1. Distribution of body fluids.

Intracellular fluid: 36 liters (80 × .45 = 36)
Extracellular fluid: 12 liters (80 × .15 = 12)
   Interstitial fluid: 8.4 liters (80 × .105 = 8.4)
   Intravascular fluid: 3.6 liters (80 × .045 = 3.6)

ELECTROLYTES

An *electrolyte* is a substance that when placed in water separates into electrically charged particles called ions. There are two types of ions: **cations** and **anions.** A *cation* is a positively charged ion, and an *anion* is a negatively charged ion (Fig. 6–2).

The major cations of the body include:

Calcium (Ca^{2+}): Calcium is the most abundant cation in the body. It is required for bone growth, metabolism, blood clotting, normal cardiac function, and the initiation of neuromuscular contractions.

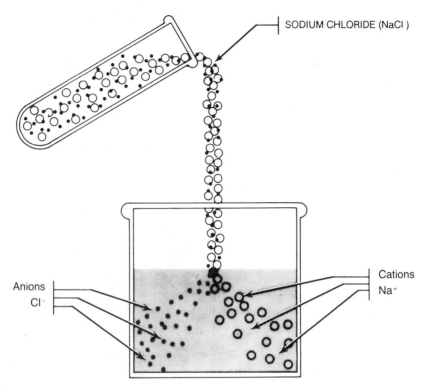

Figure 6–2. Dissociation of electrolytes. When sodium chloride (NaCl) is dissolved in water, the elements dissociate, resulting in atoms of chloride with a negative charge (anions) and atoms of sodium with a positive change (cations).

Magnesium (Mg^{2+}): Magnesium is required for body temperature regulation, protein and carbohydrate metabolism, and neuromuscular contraction.

Potassium (K^+): Potassium is the major intracellular cation. It is responsible for acid-base regulation, muscle excitability, and nerve impulse conduction.

Sodium (Na^+): Sodium is the major extracellular cation. It is responsible for fluid balance. When the body eliminates sodium, water is lost also. Conversely, when sodium levels in the body rise, water is retained. Sodium also preserves the balance between calcium and potassium.

The major anions of the body include:

Bicarbonate (HCO_3^-): Bicarbonate is the major buffer of the body. Its main function is to maintain acid-base balance.

Chloride (Cl^-): Chloride is the major extracellular anion. Its main function is to maintain fluid balance.

Phosphate ($HPO_4^=$): Phosphate is the major intracellular anion. It helps maintain acid-base balance.

Electrolytes are measured in milliequivalents (mEq). A milliequivalent is the concentration of electrolytes in a certain volume of solution, based on the number of available ionic charges. One milliequivalent of a cation will completely react with 1 milliequivalent of an anion forming a new compound. For example,

$$\left. \begin{array}{l} Na^+ \text{ (1 mEq of sodium)} \\ Cl^- \text{ (1 mEq of chloride)} \end{array} \right\} \text{Combine to form NaCl}$$

or

$$\left. \begin{array}{l} Ca^{2+} \text{ (2 mEq of calcium)} \\ Cl^- \text{ (1 mEq of chloride)} + Cl^- \text{ (1 mEq of chloride)} \end{array} \right\} \text{Combine to form } CaCl_2$$

Note that Ca^{2+} has two positive charges, or 2 milliequivalents. Therefore, it must have 2 milliequivalents of a singly charged anion ($Cl^- + Cl^-$) to combine to form calcium chloride. In practice, electrolytes are given as milliequivalents per liter (mEq/L), as in intravenous solution.

Body fluid also contains compounds with no electrical charges. These substances are called *nonelectrolytes.* Nonelectrolytes are normally measured in milligrams.

Nonelectrolytes include:

Glucose: Glucose is a carbohydrate or sugar formed during digestion. It is the most important carbohydrate in metabolism.

Urea: Urea is the major nitrogen end product of protein metabolism. It is formed in the liver.

FLUID TRANSPORT

Pharmacologists think of intracellular and extracellular fluid as occupying two separate *compartments*—the intracellular compartment and the extracellular compartment. For normal metabolism to occur, water, electrolytes, and other substances must pass between these two compartments. To do so, they must cross the cell wall, which is a **semipermeable membrane** that allows only some molecules to pass through. There are two ways in which this movement occurs: (1) passive transport and (2) active transport.

Passive Transport

Passive transport depends on three mechanisms: (1) filtration, (2) **diffusion,** and (3) **osmosis.**

Filtration

Filtration is the movement of fluid through a membrane caused by differences in hydrostatic pressure. *Hydrostatic pressure* is the force exerted by the weight of a solution; it causes the solution to move from an area of higher pressure to an area of lower pressure. In two compartments separated by a permeable or semipermeable membrane, hydrostatic pressure tends to cause fluid to move from one compartment to the other until the pressure in both compartments is equal.

Diffusion

Diffusion is the tendency of molecules in solution to distribute themselves equally. You can see diffusion at work by adding a drop of ink to a container of water (Fig. 6–3). Soon, without stirring, the ink **(solute)** spreads itself evenly throughout the water. In diffusion, molecules, atoms, or ions flow from an area of higher concentration to areas of lower concentration, until the concentration (the number of molecules of solute per amount of solution) is the same everywhere in the solution.

Osmosis

Osmosis is the diffusion of solute and/or solvent through a permeable or semipermeable membrane. It is a result of the same force that causes solute molecules or ions within a solution to flow from areas of high concentration to areas of low concentration. With two solutions separated by a semipermeable membrane, a difference in solute concentration creates **osmotic pressure,** which causes water and (if possible) solute to move across the membrane until the solutions are in equilibrium (Fig. 6–4).

Whether both solute and water cross the membrane, or just water, depends on the nature of the solution. There are two kinds of solutions, with opposite reactions to osmotic pressure: **crystalloid solutions** and **colloid solutions.**

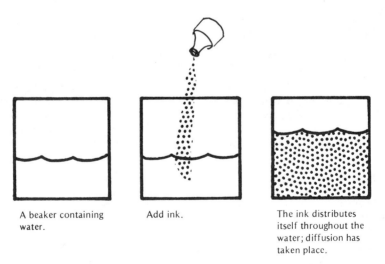

A beaker containing water.

Add ink.

The ink distributes itself throughout the water; diffusion has taken place.

Figure 6–3. Diffusion. (From Stroot, VR, Lee, CA, and Barrett, CA: Fluids and Electrolytes: A Practical Approach, ed. 3. F.A. Davis, Philadelphia, 1984, p 4, with permission.)

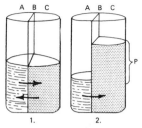

A. CHAMBER CONTAINING WATER

B. MEMBRANOUS PARTITION
 BETWEEN CHAMBERS

C. CHAMBER CONTAINING
 A SOLUTION OF SALT IN WATER

1. B IS PERMEABLE TO ALL SUBSTANCES

2. B IS SEMIPERMEABLE.
 IMPERMEABLE TO SALT PARTICLES
 BUT PERMEABLE TO WATER
 PARTICLES.

P OSMOTIC PRESSURE THAT CAUSES
 THE DIFFERENCE IN LEVELS
 BETWEEN CHAMBERS A AND C
 WHEN SEPARATED BY A
 SEMIPERMEABLE MEMBRANE.

Figure 6–4. Osmosis. The solvent (water) flows from chamber A into chamber C until the concentration (the ratio of solute to solution) in the two chambers is equal. (From Thomas, CL: Taber's Cyclopedic Medical Dictionary, ed. 15. F.A. Davis, Philadelphia, 1985, p 1183, with permission.)

A *crystalloid* is substance that truly dissolves—that is, its molecules or atoms separate and disperse completely and equally throughout the solvent. Such a solution is called a *true solution* or a *crystalloid solution.* In a crystalloid solution, the small, individual molecules or atoms of solute easily pass through (diffuse across) a semipermeable membrane. When two crystalloid solutions of unequal concentration are separated by a semipermeable membrane, the osmotic pressure will be higher in the more concentrated solution. This difference in osmotic pressure will cause the dissolved molecules or ions to cross the membrane, from the more concentrated solution to the solution with lower concentration, until the solute concentration is equal on both sides of the membrane.

Colloids are the physical opposites of crystalloids. When mixed with water, colloids do not truly dissolve. Instead, they form a suspension (sometimes called a *colloid solution*), in which groups of colloid molecules are dispersed throughout the liquid. Unlike crystalloids, colloids do not pass through semipermeable membranes. Therefore, when two colloid solutions of unequal concentration are separated by a semipermeable membrane, osmotic pressure causes the flow of *water* across the membrane, from lower concentration to higher, until the concentration of solute is equal on both sides of the membrane.

In pharmacology, the difference in behavior of the two kinds of solutions allows for different applications. When a crystalloid solution (such as lactated Ringer's, dextrose 5% in water, and normal saline) is injected into the bloodstream, both solute and water can travel across cell membrane. Crystalloid solutions, therefore, are effective ways of getting water *and* the dissolved substance into the cells. On the other hand, when a colloid solution (such as Dextran and Plasmanate) is injected into the bloodstream, the colloid cannot enter the cells, so osmotic pressure causes water to flow from the cellular compart-

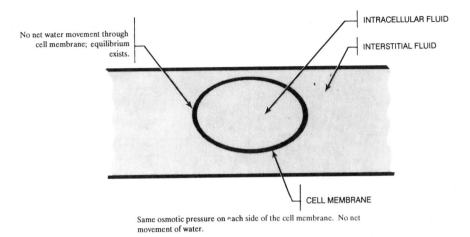

No net water movement through cell membrane; equilibrium exists.

INTRACELLULAR FLUID

INTERSTITIAL FLUID

CELL MEMBRANE

Same osmotic pressure on each side of the cell membrane. No net movement of water.

Figure 6–5. Passive transport for a cell in an isotonic solution.

ment into the bloodstream. The flow of water from cell to bloodstream helps maintain vascular volume.

Two solutions may contain different substances but have the same milliequivalence, or ionic potentials. Separated by a semipermeable membrane, each has the same osmotic pressure. Such solutions are said to be **isotonic.** For instance, normal saline solution, a common intravenous (IV) solution, is isotonic. Because osmotic pressures on both sides of cell membranes are equal, normal saline solution tends to stay in the extracellular space (primarily the bloodstream) longer than **hypotonic** or **hypertonic** solutions. Figure 6–5 illustrates the situation when intracellular and extracellular solutions are isotonic.

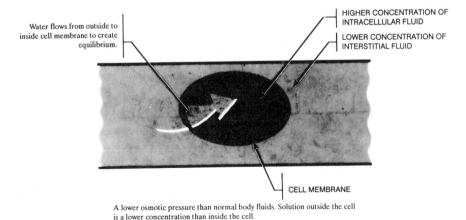

Water flows from outside to inside cell membrane to create equilibrium.

HIGHER CONCENTRATION OF INTRACELLULAR FLUID

LOWER CONCENTRATION OF INTERSTITIAL FLUID

CELL MEMBRANE

A lower osmotic pressure than normal body fluids. Solution outside the cell is a lower concentration than inside the cell.

Figure 6–6. Passive transport for a cell in a hypotonic solution.

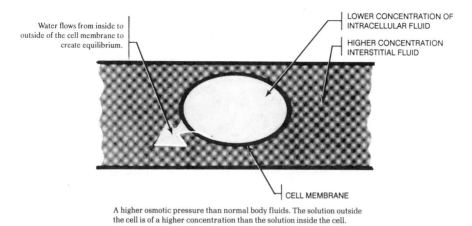

A higher osmotic pressure than normal body fluids. The solution outside
the cell is of a higher concentration than the solution inside the cell.

Figure 6–7. Passive transport for a cell in a hypertonic solution.

A *hypotonic solution* has a lower ionic potential than the solution to which
it is compared. A solution of one-half normal saline, for instance, is hypotonic
to normal body fluid. For a normal body cell surrounded by hypotonic fluid, the
osmotic pressure on the inside of the cell is greater than on the outside. Water
will tend to flow from outside the cell to inside the cell to lower the solute concentration (and therefore the ionic potential). Figure 6–6 illustrates the situation when extracellular solution is hypotonic to intracellular solution.

A hypertonic solution has a higher solute concentration and ionic potential
than the solution to which it is compared. For instance, a solution of dextrose
50% in water is hypertonic to normal body fluid. For a cell in a hypertonic solution, the osmotic pressure inside the cell is lower than outside. The higher
osmotic pressure outside the cell pulls water out of the cell to lower the solute
concentration in the extracellular fluid. Figure 6–7 illustrates this situation.

Active Transport

As we have seen, passive transport allows some solutes to travel across cell
membrane, but only from the concentrated solution to the less concentrated
solution. Cell metabolism, however, requires substances to travel "upstream,"
that is, from the less concentrated solution to the more concentrated one (Fig.
6–8). Cell health also requires that the concentration of some substances be
higher inside the cell than outside, and vice versa. For instance, under normal
conditions, the cellular fluid has more potassium ions that does the extracellular fluid. The process of moving substances across the cell wall from the less
concentrated to the more concentrated solution and keeping the concentration
of solutes higher on one side of the cell wall than on the other is called **active
transport.** Active transport requires metabolic energy. Substances that require
active transport across cell membranes include potassium, sodium, calcium,
hydrogen, chloride, and several sugars and amino acids.

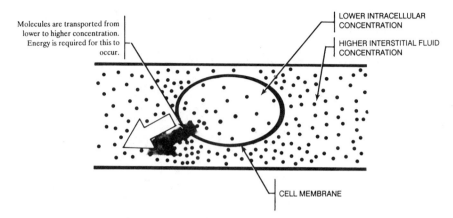

Figure 6–8. Active transport.

ACID-BASE BALANCE

We have discussed how body chemistry and metabolism work to maintain equilibrium between fluid compartments. A state of equilibrium must also be maintained between the acidity and alkalinity of body fluid. Acid-base balance is the body's way of maintaining this equilibrium.

Body fluid **potential of hydrogen (pH)** is the most frequently used measurement of acid-base balance. The pH measurement is inversely related to the body's hydrogen ion concentration. The higher the hydrogen ion concentration in a fluid, the lower the pH. Conversely, the lower the hydrogen ion concentration, the higher the pH. The pH scale ranges from 1 to 14. A pH reading of 1 means that a substance consists of only hydrogen ions. A pH of 14 means that there are no hydrogen ions present. A pH of 7 is neutral.

The normal pH of the body ranges from 7.35 to 7.45. When body fluid's pH is greater than 7.45, the body is in a state of **alkalosis.** Body fluid pH of less than 7.35 indicates a state of **acidosis.** Increases or decreases in body pH can be potentially harmful. For example, a significant decrease in the body's pH can cause diminished heart contractions, reduce the body's response to catecholamine release, and inhibit the therapeutic action of drugs. An increase in the body's pH can inhibit the release of oxygen from the red blood cells. A body fluid pH above 7.8 or below 7.0 indicates a serious, usually fatal condition.

The body regulates acid-base balance by three major mechanisms: the buffer system, the respiratory system, and the renal system.

The buffer system is the body's primary mechanism for adjusting and maintaining acid-base balance. This system's effect on acid-base balance is almost instantaneous. Two components of the buffer system include bicarbonate ion (HCO_3^-) and carbonic acid (H_2CO_3), which maintain an equilibrium with the hydrogen ion (H):

$$\underset{\text{Hydrogen ion}}{H^+} \quad + \quad \underset{\text{Bicarbonate ion}}{\overset{20}{HCO_3^-}} \quad \xleftarrow{\hspace{1cm}}\overset{:}{\longrightarrow} \quad \underset{\text{Carbonic acid}}{\overset{1}{H_2CO_3}}$$

This reaction requires 20 molecules of bicarbonate ion for every molecule of carbonic acid. For the buffer system to maintain body fluid pH, any change in this 20:1 ratio must be immediately corrected.

The respiratory system is the second mechanism for acid-base regulation. It takes approximately 1 to 3 minutes for the respiratory system to be effective. The respiratory system works to regulate acid-base balance by altering the carbon dioxide (CO_2) level in the bloodstream. When the respiration rate increases, the lungs excrete more carbon dioxide, which causes a decrease in hydrogen ions and an increase in the pH. Conversely, when there is a decrease in respirations, more carbon dioxide remains in the blood, causing hydrogen ions to increase and pH to decrease.

The renal system is the third and slowest mechanism for acid-base regulation. It takes from several hours to days for this system to correct acid-base imbalance. The kidneys regulate acid-base balance by eliminating excess hydrogen or bicarbonate ions from the bloodstream. For example, if the hydrogen ion concentration of the body increases, the body's pH falls and the kidneys eliminate more hydrogen ions to restore equilibrium. On the other hand, if the hydrogen ion concentration falls, body pH increases and the kidneys eliminate bicarbonate ions to restore equilibrium.

There are four clinical situations that result when acid-base balance is disrupted: respiratory acidosis, respiratory alkalosis, metabolic acidosis, and metabolic alkalosis.

Respiratory acidosis: This condition results from inadequate ventilations resulting in the retention of carbon dioxide and an increased level of carbonic acid in the blood. The pH of a person in respiratory acidosis falls as the carbon dioxide level increases. To reverse respiratory acidosis, improve ventilation, using 100% oxygen. This removes carbon dioxide from the circulation via the lungs.

Respiratory alkalosis: This condition occurs when excessive amounts of carbon dioxide have been eliminated from the patient. In prehospital emergency situations, respiratory alkalosis often occurs when a patient hyperventilates, blowing off more carbon dioxide than normal. When more carbon dioxide than normal is blown off, body pH increases. Prehospital treatment of respiratory alkalosis consists of increasing the carbon dioxide levels by rebreathing carbon dioxide; for instance, having the patient breath into a paper bag.

Metabolic acidosis: This condition occurs when the body produces an excessive amount of metabolic acids. This increase in acid consumes some of the bicarbonate buffer, causing a further acid buildup and a decrease in base. Metabolic acidosis causes a decrease in pH, but carbon dioxide levels remain within normal limits. In prehospital emergency situations, treat metabolic acidosis by attempting to improve ventilation by using 100% oxygen. This removes carbon dioxide and, subsequently, hydrogen ions. When the diagnosis of metabolic acidosis is documented, treatment may also include giving the patient sodium bicarbonate.

Metabolic alkalosis: In prehospital emergency medicine, this condition often occurs as a result of giving excessive amounts of sodium bicarbonate. Metabolic acidosis occurs when body pH increases but carbon dioxide levels remain normal. Patients who develop metabolic alkalosis usually breathe more slowly and more shallowly because of the body's need to retain carbon dioxide. The kidneys also try to correct the problem by retaining hydrogen ions, which aids in balancing the excess in bicarbonate. Prehospital treatment of metabolic alkalosis consists of correcting the underlying cause.

INTRAVENOUS THERAPY

There are two basic reasons for starting an intravenous line in an emergency prehospital situation: (1) as a route for fluid replacement and (2) as a route for drug administration.

Intravenous solutions are either colloid or crystalloid (see page 87). Colloid solutions are more effective for fluid replacement, because they stay in the vascular space much longer than crystalloid solutions. Colloid solutions are rarely used in prehospital medicine, however, because they are expensive and have a very short shelf life. Crystalloid solutions are usually less expensive and last longer, so they are the intravenous fluids of choice in the prehospital setting.

Dextrose 5% in water is one of the most frequently used solutions for intravenous lifeline drug administration. Table 6–1 illustrates some common intravenous solutions and their indications and contraindications.

The rate at which to run an intravenous line depends on the emergency situation, local protocols, and physician orders. All patients with an intravenous line in place should be continuously monitored, and any changes in patient condition should be immediately reported to the physician.

Procedures for establishing an intravenous line (for either fluid replacement or drug therapy) and for administering drugs via an established line are set out in Chapter 4.

CONCLUSION

You must be able to recognize and treat fluid, electrolyte, and acid-base abnormalities quickly. The major key to treatment is rapid aggressive therapy. To replenish fluids and electrolytes, the proper intravenous fluids must be chosen and given at the appropriate rate. To maintain appropriate acid-base limits or correct acid-base abnormalities, you must maintain a patent airway and improve ventilation (using 100 percent oxygen as needed). The most important drug in correcting acid-base abnormalities is oxygen. Appropriate airway support coupled with correct cardiopulmonary resuscitation, if needed, can maintain pH levels within or very close to normal limits within the lungs, heart, and brain.

STUDY QUESTIONS

1. Fluid located in the spaces between the body's cells, accounting for approximately 10.5 percent of body weight, is called _____ fluid.

Table 6–1. INDICATIONS AND CONTRAINDICATIONS FOR COMMONLY USED INTRAVENOUS SOLUTIONS

Solution	Indications	Contraindications
Colloids		
Plasma Protein Fraction	Hypovolemic shock	None
Dextran	Hypovolemic shock	Known hypersensitivity
		Patient is receiving anticoagulants
Hetastarch	Hypovolemic shock	None
Crystalloids		
Lactated Ringer's (LR)	Hypovolemic shock	CHF
		Renal failure
Dextrose 5% in water (D_5W)	Intravenous drug route	Volume replacement
	Dilution of concentrated drugs for intravenous infusion	
Dextrose 10% in water ($D_{10}W$)	Hypoglycemia	Volume replacement
Normal saline (NS; 0.9% sodium chloride)	Hypovolemia	CHF
	Heat-related emergencies	
	Freshwater drowning	
	Diabetic ketoacidosis (DKA)	
½ Normal saline (½NS; 0.45% sodium chloride)	Compromised cardiac function	Emergency rehydration
Dextrose 5% in ½ normal saline ($D_5½NS$)	Heat emergencies	Emergency rehydration
	Diabetic emergencies	
Dextrose 5% in normal saline (D_5NS)	Heat emergencies	Compromised cardiac function/renal function
	Volume replacement	
	Freshwater drowning	
Dextrose 5% in lactated Ringer's (D_5LR)	Volume replacement	Compromised cardiac function/renal function

    a. Interstitial.
    b. Intravascular.
    c. Extracellular.
    d. Intracellular.

2. Two major cations of the body are:
    a. Calcium and chloride.
    b. Sodium and bicarbonate.
    c. Potassium and phosphate.
    d. Magnesium and potassium.

3. A solution equal in milliequivalents to normal body fluid is called a[n] _____ solution.

    a. Hypotonic.
    b. Isotonic.
    c. Hypertonic.
    d. Colloid.

4. The body's primary mechanism for adjusting and maintaining acid-base balance is the _____ system.
    a. Buffer.
    b. Renal.
    c. Respiratory.
    d. Circulatory.

Unit Two

INTRODUCTION TO UNIT TWO

Not all advanced level Emergency Medical Services (EMS) systems use the same prehospital drugs. There are some drugs, however, whose use is fairly common throughout EMS. For example, the drugs atropine, dopamine, epinephrine, lidocaine, and oxygen are prehospital drugs used in most advanced EMS systems. Examples of less common prehospital drugs include dobutamine, diazoxide, morphine, and phenytoin.

Each EMS system places different priorities on each drug used in its system. To help eliminate confusion, each chapter presents the drugs in alphabetical order by generic name. At the beginning of each chapter, each drug is listed according to its therapeutic classification(s). Drugs may have more than one classification. For example, the drug verapamil is therapeutically classified as an antianginal, antihypertensive, and antiarrhythmic.

The drug monographs in this text are presented by body system affected. Some drugs can be used to treat emergencies in more than one body system. For example, the drug epinephrine is a **first-line drug** (priority drug that is initially given) used in the treatment of cardiac arrest. It is also often used to treat anaphylactic reactions and bronchial asthma. Therefore, epinephrine is presented in the chapters on cardiovascular emergencies, respiratory emergencies, and toxicologic emergencies.

Each drug monograph is designed to present the information in a logical progression that makes the material less confusing and easier to learn.

Different EMS systems have different drug protocols that are designed to meet their own specific needs. Just as protocols may vary slightly, so can drug dosages. Every attempt has been made in this text to present drug dosages and treatment protocols in accordance with accepted national standards. However, it is the responsibility of each EMS professional to know and follow the accepted standards within his own EMS system.

The goal of this unit is to make learning drugs less confusing. Each chapter opens with an introduction to the drugs presented and their relationship to treating emergencies in that specific body system. Following the introduction are the drug monographs, in alphabetical order by generic name. The most common brand names are listed immediately below the generic name. A brief summary follows the monographs, and questions and case studies end the chapter.

The questions and short case studies at the end of the chapters are designed to help you study and understand the drugs more fully. Also, each chapter will have at least one major case study to illustrate the progression of an emergency situation.

The drug monographs, questions, and case studies are designed to make prehospital pharmacology easier to learn. The book's format should also make it useful after graduation, as a reference guide.

Chapter 7

Cardiovascular Emergencies

THERAPEUTIC CLASSIFICATIONS
  OF DRUGS USED FOR
  CARDIOVASCULAR
  EMERGENCIES
Adenosine
Alteplase
Amrinone
Atropine
Bretylium Tosylate
Bumetanide
Butorphanol
Calcium Salts
Diazoxide
Digoxin
Dobutamine
Dopamine
Edrophonium
Epinephrine (1:10,000 Solution)
Ethacrynic Acid
Furosemide
Hydralazine
Hydromorphone
Isoproterenol
Labetalol

Lidocaine
Magnesium Sulfate
Meperidine
Metoprolol
Morphine
Nalbuphine
Nifedipine
Nitroglycerin
Nitroprusside
Nitrous Oxide–Oxygen Mixture
Norepinephrine
Oxygen
Pentazocine
Phenytoin
Procainamide
Propranolol
Sodium Bicarbonate
Streptokinase
Verapamil

CASE STUDIES

APPENDIX: AMERICAN HEART
  ASSOCIATION TREATMENT
  ALGORITHMS

THERAPEUTIC CLASSIFICATIONS OF DRUGS USED FOR CARDIOVASCULAR EMERGENCIES

ANALGESICS
Butorphanol
Hydromorphone
Meperidine
Morphine
Nalbuphine
Nitrous oxide–oxygen mixture
Pentazocine

ANTIANGINALS
Nifedipine
Nitroglycerin
Verapamil

ANTIARRYTHMICS
Atropine
Bretylium tosylate

Digoxin
Edrophonium
Isoproterenol
Lidocaine
Phenytoin
Procainamide
Propranolol
Verapamil

ANTICONVULSANT
Phenytoin

ANTIHYPERTENSIVES
Bumetanide
Diazoxide
Furosemide
Hydralazine
Labetalol
Metoprolol
Nitroprusside
Propranolol
Verapamil

ANTITUSSIVE
Hydromorphone

BRONCHODILATOR
Epinephrine
Isoproterenol

CARDIAC STIMULATOR
Epinephrine
Isoproterenol

CHOLINERGIC AGONIST
Edrophonium

CORONARY VASODILATOR
Nitroglycerin

DIURETICS
Bumetanide
Ethacrynic acid
Furosemide

ELECTROLYTE
Magnesium sulfate

ELECTROLYTE MODIFIER
Calcium chloride
Calcium gluceptate
Calcium gluconate

HYDROGEN ION BUFFER
Sodium bicarbonate

INOTROPIC
Amrinone
Digoxin
Dobutamine
Dopamine

MEDICINAL GAS
Nitrous oxide–oxygen mixture
Oxygen

PERIPHERAL VASCONSTRICTOR
Epinephrine

THROMBOLYTIC ENZYME
Alteplase
Streptokinase

VASODILATOR
Amrinone

VASOPRESSOR
Dopamine
Norepinephrine

The most common kind of death in the United States is death due to cardiovascular emergencies. Most of the time, when EMT-Ps give drugs, it is for cardiovascular emergencies.

This chapter focuses on drugs used in prehospital cardiovascular emergencies. Among the drugs presented are those that therapeutically correct cardiac arrhythmias. This category includes drugs that alter the rate and force of cardiac contractions and help to maintain a sufficient amount of blood to the heart muscle. For example, antiarrhythmic drugs, such as lidocaine or procainamide, suppress arrhythmias caused by imbalances in cardiac discharges that affect the ventricles. A cardiac stimulator, such as epinephrine, increases the rate and force of contractions, resulting in an increase in cardiac output.

The chapter also discusses drugs used to increase or decrease blood pressure and to relieve chest pain and drugs that aid in the elimination of salt and water from the body. For example, an EMT-P or physician may administer an antianginal such as nitroglycerin to decrease the heart's ventricular work load, to reduce the heart's oxygen demands, and to increase the coronary blood flow of the heart. Antihypertensives, such as nitroprusside, increase the capacity of the venous circulation and reduce blood pressure. Diuretics, such as furosemide, reduce edema in the lungs.

The chapter also presents alteplase and streptokinase, two thrombolytic agents. Thrombolytics are used to dissolve **thrombi** (blood clots) that obstruct a blood vessel or a cavity of the heart.

Correct administration of one or more of these drugs, in conjunction with the appropriate supportive treatment, will give the patient the best chance for a successful outcome from a cardiovascular emergency.

ADENOSINE
Adenocard

CLASSIFICATIONS
Pharmacologic: Naturally occurring nucleoside
Therapeutic: Antiarrhythmic

MECHANISM OF ACTION: Adenosine is used to slow conduction through the AV node of the heart. It may also interrupt reentry pathways through the AV node.

THERAPEUTIC BENEFIT: Adenosine can restore normal sinus rhythm (NSR) in patients experiencing paroxysmal supraventricular tachycardia (PSVT), including those associated with Wolff-Parkinson-White (WPW) syndrome (Fig. 7-1).

INDICATIONS FOR PREHOSPITAL USE: Adenosine is used to convert PSVT, including WPW, to a normal sinus rhythm (NSR).

It should be noted that adenosine should not be given until appropriate vagal maneuvers have been performed; however, you should follow your local protocols.

Note: Adenosine is *not* effective in treating other atrial dysrhythmias or arrhythmias such as atrial fibrillation or atrial flutter.

CONTRAINDICATIONS: ▪ Do not give adenosine to patients: ▪ Hypersensitive to the drug. ▪ Experiencing second- or third-degree AV heart block or sick sinus syndrome.

PRECAUTIONS: Adenosine may produce brief periods of heart block (first, second, or third degree). Approximately 50–60% of patients develop some type of cardiac arrhythmia after the administration of adenosine. However, these arrhythmias generally last only a few seconds. Arrhythmias most likely to develop include premature ventricular contractions (PVCs), pre-

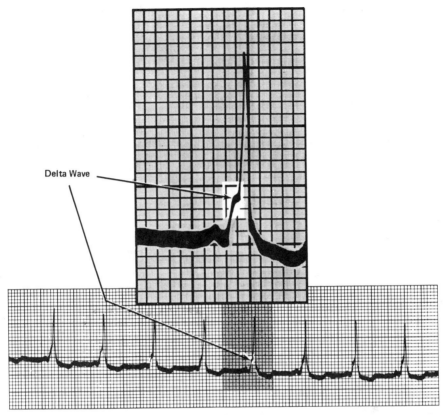

Delta Wave

Figure 7–1. Wolff-Parkinson-White syndrome is associated with a high incidence of paroxysmal tachycardia. A major defining characteristic is the initial slurring of the R wave (delta wave). Other characteristics include heart rate of about 100 beats/min, with regular rhythm; a shortened PR interval (0.06 sec); and a widened QRS complex (0.14 sec).

mature atrial contractions (PACs), sinus bradycardia, and sinus tachycardia.

ROUTE AND DOSAGE

Adult: Initially give 6 mg by rapid IV bolus, followed by a rapid IV flush of normal saline (NS). If the initial dose is unsuccessful after 1–2 min, give 12 mg rapid IV bolus followed by a rapid IV flush of NS. Another 12-mg dose may be repeated if necessary. Do not give more than 12 mg in a single dose.

Pediatric: Not recommended for prehospital use.

ADVERSE REACTIONS AND SIDE EFFECTS

- *Respiratory:* Dyspnea, may cause bronchoconstriction in asthma patients.
- *Cardiovascular:* Palpitations, hypotension, chest pain, facial flushing.

- *CNS:* Headache.
- *Gastrointestinal:* Nausea, metallic taste.

PARAMEDIC IMPLICATIONS: ▪ Assess patient vital signs frequently. ▪ Patients who develop high-degree (second- or third-degree) AV heart block should not be given additional doses of adenosine.

DRUG INTERACTIONS: Theophylline-type drugs (methylxanthines), such as aminophylline, prevent adenosine from binding to receptor sites. Asthma or COPD patients may be taking these types of drugs. Such patients may require larger doses. Dipyridamole (Persantine), a vasodilator, can potentiate adenosine's effect, and patients using this drug may require smaller doses.

ALTEPLASE, TISSUE PLASMINOGEN ACTIVATOR (t-PA)
Activase

CLASSIFICATIONS
Pharmacologic: Enzyme
Therapeutic: Thrombolytic

MECHANISM OF ACTION: Alteplase stimulates the conversion to plasmin of plasminogen trapped in **thrombi.** Plasminogen, the precursor of plasmin, is a protein important in preventing fibrin clot formation.

THERAPEUTIC BENEFIT: Alteplase dissolves thrombi, which may subsequently limit infarction size during a **myocardial infarction (MI).**

INDICATION FOR PREHOSPITAL USE: Alteplase is used to treat acute MI within 4–6 h of the onset of chest pain.

CONTRAINDICATIONS: ▪ Do not administer alteplase to patients: ▪ With active internal bleeding. ▪ With a history of a cerebral vascular accident (CVA). ▪ Who have had intracranial or spinal trauma or surgery within the past 2 mo. ▪ With severe uncontrolled hypertension. ▪ With known bleeding disorders.

PRECAUTIONS: ▪ Use caution in administering alteplase to patients: ▪ With cerebrovascular disease. ▪ With hypertension. ▪ With severe liver or kidney disease. ▪ Over 75.

ROUTE AND DOSAGE

Adult (>65 kg or 143 lb): A total of 100 mg by IV over 3 h as follows:

- 60 mg over the first hour. Administer the first 6–10 mg of the 60 mg by IV bolus over the first 1–2 min and the rest by IV infusion.
- 20 mg by IV infusion over the second h.
- 20 mg by IV infusion over the third h.

Adult (<65 kg or 143 lb): A total of 1.25 mg/kg IV over 3 h as follows:

- 0.75 mg/kg over the first h. Administer the first 0.075–0.125 mg/kg of the 0.75 mg/kg by an IV bolus over the first 1–2 min.
- 0.25 mg/kg by IV infusion over the second h.
- 0.25 mg/kg by IV infusion over the third h.

Pediatric: Not recommended for prehospital use.

ADVERSE REACTIONS AND SIDE EFFECTS

- *Central nervous system (CNS):* Intracranial bleeding, headache.
- *Cardiovascular:* Arrhythmias due to **reperfusion,** hypotension.
- *Gastrointestinal:* Gastrointestinal bleeding, retroperitoneal bleeding, nausea, vomiting.

PARAMEDIC IMPLICATIONS: ▪ Assess vital signs every 15 min. ▪ ECG should be continuously monitored. Reperfusion of the heart may cause the following arrhythmias:

- Accelerated idioventricular rhythm.
- Bradycardia.
- Asystole.
- Ventricular arrhythmia.

▪ Medical control may order prophylactic antiarrhythmic therapy concurrently with alteplase therapy. ▪ Assess patient frequently for signs of bleeding.

DRUG INTERACTIONS: Using alteplase simultaneously with aspirin, oral anticoagulants, or heparin may increase the risk of bleeding.

AMRINONE
Inocor

CLASSIFICATIONS
Pharmacologic: Bipyridine
derivative
Therapeutic: Inotropic,
vasodilator

MECHANISM OF ACTION: Amrinone is a fast acting positive inotropic drug—it increases the force and frequency of cardiac contractions. It also relaxes vascular smooth muscle. The resulting vasodilation decreases both preload and afterload.

THERAPEUTIC BENEFIT: Amrinone increases cardiac output and diminishes peripheral resistance.

INDICATIONS FOR PREHOSPITAL USE: Amrinone is used to treat severe congestive heart failure that has not responded to therapy with milder agents such as diuretics, vasodilators, and other inotropic drugs.

CONTRAINDICATIONS: Do not administer amrinone if the patient is hypersensitive to bisulfite drugs.

PRECAUTIONS: Amrinone may reduce the supply of blood to the heart, thereby causing or worsening ischemia. Therefore, use amrinone in the lowest dose possible.

ROUTE AND DOSAGE

Adult: 0.75 mg/kg by IV bolus over 2–3 min, followed by an IV infusion of 5–15 µg/kg/min **titrated** to effect.

To prepare the infusion, add 100 mg of amrinone to 500 mL of normal saline, which yields a concentration of 0.2 mg/mL.

Pediatric: Not recommended in the prehospital setting.

ADVERSE REACTIONS AND SIDE EFFECTS

- *Cardiovascular:* Arrhythmias, hypotension.
- *Gastrointestinal:* Nausea, vomiting.

PARAMEDIC IMPLICATIONS: Because amrinone can cause or aggravate cardiac ischemia, monitor the patient continuously.

DRUG INTERACTIONS: ▪ Cardiac glycoside drugs may cause additive inotropic effects if used with amrinone. ▪ Amrinone is reported to be incompatible with furosemide. A precipitate forms immediately when these two drugs are mixed. Do not inject furosemide directly into the tubing of an IV infusion of amrinone. ▪ Amrinone is also reportedly incompatible with dextrose. The manufacturer recommends that amrinone not be diluted in solutions containing dextrose. However, amrinone may be given into a free-flowing IV line that contains a dextrose solution.

ATROPINE

CLASSIFICATIONS
Pharmacologic: Anticholinergic
Therapeutic: Antiarrhythmic

MECHANISM OF ACTION: Atropine competes with the neurotransmitter acetylcholine for receptor sites, blocking the stimulation of parasympathetic nerve fibers. This blocking action enhances both sinus node automaticity and atrioventricular conduction.

THERAPEUTIC BENEFIT: Atropine improves cardiac output when its parasympathetic blocking action results in a higher heart rate.

INDICATIONS FOR PREHOSPITAL USE

1. Symptomatic sinus bradycardia (Class I: definitely helpful). Signs/symptoms can include the following:
   - Chest pain
   - Shortness of breath
   - Decreased level of consciousness
   - Hypotension

- Congestive heart failure
- PVCs in the setting of acute MI

2. AV block at the nodal level (Class IIa: acceptable, probably helpful).
3. Ventricular asystole (Class IIa: acceptable, probably helpful).
4. Slow pulseless electrical activity (Class IIa: acceptable, probably helpful); to be given if absolute bradycardia (<60 beats/min) or relative bradycardia.

CONTRAINDICATIONS: ▪ Do not administer atropine to patients with a known hypersensitivity to the drug. ▪ Do not administer atropine to patients suffering acute hemorrhage.

PRECAUTIONS: Use atropine with caution if the patient's symptoms suggest myocardial ischemia or MI, because increases in heart rate may worsen ischemia or increase the area of infarction.

ROUTE AND DOSAGE

Adult (Symptomatic Sinus Bradycardia): 0.5–1.0 mg by IV bolus. This can be repeated every 3–5 min, to a total dose of 0.04 mg/kg.

Adult (AV Block at the Nodal Level): 0.5–1.0 mg by IV bolus. This can be repeated every 3–5 min, to a total dose of 0.04 mg/kg.

Adult (Asystole):   1 mg by IV bolus. This can be repeated every 3–5 min, to a total dose of 0.04 mg/kg. Some feel shorter dosage intervals may be indicated during asystolic arrest. If shorter dosage intervals are used, atropine is Class IIb: acceptable, possibly helpful.

   Note: A total dose of 0.04 mg/kg (3 mg) of atropine causes full vagal blockage in adults.

Pediatric: 0.02 mg/kg by IV bolus. This can be repeated every 5 min, to a maximum total dose of 1.0 mg in a child and 2.0 mg in an adolescent. Minimum single dose of atropine is 0.1 mg. Maximum single dose in the child is 0.5 mg, and maximum single dose in the adolescent is 1.0 mg.

   Note: Atropine can be administered through a catheter that has been passed down and beyond the tip of an established ET tube. The dosage is 2–2.5 times the IV bolus dosage, and should be diluted in 10 mL of normal saline or distilled water for the adult patient and diluted in 1–2 mL of normal or half-normal saline in the pediatric patient.

ADVERSE REACTIONS AND SIDE EFFECTS

- *CNS:* Drowsiness, confusion.
- *Cardiovascular:* Tachycardia.
- *Eyes:* Blurred vision, dilated pupils, dry eyes.
- *Gastrointestinal:* Dry mouth.

PARAMEDIC IMPLICATIONS: ▪ Doses less than the minimum may actually *slow* the heart rate. ▪ Excessive doses may cause ventricular tachycardia or ventricular fibrillation. ▪ Atropine given to patients with nonsymptomatic bradycardia may produce adverse effects. Some feel atropine may be harmful (Class III) if used to treat AV block at the His-Purkinje level (second-degree type II AV block and third-degree block with wide-QRS complexes). Follow local protocols.

DRUG INTERACTIONS: ▪ If atropine is given with other anticholinergic drugs, additive effects may occur. ▪ Antacids slow the absorption of anticholinergic drugs such as atropine.

> ## BRETYLIUM TOSYLATE
> Bretylol
>
> *CLASSIFICATIONS*
> *Pharmacologic: Adrenergic blocker*
> *Therapeutic: Ventricular antiarrhythmic*

MECHANISM OF ACTION: Bretylium has both adrenergic blocking effects and direct effects on the heart. Bretylium's first effect is to cause a release of norepinephrine, resulting in hypertension, tachycardia, and possibly an increase in cardiac output. However, approximately 20 min after bretylium administration, it causes the adrenergic blockage of norepinephrine, resulting in hypotension and an increase in the effect of any administered catecholamines.

THERAPEUTIC BENEFIT: Bretylium is beneficial in the treatment of ventricular tachycardia and ventricular fibrillation when other drug therapy has failed.

INDICATIONS FOR PREHOSPITAL USE: Bretylium is recommended in the treatment of ventricular tachycardia, ventricular fibrillation, or wide-complex tachycardias of unknown origin in the following situations:

1. When defibrillation, epinephrine, and lidocaine have failed to convert ventricular fibrillation.
2. When ventricular fibrillation persists despite epinephrine and lidocaine therapy.
3. When lidocaine and procainamide have failed to control ventricular tachycardia that produces a pulse.
4. When lidocaine, adenosine, and procainamide have failed to control wide-complex tachycardias of uncertain type.

CONTRAINDICATIONS: None, when used for treating life-threatening ventricular arrhythmias.

PRECAUTIONS: Bretylium may cause significant hypotension.

ROUTE AND DOSAGE

Adult (Ventricular Fibrillation/Pulseless Ventricular Tachycardia): 5 mg/kg by IV bolus. This should circulate for 1–2 min by continuing CPR; then defibrillate at 360 J. If the patient remains in VF/pulseless VT after 5 min, administer 10 mg/kg by IV bolus. If necessary, this can be repeated every 5 min, to a maximum total dose of 30–35 mg/kg.

Adult (Ventricular Tachycardia/Wide-Complex Tachycardias): 5–10 mg/kg IV infusion over 8–10 min. Repeat doses may be ordered but should not exceed a total dose of 30 mg/kg in 24 h.

Pediatric: 5 mg/kg by rapid IV bolus. Repeat doses may be increased to 10 mg/kg by rapid IV bolus (Class IIb).

ADVERSE REACTIONS AND SIDE EFFECTS

- *CNS:* Dizziness, syncope, vertigo.
- *Cardiovascular:* Hypotension, bradycardia, angina, temporary hypertension.
- *Gastrointestinal:* Nausea and vomiting if given too rapidly to the conscious patient.

PARAMEDIC IMPLICATIONS: ■ If the ventricular fibrillation or tachycardia fibrillation is converted, closely monitor patient for changes in blood pressure and rhythm. ■ If hypotension develops, the patient may have to be placed in the Trendelenberg position. ■ Severe hypotension may require the infusion of intravenous replacement fluids.

DRUG INTERACTIONS: ■ Using bretylium with other antiarrhythmic drugs can cause either additive or antagonistic effects. ■ Hypotension may become more severe if bretylium is used simultaneously with procainamide or quinidine. ■ The release of norepinephrine that occurs soon after bretylium administration may worsen arrhythmias caused by digitalis toxicity.

BUMETANIDE
Bumex

CLASSIFICATIONS:
Pharmacologic: Loop diuretic
Therapeutic: Diuretic,
  antihypertensive

MECHANISM OF ACTION: Bumetanide inhibits the reabsorption of sodium and chloride in the kidneys. It increases the excretion of water, sodium, chloride, magnesium, hydrogen, calcium, and potassium. Bumetanide causes renal and peripheral vasodilation and may cause a temporary decrease in peripheral vascular resistance.

THERAPEUTIC BENEFIT: Bumetanide causes diuresis and works to lower blood pressure.

INDICATIONS FOR PREHOSPITAL USE: The two most common uses for bumetanide are:

1. Treatment of edema secondary to congestive heart failure.
2. Hypertension; bumetanide can be used alone or in combination with other antihypertensive drugs.

CONTRAINDICATIONS: Do not administer to patients with a known hypersensitivity to bumetanide.

PRECAUTIONS: Use bumetanide with caution in patients whose electrolytes are depleted or in patients who have diabetes mellitus.

ROUTE AND DOSAGE

Adult: 0.5–2 mg by IV bolus over 2 min or IM. Repeat at 2–3 h intervals if needed. The total dosage of bumetanide should not exceed 10 mg/d.

Pediatric: Not recommended for prehospital use.

ADVERSE REACTIONS AND SIDE EFFECTS

- *CNS:* Headache, dizziness.
- *Cardiovascular:* Hypotension, possible ECG changes.
- *Fluid and electrolytes:* Metabolic alkalosis, hypovolemia, dehydration.
- *Gastrointestinal:* Nausea, vomiting.

PARAMEDIC IMPLICATIONS: Excessive amounts of bumetanide can ultimately lead to circulatory collapse. Closely monitor the patient, frequently assessing vital signs and lung sounds looking for edema or signs of developing dehydration.

DRUG INTERACTIONS: Bumetanide administered with other antihypertensives or diuretics may cause additive hypotension and fluid depletion.

BUTORPHANOL
Stadol

CLASSIFICATIONS
Pharmacologic: Narcotic agonist-antagonist, opioid partial agonist
Therapeutic: Analgesic

MECHANISM OF ACTION: Butorphanol is thought to bind to the opiate receptors in the CNS, acting as an agonist to some receptors and as an antagonist to others.

THERAPEUTIC BENEFIT: Butorphanol alters the awareness of and response to pain; it also causes generalized CNS depression.

INDICATIONS FOR PREHOSPITAL USE: Butorphanol is used to treat moderate to severe pain of any cause.

CONTRAINDICATIONS: Do not use butorphanol in patients who:

- Are known to be hypersensitive to the drug.
- Are dependent on opiates.
- Have suffered head injury.
- Complain of abdominal pain.

PRECAUTIONS: ▪ Use butorphanol cautiously in patients whose respiration is impaired. ▪ The dosage of butorphanol may have to be reduced in elderly patients because they may be more sensitive to the drug. ▪ Give butorphanol with caution to patients with a history of convulsive disorders, because it may cause seizure activity.

ROUTE AND DOSAGE

Adult (IV Bolus): 0.5–2 mg every 3 h as needed.

Adult (IM): 1–4 mg every 3 h as needed.

Pediatric: Not recommended for prehospital use.

ADVERSE REACTIONS AND SIDE EFFECTS

- *CNS:* Headache, confusion, hallucinations.
- *Cardiovascular:* Hypotension or hypertension, palpitations.
- *Respiratory:* Respiratory depression.
- *Gastrointestinal:* Nausea, vomiting, dry mouth.

PARAMEDIC IMPLICATIONS: ▪ Assess patient vital signs very closely. ▪ Because butorphanol is very potent, administer with caution. For example, 2 mg of butorphanol has effects equal to 10 mg of morphine.

DRUG INTERACTIONS: ▪ Additive CNS depression may occur if butorphanol is used with alcohol, antihistamines, antidepressants, or sedative/hypnotic drugs. ▪ Use with other narcotics may diminish the analgesic effects. ▪ Butorphanol may cause acute withdrawal syndrome to patients dependent on opiate drugs.

CALCIUM SALTS (CALCIUM CHLORIDE, CALCIUM GLUCEPTATE, CALCIUM GLUCONATE)

CLASSIFICATIONS
Pharmacologic: Calcium supplement
Therapeutic: Electrolyte modifier

MECHANISM OF ACTION: Calcium salts are electrolytes; they are essential for the transmission of nerve impulses that initiate the contraction of cardiac muscle.

THERAPEUTIC BENEFIT: Calcium salts replace missing electrolytes necessary for the contractile function of the heart.

INDICATIONS FOR PREHOSPITAL USE: Calcium salts are used to balance severe excesses in the amount of potassium in the blood (hyperkalemia) or severe deficits in the amount of calcium in the blood (hypocalcemia).

CONTRAINDICATIONS: Calcium salts should not be used during resuscitative efforts unless hyperkalemia, hypocalcemia, or calcium channel blocker toxicity has been proved.

PRECAUTIONS: ▪ Calcium salts may produce arterial vasospasm in the heart and brain. ▪ Use calcium salts with caution in patients suffering from cardiac disease or respiratory insufficiency.

ROUTE AND DOSAGE
Adult

Calcium chloride: 2–4 mg/kg by slow IV bolus. Repeat every 10 min as needed. 1 mL of a 10% solution = 100 mg of calcium chloride.
Calcium gluceptate: 5–7 mL by slow IV bolus.
Calcium gluconate: 5–8 mL by slow IV bolus.

Pediatric

Calcium chloride: 5–7 mg/kg by slow IV bolus. Repeat once, 10 min after the first dose, if necessary. 1 mL of a 10% solution = 100 mg.
Calcium gluceptate: Not recommended in the prehospital setting.
Calcium gluconate: Not recommended in the prehospital setting.

ADVERSE REACTIONS AND SIDE EFFECTS

- *CNS:* Syncope.
- *Cardiovascular:* Cardiac arrest, arrhythmia, bradycardia.
- *Gastrointestinal:* Nausea, vomiting.
- *Local:* Tissue necrosis at the injection site.

PARAMEDIC IMPLICATIONS: ▪ Giving calcium salts too rapidly to a patient with a pulse may cause bradycardia. ▪ Calcium chloride is the preferred calcium salt because it produces higher and more predictable concentrations of the drug in the bloodstream.

DRUG INTERACTIONS: ▪ Do not administer calcium salts with sodium bicarbonate, because if the two substances are mixed a precipitate develops. ▪ Use calcium salts with caution and in smaller doses for patients taking digoxin, because calcium salts in the presence of digoxin increase cardiac irritability.

DIAZOXIDE
Hyperstat, Proglycem

CLASSIFICATIONS
Pharmacologic: Peripheral vasodilator
Therapeutic: Antihypertensive

MECHANISM OF ACTION: Diazoxide relaxes the vascular smooth muscles in the peripheral arterioles. It causes vasodilation and decreases peripheral vascular resistance.

THERAPEUTIC BENEFIT: Diazoxide lowers both systolic and diastolic blood pressure.

INDICATIONS FOR PREHOSPITAL USE: Diazoxide is used for the emergency treatment of malignant hypertension.

CONTRAINDICATIONS: Do not administer diazoxide to patients with known hypersensitivity to diazoxide or to thiazide diuretics.

PRECAUTIONS: ▪ Use diazoxide with caution in patients with symptomatic cardiac disease. ▪ Use with caution with diabetic patients, because diazoxide can cause an increase in blood sugar (hyperglycemia).

ROUTE AND DOSAGE

Adult: 1–3 mg/kg, up to 150 mg in a single dose, by rapid IV bolus. Repeat in 5–15 min if needed.

Pediatric: Same as adult.

ADVERSE REACTIONS AND SIDE EFFECTS

- *CNS:* Dizziness, headache, light-headedness.
- *Cardiovascular:* Tachycardia, hypotension, arrhythmia, chest pain, edema, congestive heart failure.
- *Fluid and electrolytes:* Sodium and water retention.
- *Endocrine:* Hyperglycemia.

PARAMEDIC IMPLICATIONS: ▪ Assess patient every 5 min. Adverse reactions and side effects can develop rapidly. ▪ Patient should remain supine for approximately 30 min after administration.

DRUG INTERACTIONS: ▪ Use with other antihypertensive or nitrate drugs may cause an additive hypotensive effect. ▪ Diazoxide may decrease the effectiveness of phenytoin. ▪ Simultaneous use with diuretics may increase hyperglycemic and hypotensive effects.

DIGOXIN
Lanoxin

CLASSIFICATIONS
Pharmacologic: Digitalis
glycoside
Therapeutic: Antiarrhythmic,
inotropic

MECHANISM OF ACTION: Digoxin increases both the force and velocity of ventricular contractions while simultaneously slowing conduction through the atrioventricular node.

THERAPEUTIC BENEFIT: Digoxin significantly increases both stroke volume and cardiac output.

INDICATIONS FOR PREHOSPITAL USE:

1. Digoxin is used to control the heart's ventricular rate in the management of:
   - Atrial fibrillation.
   - Atrial flutter.
   - Paroxysmal supraventricular tachycardia.
2. Digoxin is used to treat congestive heart failure.

CONTRAINDICATIONS: ▪ Do not administer digoxin to patients: ▪ Who are hypersensitive to digitalis preparations. ▪ With uncontrolled ventricular arrhythmias. ▪ With atrioventricular heart block.

PRECAUTIONS: ▪ Use digoxin with caution with patients with: ▪ Recent heart muscle damage. ▪ Lung disease. ▪ Hypoxia. ▪ Hypothyroidism. All such patients may experience increased sensitivity to the drug.

ROUTE AND DOSAGE

Adult: 10–15 μg/kg by slow IV bolus. Because of its toxicity, many local protocols do not allow the prehospital administration of digoxin. Administer digoxin in divided doses, beginning at 50% of the **loading dose,** with additional fractional doses of 25% of the loading dose. Administering digoxin in divided doses may avoid the development of toxicity.

Pediatric: Not recommended for prehospital use.

ADVERSE REACTIONS AND SIDE EFFECTS

- *CNS:* Fatigue, headache, blurred vision, yellow vision.
- *Cardiovascular:* Bradycardia and almost any cardiac arrhythmia.
- *Gastrointestinal:* Nausea, vomiting, anorexia.

PARAMEDIC IMPLICATIONS: ▪ In cases of digoxin toxicity, electrical cardioversion may cause a fatal ventricular cardiac arrhythmia. Therefore, do not attempt cardioversion unless the patient develops a life-threatening arrhythmia. If attempted, electrical cardioversion should begin at the lowest possible energy level. ▪ Digoxin may cause both severe toxicity and drug interactions in the critically ill patient. Therefore, digoxin may have a limited role in the prehospital management of congestive heart failure.

DRUG INTERACTIONS: ▪ Use of digoxin with beta-adrenergic blocking drugs may cause additive bradycardia. ▪ Diuretics, corticosteroids that cause potassium depletion, quinidine, and verapamil may increase the risk of toxicity.

DOBUTAMINE
Dobutrex

CLASSIFICATIONS
Pharmacologic: Adrenergic,
   beta$_1$-agonist
Therapeutic: Inotropic

MECHANISM OF ACTION: Dobutamine increases cardiac contractility and stroke volume with relatively little effect on the heart rate or blood vessels.

THERAPEUTIC BENEFIT: Dobutamine increases cardiac output without significantly increasing heart rate.

INDICATIONS FOR PREHOSPITAL USE: Dobutamine is used to treat:

1. Pulmonary congestion and low cardiac output.
2. Hypotension when vasodilator drugs cannot be used.

CONTRAINDICATIONS: Do not administer dobutamine to patients with bradycardia.

PRECAUTIONS: Use dobutamine with caution with patients who might be experiencing an MI, because dobutamine may aggravate or extend the infarction size.

ROUTE AND DOSAGE

Adult: 2–20 μg/kg/min by IV infusion titrated to effect.

There are two ways to prepare the IV infusion:

1. Add 250 mg of dobutamine to 500 mL of D_5W or NS to make a concentration of 500 μg/mL.
2. Add 500 mg of dobutamine to 250 mL of D_5W or NS to make a concentration of 2 mg/mL (2000 μg/mL).

Pediatric: 2–20 μg/kg/min IV infusion titrated to effect.

Infusion preparation: Multiply the patient's body weight (in kg) by 6. This equals the amount of milligrams added to D_5W, 5% dextrose in ½ NS, NS, or LR. Running the infusion at 1 mL/h will deliver 1 μg/kg/min.

ADVERSE REACTIONS AND SIDE EFFECTS

- *CNS:* Headache.
- *Cardiovascular:* Tachycardia, hypertension, premature ventricular contractions, chest pain.
- *Respiratory:* Shortness of breath.
- *Gastrointestinal:* Nausea, vomiting.

PARAMEDIC IMPLICATIONS: ■ Monitor the patient closely. An increase in systolic blood pressure of 10–20 mm Hg and an increase in heart rate of 5–15 beats/min is considered normal. ■ If the patient is hypovolemic, treat hypovolemia with IV volume expanders before giving dobutamine.

DRUG INTERACTIONS: ■ Use with nitroprusside may have a synergistic effect on increasing cardiac output. ■ Beta-adrenergic blocking agents may cause dobutamine to be ineffective. ■ The hypertensive potential of dobutamine may be enhanced by oxytocics or tricyclic antidepressants.

DOPAMINE
Dopastat, Intropin

CLASSIFICATIONS
Pharmacologic: Adrenergic
Therapeutic: Inotropic,
  vasopressor

MECHANISM OF ACTION: Dopamine stimulates both alpha- and beta-adrenergic receptors and dopaminergic receptors in a **dose-dependent** fashion. Table 7–1 lists the various dose levels of dopamine, the receptors stimulated, and the actions produced on the body.

THERAPEUTIC BENEFIT: Dopamine increases blood pressure and cardiac output and improves blood flow through the kidneys.

Table 7-1. DOSAGE-RELATED RESPONSES TO DOPAMINE

Dose	Major Receptors Stimulated	Response
1-2 μg/kg/min	Dopaminergic	Vasodilation of renal, mesenteric, and cerebral arteries. No effect on heart or blood pressure
2-10 μg/kg/min	Beta$_1$-adrenergic	Increased cardiac output (beta)
	Alpha-adrenergic	Vasoconstriction (alpha)
10-20 μg/kg/min	Alpha-adrenergic	Renal, mesenteric, and peripheral arterial and venous vasoconstriction, producing marked increase in systemic vascular resistance and preload
>20 μg/kg/min	Alpha-adrenergic	Similar to the response to norepinephrine, i.e., vasoconstriction; positive inotropism

INDICATIONS FOR PREHOSPITAL USE: Dopamine is used to treat hemodynamically significant hypotension in the absence of hypovolemia.

CONTRAINDICATIONS: Do not administer dopamine to patients with tachyarrhythmias or to patients with pheochromocytoma. (Pheochromocytoma is a usually benign catecholamine-producing tumor that causes hypertension in the patient.)

PRECAUTIONS: Use caution in administering dopamine to patients with occlusive vascular disease.

Depending on the infusion rate, you will prepare one of several different concentrations:

1. 200 mg diluted in 250 mL of D$_5$W = 800 μg/mL.
2. 400 mg diluted in 250 mL of D$_5$W = 1600 μg/mL.
3. 800 mg diluted in 250 mL of D$_5$W = 3200 μg/mL.
4. 800 mg diluted in 500 mL of D$_5$W = 1600 μg/mL.

ROUTE AND DOSAGE

Adult: 2.5-5 μg/kg/min IV infusion. If necessary, increase infusion rate until there is a therapeutic effect.

Pediatric: 2-20 μg/kg/min IV infusion. To administer the pediatric dosage, use the following shortcut: Multiply the patient's body weight (in kg) by 6. That product equals the number of mg of dopamine to dilute in 100 mL of D$_5$W; the resulting solution, administered at the rate of 1 mL/h, will yield the required dosage (1 μg/kg/min).

ADVERSE REACTIONS AND SIDE EFFECTS

- *CNS:* Headache.
- *Cardiovascular:* Arrhythmias, hypotension, palpitations, chest pain.
- *Respiratory:* Dyspnea.
- *Eyes:* Dilated pupils.
- *Gastrointestinal:* Nausea, vomiting.
- *Local:* Tissue necrosis at IV site.

PARAMEDIC IMPLICATIONS: ▪ Correct hypovolemia with IV volume expanders before giving dopamine. ▪ If dopamine is to be discontinued, do so gradually, because sudden cessation can result in acute hypotension.

DRUG INTERACTIONS: ▪ Do not mix dopamine with alkaline drugs, because alkaline solutions may deactivate dopamine. ▪ Using dopamine with phenytoin may produce hypotension and bradycardia. ▪ Dopamine has an advantage over isoproterenol in that dopamine does not increase myocardial oxygen demand as much as isoproterenol.

EDROPHONIUM
Tensilon

CLASSIFICATIONS
Pharmacologic: Cholinesterase
* inhibitor*
Therapeutic: Antiarrhythmic,
* cholinergic agonist*

MECHANISM OF ACTION: Edrophonium inhibits the breakdown of the neurotransmitter acetylcholine, causing increased cholinergic receptor stimulation.

THERAPEUTIC BENEFIT: Edrophonium produces stimulation of the vagus nerve, causing bradycardia.

INDICATIONS FOR PREHOSPITAL USE: Edrophonium is used to treat paroxysmal atrial tachycardia resistant to vagal maneuvers.

CONTRAINDICATIONS: ▪ Do not administer edrophonium to patients who: ▪ Are hypersensitive to the drug. ▪ Are hypotensive. ▪ Have bradycardia.

PRECAUTIONS: Administer edrophonium cautiously to patients with a history of bronchial asthma, because it may cause an asthma attack.

ROUTE AND DOSAGE

Adult: 5–10 mg by IV bolus.

Pediatric: Not recommended for prehospital use.

ADVERSE REACTIONS AND SIDE EFFECTS

- *CNS:* Dizziness, weakness, seizures.
- *Cardiovascular:* Hypotension, bradycardia.
- *Respiratory:* Increased secretions, bronchospasm.
- *Gastrointestinal:* Abdominal cramps, nausea, vomiting, excessive salivation.

PARAMEDIC IMPLICATIONS: Monitor patient vital signs before and frequently after administration. Bradycardia and hypotension may develop rapidly.

DRUG INTERACTIONS: ▪ Edrophonium's actions are opposed by anticholinergic drugs, including antihistamines, antidepressants, atropine, haloperidol, phenothiazines, and quinidine. ■ Severe bradycardia may develop in patients using digitalis glycosides.

EPINEPHRINE (1:10,000 SOLUTION)
Adrenalin

CLASSIFICATIONS
Pharmacologic: Beta-adrenergic agonist
Therapeutic: Bronchodilator, cardiac stimulator, peripheral vasoconstrictor

MECHANISM OF ACTION: Epinephrine is a catecholamine that stimulates both alpha- and beta-adrenergic receptors in the sympathetic nervous system. Stimulation of $beta_1$-receptors in the heart increases the rate and force of contraction, resulting in an increase in cardiac output. Stimulation of $beta_2$-receptors causes the bronchial smooth muscles to relax, thereby increasing vital lung capacity. Epinephrine's stimulation of alpha-adrenergic receptors causes the arterioles of the bronchioles to constrict, which reduces edema. The constriction of the arterioles also produces peripheral vasoconstriction, which aids in raising arterial blood pressure.

THERAPEUTIC BENEFIT: The therapeutic benefits of epinephrine include:

- Increase in heart rate
- Increase in contractility of the heart
- Increase in automaticity of the heart
- Bronchodilation
- Increase in arterial blood pressure
- Increase in systemic vascular resistance

INDICATIONS FOR PREHOSPITAL USE: Epinephrine is a first-line drug used for all forms of cardiopulmonary arrest, including:

- Ventricular fibrillation
- Ventricular tachycardia without a pulse (to be treated as ventricular fibrillation)
- Pulseless electrical activity (PEA) [electromechanical dissociation (EMD)]
- Asystole

Epinephrine can also be used as a vasopressor when treating symptomatic sinus bradycardia.

CONTRAINDICATIONS: None, during cardiopulmonary arrest. Otherwise, do not administer epinephrine to patients hypersensitive to sympathomimetic amines.

PRECAUTIONS: ■ Administer epinephrine with caution to elderly patients with: ■ Heart disease. ■ Diabetes. ■ Hypertension.

ROUTE AND DOSAGE

Adult (Cardiac Arrest): 1 mg by IV bolus, followed by a 20-mL flush of IV solution. This dosage should be repeated every 3–5 min during the arrest. If this approach fails, the following Class IIb (acceptable, possibly helpful) options can be administered:

- *Intermediate dosage*: 2–5 mg by IV bolus every 3–5 min.
- *Escalating dosage*: 1 mg–3 mg–5 mg by IV bolus 3 min apart.
- *High dosage*: 0.1 mg/kg by IV bolus every 3–5 min.

During cardiac arrest, epinephrine may be administered as a continuous IV infusion. If this method of treatment is chosen, the infusion is prepared by adding 30 mg (30 mL) of a 1:1000 solution to 250 mL of normal saline or D_5W and running at 100 mL/h, titrating to effect.

Adult (Symptomatic Sinus Bradycardia): 1 μg/min IV infusion titrated to effect. Desired response is generally seen at a dosage range of 2–10 μg/min.
Infusion preparation: Add 1 mg (1 mL) of a 1:1000 solution to 500 mL of normal saline or D_5W.

Pediatric (Asystolic and Pulseless Arrest): Initially, administer 0.01 mg/kg of a 1:10,000 solution by IV bolus or IO. If the initial dosage is administered via the ET tube, the dose is 0.1 mg/kg of a 1:1000 solution. All subsequent dosages (IV, IO, and ET) should be given at 0.1 mg/kg of a 1:1000 solution every 3–5 min. Repeat dosages of 0.2 mg/kg of a 1:1000 solution may be effective. Follow local protocols.

Pediatric (Bradycardia): 0.01 mg/kg of a 1:10,000 solution should be administered by IV bolus or IO. Dosages of 0.1 mg/kg of a 1:1000 solution should be administered via the ET tube; however, doses of up to 0.2 mg/kg of a 1:1000 solution may be effective. Follow local protocols.

If an epinephrine infusion is ordered by medical control, the initial dosage is 0.1 μg/kg/min titrated to effect.

Infusion preparation: 0.6 times the body weight (in kg) equals the amount of milligrams added to 100 mL of D_5W, 5% dextrose in ½ NS, NS, or LR. Running the infusion at 1 mL/h delivers 0.1 μg/kg.

Note: Epinephrine can be administered through a catheter that has been passed down and beyond the tip of an established ET tube. The dosage for adults is 2–2.5 times that of the recommended IV bolus dosage and should be diluted in 10 mL of normal saline or distilled water. The dosage for pediatric patients can be increased up to 10 times the IV bolus or IO dosage and should be diluted in 1–2 mL of normal or half-normal saline to aid in drug delivery. Follow local protocols.

ADVERSE REACTIONS AND SIDE EFFECTS: None, during cardiopulmonary resuscitation. Otherwise:

- *CNS:* Nervousness, restlessness, headache, tremor.
- *Cardiovascular:* Arrhythmia, angina, hypertension.
- *Gastrointestinal:* Nausea, vomiting.

PARAMEDIC IMPLICATIONS: ▪ Epinephrine's therapeutic effects usually begin about 90 s after administration. However, because these effects are short-lived, epinephrine must be given every 5 min during resuscitative efforts to maintain therapeutic levels. ▪ The beta-adrenergic effects of epinephrine may cause or aggravate myocardial ischemia due to the increased work load and oxygen demand that beta-adrenergic stimulation places on the heart. Therefore, the patient must be adequately ventilated using 100% oxygen to minimize myocardial ischemia. ▪ Epinephrine may cause or increase the severity of ventricular ectopic activity. This is of special concern if the patient is taking digitalis, because digitalis causes the heart to become sensitive to the effects of epinephrine.

DRUG INTERACTIONS: ▪ Beta-adrenergic blocking drugs may block the therapeutic response to epinephrine. ▪ The use of epinephrine with oxytocics can cause severe hypertension. ▪ Combination of epinephrine with other beta-adrenergic agonists can cause severe arrhythmias.

ETHACRYNIC ACID
Edecrin

CLASSIFICATIONS
Pharmacologic: Loop diuretic
Therapeutic: Diuretic

MECHANISM OF ACTION: Ethacrynic acid inhibits the reabsorption of sodium and chloride in the kidneys, enhancing the excretion of sodium, chloride, potassium, calcium, and magnesium.

THERAPEUTIC BENEFIT: The diuretic action of ethacrynic acid reduces the edema and lowers blood pressure.

INDICATIONS FOR PREHOSPITAL USE

1. Management of edema secondary to congestive heart failure.
2. Hypertension.

CONTRAINDICATIONS: Do not administer ethacrynic acid to patients with hypersensitivity to the drug or to patients with hypotension.

PRECAUTIONS: Use caution in administering ethacrynic acid to patients with electrolyte depletion and diabetes.

ROUTE AND DOSAGE

Adult: 0.5–1 mg/kg or 50–100 mg by IV bolus. A single dose should not exceed 100 mg.

Pediatric: Not recommended for prehospital use.

ADVERSE REACTIONS AND SIDE EFFECTS

- *CNS:* Dizziness, headache.
- *Cardiovascular:* Hypotension.
- *Fluid and electrolytes:* Hypovolemia, metabolic alkalosis, dehydration.
- *Gastrointestinal:* Nausea, vomiting, dry mouth.

PARAMEDIC IMPLICATIONS: Monitor the patient, being alert for the development of dehydration, hypotension, or electrolyte depletion.

DRUG INTERACTIONS: ▪ Use with antihypertensive or nitrate drugs may cause an additive hypotensive effect. ▪ Use with other diuretics may cause additive hypokalemia. ▪ Hypokalemia may cause or increase digitalis toxicity.

FUROSEMIDE
Lasix

CLASSIFICATIONS
Pharmacologic: Loop diuretic
Therapeutic: Antihypertensive,
diuretic

MECHANISM OF ACTION: Furosemide inhibits the reabsorption of sodium and chloride in the kidneys. It also causes vasodilation, which decreases venous return to the heart. Furosemide's diuretic effect results in excretion of sodium chloride, potassium, hydrogen, calcium, and magnesium.

THERAPEUTIC BENEFIT: The therapeutic benefits of furosemide include reduction of pulmonary edema and lowering of blood pressure.

INDICATIONS FOR PREHOSPITAL USE: Furosemide is given in cardiac emergencies for the treatment of lung congestion associated with inadequate ventricular function.

CONTRAINDICATIONS: ▪ Do not administer furosemide to patients with: ▪ Hypovolemia. ▪ Hypotension. ▪ Hypokalemia. Suspect hypokalemia if the patient is on long-term diuretic therapy or if the ECG shows prominent P waves, diminished T waves, or the presence of U waves.

PRECAUTIONS: ▪ Furosemide administration may result in dehydration and hypotension. ▪ Patients who are sensitive to sulfonamides may develop an allergic reaction.

ROUTE AND DOSAGE

Adult: 0.5–1.0 mg/kg by slow IV bolus.

Pediatric: Not recommended for prehospital use.

ADVERSE REACTIONS AND SIDE EFFECTS
- *CNS:* Dizziness, headache.
- *Cardiovascular:* Hypotension, arrhythmias.
- *Fluids and electrolytes:* Potassium depletion, metabolic alkalosis.
- *Gastrointestinal:* Nausea, vomiting, diarrhea.

PARAMEDIC IMPLICATIONS: ▪ Because of furosemide's diuretic effect, monitor the patient's blood pressure closely. ▪ Assess lung sounds before giving furosemide and monitor them closely after administration.

DRUG INTERACTIONS: ▪ Antihypertensive and nitrate drugs may worsen hypotension. ▪ Furosemide given with other diuretic drugs may cause severe fluid and electrolyte loss. ▪ Severe potassium loss may increase digitalis toxicity in patients taking digoxin.

HYDRALAZINE
Apresoline

CLASSIFICATIONS
Pharmacologic: Peripheral vasodilator
Therapeutic: Antihypertensive

MECHANISM OF ACTION: Hydralazine causes dilation of peripheral arterioles.

THERAPEUTIC BENEFIT: The vasodilator action of hydralazine decreases afterload, which lowers blood pressure.

INDICATIONS FOR PREHOSPITAL USE: Hydralazine is used to treat moderate to severe hypertension and congestive heart failure that is resistant to more conventional therapy using digitalis glycosides and diuretics.

CONTRAINDICATIONS: ■ Do not administer hydralazine to patients with: ■ Hypersensitivity to the drug. ■ Coronary artery disease. ■ Mitral-valve rheumatic heart disease.

PRECAUTIONS: ■ Use caution in administering hydralazine to patients with: ■ Cardiovascular disease. ■ Cerebrovascular disease. ■ Renal disease.

ROUTE AND DOSAGE

Adult: 20–40 mg by slow IV bolus or IM. Repeated after 4–6 h as needed.

Pediatric: Not recommended for prehospital use.

ADVERSE REACTIONS AND SIDE EFFECTS

- *CNS:* Headache, dizziness, drowsiness.
- *Cardiovascular:* Tachycardia, arrhythmias, orthostatic hypotension, chest pain.
- *Gastrointestinal:* Nausea, vomiting.

PARAMEDIC IMPLICATIONS: Monitor the patient closely, especially blood pressure and pulse, during and after administration.

DRUG INTERACTIONS: ■ Use with other antihypertensives and nitrate drugs may produce additive hypotensive effects, which can be particularly severe in the case of diazoxide. ■ Hydralazine may reduce the stimulation and blood-pressure effects of epinephrine.

HYDROMORPHONE
Dilaudid

CONTROLLED SUBSTANCE—
SCHEDULE II
CLASSIFICATIONS
Pharmacologic: Opioid
Therapeutic: Analgesic, antitussive

MECHANISM OF ACTION: Hydromorphone binds to opiate receptors in the CNS and acts directly on the cough center in the medulla of the brain.

THERAPEUTIC BENEFIT: Hydromorphone alters the awareness of and response to pain, causes generalized CNS depression, and suppresses cough.

INDICATIONS FOR PREHOSPITAL USE: Hydromorphone is used for the treatment of moderate to severe pain.

CONTRAINDICATIONS: ■ Do not administer hydromorphone to patients with: ■ Hypersensitivity to the drug. ■ Head trauma. ■ Abdominal pain. ■ Pulmonary disease.

PRECAUTIONS: ■ Use caution in administering hydromorphone to patients who have a history of convulsive disorders, because it may cause seizure activity. ■ Use caution in administering hydromorphone to elderly patients, because they are usually more sensitive to both the therapeutical action and the side effects of the drug.

ROUTE AND DOSAGE

Adult (IV Bolus): 1 mg by slow IV bolus. Repeat IV bolus of 0.5–1 mg every 5 min until adequate pain relief or respiratory depression occurs.

Adult (IM): 2–4 mg every 4–6 h as needed.

Pediatric: Not recommended for prehospital use.

ADVERSE REACTIONS AND SIDE EFFECTS

- *CNS:* headache, confusion, dizziness, sedation.
- *Cardiovascular:* Hypotension, bradycardia.
- *Respiratory:* Respiratory depression.
- *Gastrointestinal:* Nausea, vomiting.

PARAMEDIC IMPLICATIONS: ■ Assess patient vital signs frequently, being alert for the development of respiratory depression. ■ Ensure that naloxone is available in case severe respiratory depression develops.

DRUG INTERACTIONS: ■ Additive CNS depression may develop if hydromorphone is used with alcohol, antidepressants, antihistamines, or sedative/hypnotics. ■ Patients dependent on hydromorphone may experience acute withdrawal syndrome if they are given a narcotic antagonist agent.

ISOPROTERENOL
Isuprel

CLASSIFICATIONS
Pharmacologic: Beta-adrenergic
  agonist
Therapeutic: Antiarrhythmic,
  bronchodilator, cardiac
  stimulator

MECHANISM OF ACTION: Isoproterenol's adrenergic effects on $beta_1$-adrenergic receptors cause an increase in the rate and force of heart contractions. Isoproterenol's effects on $beta_2$-adrenergic receptors cause a marked relaxation of bronchial smooth muscles including the muscles of the small bronchi.

THERAPEUTIC   BENEFIT: Isoproterenol's   nonselective   beta-adrenergic effects increase cardiac output, improve blood return to the heart, and cause bronchodilation.

INDICATIONS FOR PREHOSPITAL USE: Isoproterenol may be used as a Class IIa (acceptable, probably helpful) drug for:

1. Refractory torsade de pointes (Fig. 7–2).
2. Immediate temporary control of hemodynamically significant bradycardia of heart transplant patients.

CONTRAINDICATIONS: Isoproterenol should not be used in patients who have ischemic heart disease, hypotension, or cardiac arrest.

PRECAUTIONS: Isoproterenol may aggravate arrhythmias and cause ventricular tachycardia or ventricular fibrillation.

ROUTE AND DOSAGE

Adult: 2–10 µg/min IV infusion, titrated to heart rate and rhythm response.
   Infusion preparation: Add 1 mg of isoproterenol to 500 mL of D_5W, which produces a concentration of 2 µg/mL.

Pediatric: Not recommended for prehospital use.

ADVERSE REACTIONS AND SIDE EFFECTS

- *CNS:* Nervousness, tremors, headache
- *Cardiovascular:* Arrhythmia, hypertension, angina. Isoproterenol can produce serious arrhythmias, including ventricular tachycardia and ventricular fibrillation.
- *Gastrointestinal:* Nausea, vomiting.

PARAMEDIC IMPLICATIONS: ■ Isoproterenol increases the oxygen demand of the heart, which may worsen ischemia or increase infarction size. ■ Ensure

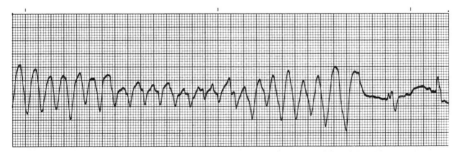

Figure 7–2. Torsade de pointes variation of ventricular tachycardia converting spontaneously to sinus rhythm. (From Brown, KR and Jacobson, S: Mastering Dysrhythmias: A Problem-Solving Guide. F.A. Davis, Philadelphia, 1988, p 124, with permission.)

that lidocaine is readily available in case ventricular irritability develops. ■ Isoproterenol is a temporary treatment until pacemaker therapy can be started. If pacemaker therapy is available in the prehospital setting, use it instead of isoproterenol.

DRUG INTERACTIONS: ■ Beta-blockers may block isoproterenol's therapeutic effects. ■ Isoproterenol may aggravate tachyarrhythmias due to digitalis toxicity.

LABETALOL
Normodyne, Trandate

CLASSIFICATIONS
Pharmacologic: Alpha- and beta-adrenergic blocking agent
Therapeutic: Antihypertensive

MECHANISM OF ACTION: Labetalol blocks the stimulation of myocardial, pulmonary, and vascular receptors.

THERAPEUTIC BENEFIT: The blocking actions of labetalol cause a decrease in heart rate and blood pressure.

INDICATIONS FOR PREHOSPITAL USE: Labetalol is used for the treatment of hypertension.

CONTRAINDICATIONS: ■ Do not administer labetalol to patients with: ■ Congestive heart failure. ■ Pulmonary edema. ■ Cardiogenic shock. ■ Bradycardia. ■ Heart block. ■ Do not administer labetalol during pregnancy, because its use can result in apnea, low Apgar scores, bradycardia, or hypoglycemia in newborns.

PRECAUTIONS: ■ Reduce labetalol dosage for patients with diminished renal function. ■ The beta-blocking action of labetalol may cause congestive heart failure in patients with coronary insufficiency. ■ Use caution in administering labetalol to patients with diabetes mellitus because labetalol may mask tachycardia caused by hypoglycemia.

ROUTE AND DOSAGE

Adult (IV Bolus): Administer 20 mg over 2 min. Administer subsequent doses of 40–80 mg at 10-min intervals if needed. Total dose should not exceed 300 mg.

Adult (IV Infusion): 2 mg/min.
To prepare IV infusion, add 200 mg labetalol to 250 mL of D_5W; this results in a drug concentration of 0.8 mg/mL. Run at 150 μgtts/min to yield an infusion rate of 2 mg/min.

Pediatric: Not recommended for prehospital use.

ADVERSE REACTIONS AND SIDE EFFECTS

- *CNS:* Fatigue, weakness, depression.
- *Cardiovascular:* Bradycardia, congestive heart failure, pulmonary edema, hypotension.

- *Respiratory:* Bronchospasm, wheezing.
- *Eyes:* Blurred vision, dry eyes.
- *Gastrointestinal:* Nausea, diarrhea.

PARAMEDIC IMPLICATIONS: ▪ Monitor patient closely for changes in blood pressure, heart rate and pattern, and respiratory rate. ▪ Patients should remain supine during administration, because labetalol may cause orthostatic hypotension.

DRUG INTERACTIONS: ▪ Use with digitalis glycosides may produce additive bradycardia. ▪ Using labetalol with other hypertensive and nitrate drugs may cause additive hypotension. ▪ Labetalol may antagonize beta-adrenergic bronchodilator drugs.

LIDOCAINE
Xylocaine

CLASSIFICATIONS
Pharmacologic: Antiarrhythmic, local anesthetic
Therapeutic: Ventricular antiarrhythmic

MECHANISM OF ACTION: Lidocaine works by decreasing the excessive spontaneous activity of ectopic pacemaker sites in the His-Purkinje fibers.

THERAPEUTIC BENEFITS: Lidocaine actions make it the drug of choice in the management of ventricular ectopy in the presence of an acute MI, ventricular tachycardia, and ventricular fibrillation.

INDICATIONS FOR PREHOSPITAL USE

1. Ventricular ectopy in the presence of an acute MI.
    Note: The prophylactic administration of lidocaine in an uncomplicated acute MI without ventricular ectopy is not recommended. Under these circumstances, lidocaine is considered in the Class IIb category (acceptable, possibly helpful). Follow local protocols.
2. Ventricular tachycardia.
3. Ventricular fibrillation/pulseless ventricular tachycardia. Class IIa (acceptable, probably helpful).

CONTRAINDICATIONS: ▪ Do not administer lidocaine to patients with: ▪ Severe heart block. ▪ Adams-Stokes syndrome. ▪ Wolff-Parkinson-White syndrome (see Fig. 7-1).

PRECAUTIONS: ▪ Use caution in administering lidocaine to patients who have bradycardia or incomplete heart block, because it can increase the severity of these conditions or cause other serious arrhythmias. ▪ Use caution in administering lidocaine in the presence of respiratory depression and shock.

ROUTE AND DOSAGE

Adult (Ventricular Fibrillation/Pulseless Ventricular Tachycardia): 1.5 mg/kg by IV bolus. This can be repeated in 3–5 min, to a total loading dose of 3 mg/kg. Only IV bolus therapy should be administered during cardiac arrest. When spontaneous circulation returns, begin a lidocaine infusion at 2–4 mg/min to maintain therapeutic levels of the drug.

Adult (Ventricular Tachycardia):   1–1.5 mg/kg by IV bolus. Repeat IV bolus doses of 0.5–0.75 mg/kg can be administered every 5–10 min if necessary, to a total loading dose of 3 mg/kg.

When the arrhythmia has been corrected, therapy should be continued by a lidocaine infusion at 2–4 mg/min.

Adult (Wide-Complex Tachycardia of Uncertain Type):   1–1.5 mg/kg by IV bolus. Repeat IV bolus doses of 0.5–0.75 mg/kg can be administered every 5–10 min if necessary, to a total loading dose of 3 mg/kg.

When the arrhythmia has been corrected, therapy should be continued by a lidocaine infusion at 2–4 mg/min.

Infusion preparation: Add 2 g of lidocaine to 500 mL of D_5W for a concentration of 4 mg/mL. The dosage rates for this 4:1 infusion are:

- 1 mg/min—15 μgtts/min.
- 2 mg/min—30 μgtts/min.
- 3 mg/min—45 μgtts/min.
- 4 mg/min—60 μgtts/min.

Adult (PVCs in the Presence of an Acute MI):   0.5 mg/kg by IV bolus. May be repeated to a total dose of 2 mg/kg unless the arrhythmia persists. Follow local protocols.

Pediatric: 1 mg/kg per dose. If prolonged therapy is needed, an IV infusion should be started at a rate of 20–50 μg/kg/min.

Preparation of infusion: Add 120 mg of lidocaine to an amount of D_5W that produces a total volume of solution of 100 mL. An infusion rate of 1–2.5 mL/kg/hr will deliver the required dosage.

Note: Lidocaine can be administered through a catheter that has been passed down and beyond the tip of an established ET tube. The dosage is 2–2.5 times that of the recommended IV bolus dosage and should be diluted in 10 mL of normal saline or distilled water for the adult patient, and diluted in 1–2 mL of normal or half-normal saline for the pediatric patient.

ADVERSE REACTIONS AND SIDE EFFECTS

- *CNS:* Anxiety, drowsiness, confusion, seizures, respiratory arrest.
- *Cardiovascular:* Hypotension, bradycardia, arrhythmias, cardiac arrest.
- *Gastrointestinal:* Nausea, vomiting.
- *Other:* **Anaphylaxis**—rare.

PARAMEDIC IMPLICATIONS: ▪ The therapeutic levels from a bolus dose of lidocaine last approximately 20 min. Once a bolus dose achieves therapeutic levels, an IV infusion of lidocaine is required to maintain the desired therapeutic level. However, the infusion should not be started until the return of spontaneous circulation or the correction of the arrhythmia. ▪ Too-rapid administration of lidocaine can result in hypotension, bradycardia, tachycardia, or seizures. If the patient develops seizure activity, discontinue the lidocaine and administer diazepam. ▪ Defibrillation causes ventricular irritability, and ventricular irritability can produce ventricular ectopic activity. The administration of lidocaine after a successful defibrillation may be ordered to prevent ventricular ectopic activity. ▪ Patients over 70 have a reduced volume of distribution,

which makes it necessary to reduce the IV infusion dosage of lidocaine by 50%.
■ When administering lidocaine, closely monitor the patient's cardiac function, respiratory status, and blood pressure.

Some publications have indicated that a contraindication for the use of lidocaine is hypersensitivity to amide-type local anesthetics. Adverse reactions associated with local anesthetics occur rarely (less than 1%). The incidence of adverse reactions may be even less, because most alleged allergic reactions may be due to an extension of pharmacologic actions or preservatives present in multidose vials (local anesthetic solutions). Life-threatening anaphylactic reactions occur *very* infrequently. On a practical basis, the incidence of adverse reactions is so rare that there would be a greater risk of withholding lidocaine if the drug is indicated.

DRUG INTERACTIONS: ■ Simultaneous use of lidocaine and beta-blockers may cause lidocaine toxicity. ■ Lidocaine used simultaneously with phenytoin, procainamide, propranolol, or quinidine can have additive, antagonistic, or toxic effects.

MAGNESIUM SULFATE

CLASSIFICATIONS
Pharmacologic: Electrolyte
Therapeutic: Magnesium
supplement

MECHANISM OF ACTION: Magnesium sulfate is one of the major cations of the body. It is one of the electrolytes responsible for neurotransmission and muscular excitability.

THERAPEUTIC BENEFIT: Magnesium sulfate resolves magnesium-deficient states, which are associated with cardiac arrhythmias and sudden cardiac death.

INDICATIONS FOR PREHOSPITAL USE: Magnesium sulfate is given to correct hypomagnesemia in the following:

1. Torsade de pointes (see Fig. 7-2).
2. Severe refractory ventricular fibrillation/pulseless ventricular tachycardia.

Hypomagnesemia can cause refractory ventricular fibrillation as well as impede the replenishment of intracellular potassium. Potassium is the major intracellular cation of the body.

CONTRAINDICATIONS: Do not administer magnesium sulfate to patients with: ■ hypocalcemia ■ heart block.

PRECAUTIONS: Use caution in administering magnesium sulfate to patients with decreased renal function.

ROUTE AND DOSAGE

Adult: Dilute 1–2 g in 100 mL of D_5W and administer over 1–2 min.

Pediatric: Not recommended in the prehospital setting.

ADVERSE REACTIONS AND SIDE EFFECTS

- *CNS:* Drowsiness.
- *Respiratory:* Respiratory depression.
- *Cardiovascular:* Bradycardia, arrhythmias, hypotension.
- *Skin:* Rash.
- *Metabolic:* Hypothermia.

PARAMEDIC IMPLICATIONS: ▪ Rapid IV administration may cause respiratory or cardiac arrest. ▪ An overdose of magnesium sulfate may cause respiratory depression and heart block. To reverse these effects, hyperventilate the patient using 100% oxygen and administer an IV bolus of 10% calcium gluconate at 5–10 mEq (10–20 mL).

DRUG INTERACTIONS: Cardiac conduction changes may occur if magnesium sulfate is administered with cardiac glycosides.

MEPERIDINE
Demerol

CONTROLLED SUBSTANCE—
  SCHEDULE II
CLASSIFICATIONS
Pharmacologic: Opioid
Therapeutic: Analgesic

MECHANISM OF ACTION: Meperidine is a narcotic agonist that binds to opiate receptors in the CNS. It is a synthetic substitute for morphine, but is not as potent. For example, it takes approximately 70 mg of meperidine to equal the effect of 10 mg of morphine.

THERAPEUTIC BENEFIT: Meperidine alters the awareness of and response to pain and causes generalized depression of the CNS.

INDICATIONS FOR PREHOSPITAL USE: Meperidine is given for the treatment of moderate to severe pain.

CONTRAINDICATIONS: ▪ Meperidine should not be given to patients with: ▪ Hypersensitivity to the drug. ▪ Head injury. ▪ Undiagnosed abdominal pain.

PRECAUTIONS: ▪ Use caution in administering meperidine to patients with a history of seizure disorders, because it may cause seizure activity. ▪ Use caution in administering meperidine to patients with pulmonary disease, because it may depress respirations.

ROUTE AND DOSAGE

Adult (IV Infusion): 15–35 mg/h.
  Prepare infusion by adding 50 mg of meperidine to 500 mL of D_5W, making a drug concentration of 0.1 mg/mL.

Adult (IM): 50–100 mg every 3–4 h.

Pediatric: 1.1–1.8 mg/kg IM every 3–4 h. Maximal single dose is 100 mg.

ADVERSE REACTIONS AND SIDE EFFECTS

- *CNS:* Headache, confusion, sedation, hallucinations.
- *Cardiovascular:* Hypotension, bradycardia.
- *Respiratory:* Respiratory depression.
- *Gastrointestinal:* Nausea, vomiting.

PARAMEDIC IMPLICATIONS: ▪ Closely monitor the patient for signs of developing respiratory depression. ▪ Ensure that naloxone is available to reverse respiratory depression, should it occur.

DRUG INTERACTIONS: Using meperidine with antihistamines and sedative/ hypnotics may cause additive CNS depressant effects.

METOPROLOL
Lopressor

CLASSIFICATIONS
Pharmacologic: Beta-adrenergic
   blocker
Therapeutic: Antihypertensive

MECHANISM OF ACTION: Metoprolol blocks the stimulation of cardiac and, to a lesser degree, pulmonary adrenergic receptors.

THERAPEUTIC BENEFIT: Metoprolol decreases heart rate and blood pressure.

INDICATIONS FOR PREHOSPITAL USE: Metoprolol is used to treat hypertension and angina pectoris and for early intervention in acute MI.

CONTRAINDICATIONS: ▪ Do not administer metoprolol to patients with: ▪ Hypersensitivity to the drug. ▪ Congestive heart failure. ▪ Second- or third-degree heart block. ▪ Bradycardia.

PRECAUTIONS: ▪ Use caution in administering metoprolol to patients with coronary insufficiency, because it may cause congestive failure. ▪ Use metoprolol cautiously with patients with diabetes mellitus because it may mask a tachycardia associated with hypoglycemia.

ROUTE AND DOSAGE

Adult: 5 mg by slow IV bolus every 2 min for up to 3 doses or as long as vital signs remain stable.

Pediatric: Not recommended for prehospital use.

ADVERSE REACTIONS AND SIDE EFFECTS

- *CNS:* Weakness, dizziness, depression.
- *Cardiovascular:* Bradycardia, pulmonary edema, congestive heart failure.
- *Respiratory:* Bronchospasm, wheezing.
- *Eyes:* Blurred vision.
- *Gastrointestinal:* Nausea.

PARAMEDIC IMPLICATIONS: Assess patient vital signs frequently during administration. Side effects can develop rapidly.

DRUG INTERACTIONS: ▪ Use with phenytoin and verapamil may produce additive cardiac depression. ▪ Use with digitalis glycosides may cause additive bradycardia. ▪ Excessive alpha-adrenergic stimulation may be produced if metoprolol is used with epinephrine.

MORPHINE
Duramorph, Roxanol

CONTROLLED SUBSTANCE—
SCHEDULE II
CLASSIFICATIONS
Pharmacologic: Opioid
Therapeutic: Narcotic analgesic

MECHANISM OF ACTION: Morphine is a powerful CNS depressant. It also increases the capacity of the venous circulation, pooling blood and decreasing blood return to the heart, thereby reducing the heart's oxygen requirement and relieving lung congestion. Morphine also decreases systemic vascular resistance, which aids in reducing the oxygen requirements of the heart.

THERAPEUTIC BENEFIT: Morphine relieves pain caused by cardiac ischemia and helps to relieve acute congestion in the lungs.

INDICATIONS FOR PREHOSPITAL USE: Morphine is used to treat pain and anxiety associated with acute MI and in treating acute cardiogenic pulmonary edema.

CONTRAINDICATIONS: ▪ Do not administer morphine to patients with: ▪ Hypersensitivity to the drug. ▪ Hypotension. ▪ Respiratory depression not associated with pulmonary edema. ▪ Head injury. ▪ Undiagnosed abdominal pain. ▪ Do not administer to patients who are taking depressant drugs.

PRECAUTIONS: Use extreme caution in administering morphine to patients with chronic obstructive pulmonary disease, because it may depress respirations and suppress the cough reflex.

ROUTE AND DOSAGE

Adult: 1–3 mg by slow IV bolus every 5–30 min until it has desired effect. Do not exceed 15 mg in the prehospital setting.

Pediatric: Not recommended for prehospital use.

ADVERSE REACTIONS AND SIDE EFFECTS
- *CNS:* Confusion, sedation, headache.
- *Cardiovascular:* Hypotension, bradycardia.
- *Respiratory:* Respiratory depression.
- *Eyes:* Dry eyes, blurred vision.

- *Gastrointestinal:* Nausea, vomiting.
- *Skin:* Rashes.

PARAMEDIC IMPLICATIONS: ▪ Morphine is less likely to cause serious respiratory depression if given slowly and in small amounts. ▪ Naloxone should be available in case the patient shows any signs of overdose. ▪ Monitor patient vital signs closely after administering morphine.

DRUG INTERACTIONS: Additive CNS depression may occur when morphine is used with: ▪ Alcohol. ▪ Antihistamines. ▪ Sedative/hypnotics. ▪ Antidepressants. ▪ Barbiturates.

NALBUPHINE
Nubain

CLASSIFICATIONS
Pharmacologic: Narcotic agonist-antagonist
Therapeutic: Analgesic

MECHANISM OF ACTION: Nalbuphine produces an agonist effect by binding to opiate receptors in the CNS. It produces partial antagonist effects by competitive inhibition at opiate receptors in the CNS. Nalbuphine is as strong as morphine.

THERAPEUTIC BENEFIT: Nalbuphine alters the awareness of and response to pain.

INDICATIONS FOR PREHOSPITAL USE: Nalbuphine is used to treat moderate to severe pain.

CONTRAINDICATIONS: ▪ Do not administer nalbuphine to patients with: ▪ Head trauma. ▪ Increased intracranial pressure. ▪ Undiagnosed abdominal pain.

PRECAUTIONS: ▪ Use caution in administering nalbuphine to patients with pulmonary disease. ▪ Administer with caution and in reduced dosages to elderly patients.

ROUTE AND DOSAGE

Adult: 5–10 mg by IV bolus initially. Repeat with 2-mg doses if needed.

Pediatric: Not recommended for prehospital use.

ADVERSE REACTIONS AND SIDE EFFECTS

- *CNS:* Headache, dizziness, vertigo, confusion.
- *Cardiovascular:* Hypotension, hypertension, palpitations.
- *Respiratory:* Respiratory depression.
- *Gastrointestinal:* Nausea, vomiting, dry mouth.

PARAMEDIC IMPLICATIONS: Assess the patient's vital signs frequently, because nalbuphine may cause respiratory depression. Note, however, that the respiratory depression does not necessarily worsen with increased doses of the drug.

DRUG INTERACTIONS: ▪ Antihistamines, antidepressants, and sedative/hypnotic drugs may cause additive CNS depression. ▪ Simultaneous use with other narcotic agents may diminish nalbuphine's analgesic effects.

NIFEDIPINE
Adalat, Procardia

CLASSIFICATIONS
Pharmacologic: Calcium channel blocker
Therapeutic: Antianginal

MECHANISM OF ACTION: Nifedipine dilates both systemic and coronary arteries by acting on slow calcium channels. It decreases peripheral vascular resistance, reducing systemic blood pressure and afterload. By reducing afterload, nifedipine decreases myocardial oxygen consumption.

THERAPEUTIC BENEFITS: Nifedipine causes coronary vasodilation, which decreases the frequency and severity of angina pectoris.

INDICATIONS FOR PREHOSPITAL USE: Nifedipine is used to treat angina pectoris.

CONTRAINDICATIONS: Do not administer nifedipine to patients who are hypersensitive to the drug.

PRECAUTIONS: Use caution in administering nifedipine to patients with congestive heart failure (CHF), because it may worsen the heart failure.

ROUTE AND DOSAGE

Adult (PO): 10–40 mg three to four times daily, not to exceed 180 mg/d.

Adult (SL): 5–10 mg. Repeat every 30–60 min as needed.

Pediatric: Not recommended for prehospital use.

ADVERSE REACTIONS AND SIDE EFFECTS

- *CNS:* Headache, dizziness, nervousness.
- *Respiratory:* Dyspnea, cough, wheezing.
- *Cardiovascular:* Congestive heart failure, MI, ventricular arrhythmias, hypotension, syncope.
- *Gastrointestinal:* Nausea, abdominal discomfort, diarrhea.

PARAMEDIC IMPLICATIONS: ▪ Monitor patient blood pressure and pulse both before and during administration. ▪ Assess the patient frequently for signs of CHF, which include peripheral edema, rales, dyspnea, and jugular vein distension.

DRUG INTERACTIONS: ▪ Simultaneous use of nifedipine with beta-adrenergic blockers or digoxin increases the risk of cardiac conduction defects or CHF. ▪ Severe hypotension may occur if nifedipine is used with beta-adrenergic blockers. ■ Additive hypotension may occur if nifedipine is used with antihypertensives.

NITROGLYCERIN
Nitrostat, Nitro-bid, Nitro-Dur, Nitrolingual, Nitrol, Tridil

CLASSIFICATIONS
Pharmacologic: Nitrate
Therapeutic: Antianginal,
coronary vasodilator

MECHANISM OF ACTION: Nitroglycerin increases coronary blood flow by relaxing vascular smooth muscle. This vasodilation also causes venous pooling, resulting in decreased blood return to the heart.

THERAPEUTIC BENEFIT: Nitroglycerin decreases the heart's ventricular work load, reduces the heart's oxygen demands, increases coronary blood flow, and acts as an antagonist against vasospasm.

INDICATIONS FOR PREHOSPITAL USE: Nitroglycerin is used to treat angina pectoris and CHF.

CONTRAINDICATIONS: ■ Do not administer nitroglycerin to patients with: ■ Hypersensitivity to the drug. ■ Head trauma. ■ Hypotension.■ Hypovolemia. ■ Do not administer to patients in shock.

PRECAUTIONS: Nitroglycerin often causes a rapid decrease in blood pressure. Therefore, patients should remain lying down while taking the drug.

ROUTE AND DOSAGE

Adult (Sublingual): 0.3–0.4 mg tablet. Repeat at 5-min intervals as needed, to a total dose of 0.9–1.2 mg, if necessary.

Adult (IV Bolus): 50 μg, followed by IV infusion.

Adult (IV Infusion): 10–20 μg/min, increasing by 5–10 μg/min every 5–10 min, given to effect.

Adult (Lingual Spray): 0.4 mg/spray, sprayed directly under the tongue; additional one to two sprays every 3–5 min for a total of three sprays.

Adult (Ointment): 1–2 in (15–30 mg) every 8 h, up to 5 in every 4 h.

Adult (Transdermal Patch): 2.5–15 mg/24 h.

Pediatric: Not recommended for prehospital use.

ADVERSE REACTIONS AND SIDE EFFECTS

- *CNS:* Headache, dizziness, weakness.
- *Cardiovascular:* Hypotension, tachycardia, fainting.
- *Gastrointestinal:* Nausea, vomiting, dry mouth.

PARAMEDIC IMPLICATIONS: ■ Assess the patient's blood pressure before and after administering nitroglycerin. ■ Nitroglycerin is unstable and may rapidly deteriorate if exposed to the air, light, or temperature extremes. Therefore, it should be stored in a dark, room-temperature area. ▪ Nitroglycerin tablets taste bitter and sting the tongue. If the bitter taste is not present, the tablet may have lost its strength. Check the expiration date. ▪ Nitroglycerin may cause significant hypotension. Patients with impaired arterial perfusion are more susceptible to this side effect. Severe hypotension may require IV fluid replacement. ▪ Standard IV infusion tubing may absorb up to 80% of the nitroglycerin; therefore, you should administer nitroglycerin from glass bottles and use the special tubing provided by the manufacturer.

DRUG INTERACTIONS: ▪ Nitroglycerin may produce additive hypotensive effects in the presence of: ▪ Alcohol. ▪ Beta-adrenergic blockers. ▪ Calcium channel blockers. ▪ Phenothiazines.

NITROPRUSSIDE
Nipride, Nitropress

CLASSIFICATIONS
Pharmacologic: Vasodilator
Therapeutic: Antihypertensive

MECHANISM OF ACTION: Nitroprusside has a direct vasodilating effect on both peripheral venous and arterial smooth muscles, which reduces both preload and afterload.

THERAPEUTIC BENEFIT: Nitroprusside increases the capacity of the venous circulation and reduces blood pressure.

INDICATIONS FOR PREHOSPITAL USE: Nitroprusside is used in the treatment of hypertensive crisis. It can also be used to treat acute heart failure and cardiogenic shock.

CONTRAINDICATIONS: ▪ Do not administer nitroprusside to patients with: ▪ Hypersensitivity to the drug. ▪ Decreased cerebral perfusion. (According to some local protocols, however, there are no contraindications to nitroprusside in a life-threatening hypertensive crisis.)

PRECAUTIONS: ▪ Use caution in administering nitroprusside to patients with renal or liver disease. ▪ Excessive doses can produce cyanide toxicity, which can worsen any side effects that develop.

ROUTE AND DOSAGE

Adult: Begin IV infusion at 0.1–5.0 μg/kg/min. Doses of up to 10 μg/kg/min may be needed.

To prepare infusion, add 50 mg of nitroprusside to 250–500 mL of D_5W. The amount of D_5W depends on the desired concentration ordered. For example:

- 50 mg added to 250 mL of D_5W yields 200 μg/mL.
- 50 mg added to 500 mL of D_5W yields 100 μg/mL.

Once the infusion is prepared, immediately wrap the container in aluminum foil or other opaque material to avoid deterioration from exposure to light.

Pediatric: Not recommended for prehospital use.

ADVERSE REACTIONS AND SIDE EFFECTS

- *CNS:* Headache, dizziness.
- *Cardiovascular:* Palpitations, dyspnea, hypotension.
- *Gastrointestinal:* Nausea, vomiting.

PARAMEDIC IMPLICATIONS: Closely monitor the patient, assessing blood pressure every 3 min. Once the patient is stabilized, assess blood pressure at 5-min intervals. The desired end-point blood pressure can be determined with either of two ways (consult local protocols):

1. Maintain blood pressure between 80–100 mm Hg.
2. Maintain blood pressure at 30–40 mm Hg below previously existing systolic pressure.

DRUG INTERACTIONS: Use with other antihypertensives may cause additive hypotensive effects.

NITROUS OXIDE–OXYGEN MIXTURE
Nitronox, Entonox

CLASSIFICATIONS
Pharmacologic: Medicinal gas
Therapeutic: Analgesic

MECHANISM OF ACTION: Inhalation of a 50% mixture of nitrous oxide and oxygen produces CNS depression as well as rapid pain relief.

THERAPEUTIC BENEFIT: A nitrous oxide–oxygen mixture produces rapid but reversible relief from pain.

INDICATIONS FOR PREHOSPITAL USE: Nitrous oxide–oxygen mixture is used for the relief of moderate to severe pain from any cause.

CONTRAINDICATIONS: Do not administer a nitrous oxide–oxygen mixture if any of the following exist:

1. The patient has a decreased level of consciousness.
2. The patient has taken any depressant drug.
3. The patient has sustained thoracic trauma.
4. The patient has respiratory compromise from any cause.
5. Cyanosis develops during administration.
6. The patient is unable to follow simple instructions.
7. The patient has sustained abdominal distension or trauma.
8. The patient is pregnant.

PRECAUTIONS: Monitor the patient closely during administration. Some patients develop severe nausea and may vomit during administration. Also, patients sometimes pass out while receiving this medication.

ROUTE AND DOSAGE

Adult: Self-administration by the patient until the pain is relieved.

Pediatric: Same as the adult.

ADVERSE REACTIONS AND SIDE EFFECTS

- *CNS:* Light-headedness, drowsiness, decreased respirations.
- *Gastrointestinal:* Nausea, vomiting.

PARAMEDIC IMPLICATIONS: ■ For patients with respiratory compromise, use 100% oxygen to prevent nitrous oxide from collecting in dead air spaces and further aggravating chest injuries. ■ For patients with myocardial pain, administer oxygen when the nitrous oxide–oxygen mixture is not being given. ■ If intestinal blockage is present, nitrous oxide may collect in the obstructed space, aggravating the blockage. Do not administer a nitrous oxide–oxygen mixture to patients with abdominal pain unless it is certain that intestinal blockage is not present.

DRUG INTERACTIONS: Administration of a nitrous oxide–oxygen mixture in the presence of other drugs that cause CNS depression can produce additive effects.

NOREPINEPHRINE
Levophed

CLASSIFICATIONS
Pharmacologic: Adrenergic
Therapeutic: Vasopressor

MECHANISM OF ACTION: Norepinephrine's $beta_1$-adrenergic effect increases myocardial contractility, while its potent alpha-adrenergic effect causes arterial and venous vasoconstriction.

THERAPEUTIC BENEFIT: Norepinephrine increases both blood pressure and cardiac output.

INDICATIONS FOR PREHOSPITAL USE: Norepinephrine is used to treat hemodynamically significant hypotension.

CONTRAINDICATIONS: ■ Do not administer norepinephrine to patients with: ■ Hypotension due to hypovolemia. ■ Myocardial ischemia or infarction.

PRECAUTIONS: Use caution in administering norepinephrine to patients with hypertension or cardiac disease. Norepinephrine increases the heart's oxygen requirements without increasing coronary blood flow.

ROUTE AND DOSAGE

Adult: Begin IV infusion at 0.5–1.0 μg/min. Increase until there is a therapeutic effect while maintaining blood pressure at 90 mm Hg. The average infusion rate is 2–12 μg/min. However, patients in refractory shock may need 8–30 μg/min.

To prepare infusion, add 4 mg of norepinephrine to 250 mL of D_5W or normal saline, which yields a drug concentration of 16 μg/mL.

Pediatric: Not recommended for prehospital use.

ADVERSE REACTIONS AND SIDE EFFECTS

- *CNS:* Headache, anxiety, dizziness, restlessness.
- *Cardiovascular:* Bradycardia, hypertension, arrhythmias, chest pain.

- *Respiratory:* Dyspnea.
- *Local:* Necrosis at the IV site.

PARAMEDIC IMPLICATIONS: ▪ Give norepinephrine in the largest vein possible, because infiltration can cause necrosis of the surrounding tissue. If infiltration should occur, the drug phentolamine (Regitine) in doses of 5–10 mg diluted in 10–15 mL of saline solution will minimize tissue necrosis. ▪ Monitor ECG and blood pressure constantly. Assess blood pressure every 2–3 min until it stabilizes, then every 5 min thereafter.

DRUG INTERACTIONS: ▪ Beta-blockers used concurrently with norepinephrine can result in high elevations in blood pressure or block cardiac stimulation. ▪ Administering norepinephrine with atropine blocks reflex bradycardia and enhances norepinephrine's therapeutic effects.

OXYGEN

CLASSIFICATIONS
Pharmacologic: Medicinal gas
Therapeutic: Medicinal gas

MECHANISM OF ACTION: Oxygen is required to enable cells to break down glucose into a usable energy form. Oxygen is a colorless, odorless, tasteless gas, essential to respiration. At sea level, oxygen makes up approximately 10%–16% of venous blood and 17%–21% of arterial blood. Oxygen is carried from the lungs to the body's tissues by hemoglobin in the red blood cells.

THERAPEUTIC BENEFIT: The administration of oxygen increases **arterial oxygen tension (PaO₂)** and hemoglobin saturation. This improves tissue oxygenation when circulation is adequately maintained.

INDICATIONS FOR PREHOSPITAL USE: Oxygen is used:

1. To treat severe chest pain that may be due to cardiac ischemia.
2. To treat hypoxemia from any cause.
3. In the treatment of cardiac arrest.

CONTRAINDICATIONS: None, for emergency use.

PRECAUTIONS: If the patient has a history of chronic obstructive pulmonary disease (COPD) begin oxygen administration at low flow rates, increasing flow rate as necessary.

ROUTE AND DOSAGE

Adult: (Inhalation): There are several devices used to administer oxygen, including masks, nasal cannulas, positive pressure devices, and volume-regulated ventilators. Some of the more common oxygen devices and their delivery capacities include:

- *Nasal cannula:* O₂ concentrations of 24%–44% at flow rates of 1–6 L/min.
- *Face mask:* O₂ concentrations of 40%–60% at flow rates of 8–10 L/min.
- *Face mask with oxygen reservoir:* O₂ concentration of 60% at a flow rate of

6 L/min. An O_2 concentration of almost 100% can be achieved with a flow rate of 10 L/min.

- *Venturi mask:* O_2 concentrations:
  24% at 4L/min
  28% at 4 L/min
  35% at 8 L/min
  40% at 8 L/min
- *Mouth-to-mask:* With supplemental O_2 at 10 L/min, O_2 concentration can reach 50%. Without supplemental O_2, concentration reaches only approximately 17%.

Pediatric: Same as the adult.

ADVERSE REACTIONS AND SIDE EFFECTS

- *Respiratory:* In some cases of COPD, oxygen administration may reduce respiratory drive. This is not a reason to withhold oxygen, but be prepared to assist ventilations.
- *Miscellaneous:* Oxygen that is not humidified may dry out or be irritating to mucous membranes.

PARAMEDIC IMPLICATIONS: ▪ Use humidified oxygen whenever possible. Nonhumidified oxygen may dry and irritate mucous membranes. ▪ Oxygen therapy may reduce respiratory drive in patients with COPD. If this should happen, it may be necessary to assist ventilations. If it is indicated, oxygen therapy should never be withheld. ▪ Reassure patients who are anxious about face masks but who require high concentrations of oxygen.

DRUG INTERACTIONS: A 50:50 nitrous oxide–oxygen mixture is an analgesic medicinal gas for use in the prehospital setting for pain relief.

PENTAZOCINE
Talwin

CONTROLLED SUBSTANCE—
SCHEDULE IV
CLASSIFICATIONS
Pharmacologic: Narcotic agonist-
antagonist
Therapeutic: Analgesic

MECHANISM OF ACTION: Pentazocine is a strong analgesic and weak antagonist. It binds to opiate receptors in the CNS, producing CNS depression.

THERAPEUTIC BENEFIT: Pentazocine alters the awareness of and response to pain.

INDICATIONS FOR PREHOSPITAL USE: Pentazocine is used to treat moderate to severe pain.

CONTRAINDICATIONS: ▪ Do not administer pentazocine to patients with: ▪ Hypersensitivity to the drug. ▪ Head injury. ▪ Undiagnosed abdominal pain.

PRECAUTIONS: ■ Use caution in administering pentazocine to patients with pulmonary disease. ■ Use caution in administering pentazocine to older patients, who may also require lower doses.

ROUTE AND DOSAGE

Adult (IV Bolus):   30 mg initially. Repeat the dose every 3–4 h as needed, not to exceed 360 mg.

Adult (IM):   30–60 mg initially. Repeat the dose every 3–4 h as needed, not to exceed 360 mg/d.

Pediatric: Not recommended for prehospital use.

ADVERSE REACTIONS AND SIDE EFFECTS

- *CNS:* Headache, dizziness, sedation, hallucinations, euphoria.
- *Cardiovascular:* Hypotension or hypertension, palpitations.
- *Respiratory:* Respiratory depression.
- *Gastrointestinal:* Nausea, vomiting.

PARAMEDIC IMPLICATIONS: ■ Although pentazocine can be administered full-strength by IV bolus, it is preferable to dilute each 5 mg with 1 mL of sterile water. ■ Narcotic-dependent patients may experience withdrawal symptoms following administration. ■ Assess patient vital signs before and frequently after administration.

DRUG INTERACTIONS: ■ Antihistamines, antidepressants, and sedative/hypnotic agents may cause additive CNS depression. ■ Simultaneous use with other narcotic drugs may diminish the analgesic effect of pentazocine.

PHENYTOIN
Dilantin

CLASSIFICATIONS:
Pharmacologic: Hydantoin
derivative
Therapeutic: Anticonvulsant,
antiarrhythmic

MECHANISM OF ACTION: Phenytoin depresses ventricular automaticity at ectopic pacemaker sites within the heart.

THERAPEUTIC BENEFIT: Phenytoin's antiarrhythmic action improves the heart's atrioventricular conduction.

INDICATIONS FOR PREHOSPITAL USE: Phenytoin is used for the treatment of ventricular arrhythmias, especially those caused by digitalis glycoside toxicity.

CONTRAINDICATIONS: ■ Do not administer phenytoin to patients with: ■ Hypersensitivity to the drug. ■ Bradycardia. ■ Sinoatrial or atrioventricular block. ■ Stokes-Adams syndrome.

PRECAUTIONS: ■ Use caution in administering phenytoin to patients with inadequate cardiac or respiratory function. ▪ Use with caution with elderly patients.

ROUTE AND DOSAGE

Adult: 100 mg by slow (50 mg/min) IV bolus every 5 min, or 50–100 mg by slow IV bolus until:

- The arrhythmia has been abolished.
- Total dose has reached 1000 mg.
- Toxicity has occurred.

Pediatric: Not recommended for pediatrics in the prehospital setting.

ADVERSE REACTIONS AND SIDE EFFECTS

- *CNS:* Poor muscle coordination, drowsiness, dizziness, headache, nervousness.
- *Cardiovascular:* Hypotension.
- *Fluid and Electrolyte:* Hypocalcemia.
- *Gastrointestinal:* Nausea, vomiting.

PARAMEDIC IMPLICATIONS: ▪ Slow administration of phenytoin helps prevent toxicity. ▪ Elderly patients usually develop toxicity more rapidly. ▪ Closely monitor patients for hypotension and for respiratory and cardiac problems.

DRUG INTERACTIONS: ▪ The simultaneous use of phenytoin with dopamine may result in additive hypotension. ▪ Phenytoin may increase the metabolism of lidocaine, quinidine, theophylline, and corticosteroids. ▪ Barbiturates and alcohol may stimulate the metabolism of phenytoin.

PROCAINAMIDE
Pronestyl, Promine, Procan
  SR, Pronestyl-SR

CLASSIFICATIONS
Pharmacologic: Procaine
  derivative
Therapeutic: Antiarrhythmic

MECHANISM OF ACTION: Procainamide slows conduction velocity in the bundle of His, which decreases cardiac excitability. It also may terminate reentry.

THERAPEUTIC BENEFIT: Procainamide is effective in the suppression of ventricular ectopy and arrhythmias.

INDICATIONS FOR PREHOSPITAL USE: Procainamide is classified as Class IIa: acceptable, probably helpful for the following:

1. Refractory ventricular fibrillation.
2. Paroxysmal supraventricular tachycardia (PSVT).
3. Wide-complex tachycardia of uncertain type.
4. Ventricular tachycardia.

CONTRAINDICATIONS: Procainamide should not be used in patients presenting with preexisting QT prolongation and torsade de pointes (see Fig. 7-2).

PRECAUTIONS: ■ Use caution in administering procainamide to patients who may be experiencing: ■ MI. ■ Digitalis toxicity. ■ Renal failure.

ROUTE AND DOSAGE

Adult: 20–30 mg/min by IV infusion until:

1. The arrhythmia has been suppressed.
2. Hypotension develops.
3. The QRS segment widens by 50% of its original width.
4. A total dose of 17 mg/kg has been administered.

A maintenance infusion may be given at a rate of 1–4 mg/min.

Pediatric: Not recommended for prehospital use.

ADVERSE REACTIONS AND SIDE EFFECTS

- *CNS:* Confusion, seizures.
- *Cardiovascular:* Hypotension, ventricular arrhythmias, heart block, asystole.
- *Gastrointestinal:* Nausea, vomiting.

PARAMEDIC IMPLICATIONS: ■ Monitor patients closely during administration. ■ Giving procainamide too rapidly increases the probability of severe hypotension or life-threatening arrhythmias.

DRUG INTERACTIONS: ■ Hypotensive effect may be increased if procainamide is administered with other antihypertensives. ■ Neurologic toxicity may be increased if procainamide is administered with lidocaine.

PROPRANOLOL
Inderal

CLASSIFICATIONS
Pharmacologic: Beta-adrenergic
blocking agent
Therapeutic: Antihypertensive,
antiarrhythmic

MECHANISM OF ACTION: Propranolol, a nonselective beta-blocking agent, blocks the stimulation of myocardial and pulmonary receptor sites.

THERAPEUTIC BENEFIT: Propranolol's blocking action reduces the rate and force of the heart's contractions and blood pressure, thus decreasing myocardial oxygen consumption.

INDICATIONS FOR PREHOSPITAL USE: Propranolol is used for:

1. Control of recurrent ventricular tachycardia and recurrent ventricular fibrillation not responsive to lidocaine or bretylium.
2. Control of rapid supraventricular arrhythmias.

3. Prevention of angina pectoris.
4. Treatment of hypertension.

CONTRAINDICATIONS: ▪ Do not administer propranolol to patients with: ▪ Depressed cardiac function. ▪ Congestive heart failure. ▪ Asthma or chronic obstructive pulmonary disease.

PRECAUTIONS: ▪ Stopping propranolol treatment abruptly may cause angina, severe arrhythmias, or an MI. ▪ Use caution in administering propranolol to diabetic patients, because it can mask the symptoms of hypoglycemia.

ROUTE AND DOSAGE

Adult: 1–3 mg by IV bolus every 5 min. Total dose should not exceed 0.1 mg/kg.

For easier and safer administration, dilute 1 mg of propranolol in 9 mL of D_5W or normal saline.

Pediatric: 0.01 mg/kg by slow IV bolus.

ADVERSE REACTIONS AND SIDE EFFECTS

- *CNS:* Weakness, depression, fatigue.
- *Cardiovascular:* Bradycardia, congestive heart failure, hypotension.
- *Respiratory:* Bronchospasm, wheezing.
- *Endocrine:* Hypoglycemia or hyperglycemia.
- *Gastrointestinal:* Nausea, vomiting, diarrhea.

PARAMEDIC IMPLICATIONS: Monitor the patient constantly during administration. Propranolol may cause a rapid onset of bradycardia or heart block.

DRUG INTERACTIONS: ▪ Simultaneous use of propranolol with digitalis glycosides may produce an additive bradycardia effect. ▪ Use with other antihypertensive drugs may cause severe hypotension. ▪ Propranolol may oppose the action of bronchodilators.

SODIUM BICARBONATE

CLASSIFICATIONS
Pharmacologic: Alkalinizing agent
Therapeutic: Systemic hydrogen
ion buffer

MECHANISM OF ACTION: Sodium bicarbonate buffers acid buildup in the body caused by severe hypoxia. Severe hypoxia results in anaerobic metabolism, which produces lactic acid and metabolic acidosis.

THERAPEUTIC BENEFIT: Sodium bicarbonate helps correct metabolic acidosis in conjunction with adequate ventilation, using 100% oxygen to blow off the increasing amounts of carbon dioxide. During cardiac arrest, adequate ventilation with 100% oxygen is the main concern in controlling acid-base balance. Adequate ventilation with oxygen in conjunction with properly performed cardiopulmonary resuscitation (CPR) maintains pH in the coronary and pulmonary circulations very close to, if not at, normal. Therefore, the use of sodium bicarbonate to treat cardiac arrest is not recommended unless there is documented preexisting metabolic acidosis.

INDICATIONS FOR PREHOSPITAL USE: Possibly for the management of metabolic acidosis during CPR. Sodium bicarbonate, however, should only be used after more appropriate treatment has been attempted, such as:

- Prompt defibrillation.
- Effective chest compressions.
- ET intubation and hyperventilation using 100% oxygen.
- Administration of at least two trials of epinephrine.

CONTRAINDICATIONS: None, when used in the treatment of documented metabolic acidosis.

PRECAUTIONS: In an increasing number of EMS settings, protocols do not include the use of sodium bicarbonate. Sodium bicarbonate administration can result in metabolic alkalosis or sodium overload.

ROUTE AND DOSAGE

Adult: 1 mEq/kg by IV bolus to begin, followed by 0.5 mEq/kg every 10 min during the arrest, if ventilations are adequate.

Pediatric: 1 mEq/kg per dose if ventilations are adequate.

ADVERSE REACTIONS AND SIDE EFFECTS

- *Cardiovascular:* Fluid retention.
- *Fluid and electrolyte:* Metabolic alkalosis, hypokalemia, hypocalcemia.
- *Local:* Tissue necrosis at the IV site.

PARAMEDIC IMPLICATIONS: ■ Do not let sodium bicarbonate come in contact with catecholamines or calcium agents. ■ Monitor patients closely for the development of fluid overload (rales; peripheral edema; pink, frothy sputum).

DRUG INTERACTIONS: Sodium bicarbonate may inactivate catecholamines and form a precipitate with calcium agents.

STREPTOKINASE
Kabikinase, Streptase

CLASSIFICATIONS
Pharmacologic: Plasminogen
* activator*
Therapeutic: Thrombolytic

MECHANISM OF ACTION: Streptokinase activates plasminogen, which then acts to dissolve fibrin deposits.

THERAPEUTIC BENEFIT: Streptokinase dissolves thrombi or emboli, preserving left ventricular function after MI.

INDICATIONS FOR PREHOSPITAL USE: Streptokinase is used to treat coronary thrombosis associated with MI and to treat **pulmonary emboli.**

CONTRAINDICATIONS: ▪ Do not administer streptokinase to patients with: ▪ Hypersensitivity to the drug. ▪ Active internal bleeding. ▪ A cerebrovascular accident (CVA) within 2 mo. ▪ Uncontrolled severe hypertension.

PRECAUTIONS: ▪ Use caution in administering streptokinase to patients: ▪ Who have sustained trauma or surgery within the past 2 mo. ▪ With cerebrovascular disease. ▪ Who have had recent streptokinase therapy.

ROUTE AND DOSAGE

Adult (MI): 1,500,000 International Units (IU) by IV infusion over 60 min.

Adult (Pulmonary Emboli): 250,000 IU by IV infusion over 30 min, followed by 100,000 IU/h for 24 h.

Pediatric: Not recommended for prehospital use.

ADVERSE REACTIONS AND SIDE EFFECTS

- *Respiratory:* Bronchospasm.
- *Cardiovascular:* Arrhythmias due to reperfusion.
- *Miscellaneous:* Anaphylaxis.

PARAMEDIC IMPLICATIONS: ▪ Assess patient vital signs every 15 min. ▪ Monitor ECG continuously. ▪ Prophylactic IV lidocaine or procainamide may be ordered to control reperfusion arrhythmias.

DRUG INTERACTIONS: Using streptokinase with anticoagulants or any drug affecting platelet function increases the risk of bleeding.

VERAPAMIL
Calan, Isoptin

CLASSIFICATIONS
Pharmacologic: Calcium channel blocker
Therapeutic: Antianginal, antiarrhythmic, antihypertensive

MECHANISM OF ACTION: Verapamil inhibits the transport of calcium into cardiac and vascular smooth muscle, which inhibits cardiac contraction and causes coronary vasodilation, decreased vascular resistance, and a reduction of myocardial oxygen consumption.

THERAPEUTIC BENEFIT: Verapamil slows conduction in the sinoatrial and atrioventricular nodes and slows ventricular response. The coronary vasodilation effect of verapamil decreases the frequency and the severity of cardiac chest pain.

INDICATIONS FOR PREHOSPITAL USE: Verapamil is used to stop narrow-complex paroxysmal supraventricular tachycardia (PSVT) not requiring cardioversion and not responsive to adenosine. It may also be used for the temporary control of rapid ventricular response due to atrial fibrillation.

CONTRAINDICATIONS: ▪ Do not administer verapamil to patients with: ▪ Hypersensitivity to the drug. ▪ Sinus bradycardia. ▪ Severe CHF. ▪ High-degree heart block. ▪ Verapamil is also contraindicated for patients with Wolff-Parkinson-White syndrome (see Fig. 7–1), atrial fibrillation, or atrial flutter, because verapamil may accelerate the heart's ventricular rate.

PRECAUTIONS: Use caution in administering verapamil to patients with: ▪ Mild CHF. ▪ Sick sinus syndrome.

ROUTE AND DOSAGE

Adult: 2.5–5 mg IV given over 5 min. If necessary, repeat doses of 5–10 mg IV can be administered every 15–30 min given over a 5-min period. The maximum total dose of verapamil should not exceed 20 mg.

Pediatric: Not recommended for the prehospital setting.

ADVERSE REACTIONS AND SIDE EFFECTS

- *CNS:* Dizziness, headache.
- *Cardiovascular:* Sinus arrest, asystole, heart block, bradycardia, hypotension.
- *Respiratory:* Pulmonary edema.
- *Gastrointestinal:* Nausea.

PARAMEDIC IMPLICATIONS: ▪ Giving verapamil can cause a decease in blood pressure. If this should become a concern, calcium chloride can reverse the decreasing blood pressure when 0.5–1 g are given by slow IV. It is acceptable to administer an IV infusion of calcium chloride over a 5–10 min period (dosage to be determined by medical control) prior to giving verapamil to decrease the chances of falling blood pressure during verapamil administration. Follow local protocols. ▪ Assess the patient's vital signs frequently and monitor the ECG continuously.

DRUG INTERACTIONS: ▪ There may be additive hypotension if verapamil is used with antihypertensives, nitrates, or quinidine. ▪ Verapamil should not be used simultaneously with intravenous beta-adrenergic blockers because of the increased risk of bradycardia, CHF, and arrhythmias.

CONCLUSION

Some of the medications in this chapter do not appear, at first glance, to be intended primarily for use in cardiovascular emergencies. Each of them, however, by nature of its classification and mechanism of action, can be of use in various cardiovascular emergencies. Most drugs used by EMS professionals are employed in the treatment of cardiovascular emergencies. As a paramedic, you will encounter patients whose needs vary from the "norm," and it will be up to you to know the available drugs and to have the flexibility to meet the patient's needs while following local protocols.

STUDY QUESTIONS

1. The correct dosage of atropine to be given to the patient with symptomatic bradycardia is

   a. 1–5 mg by IV bolus initially. This can be repeated every 3–5 min to a total dose of 20 mg.
   b. 0.5 mg by IV bolus initially. This may be repeated every 3–5 min to a total dose of 2.0 mg.
   c. 0.5–1.0 mg by IV bolus. This may be repeated every 3–5 min, to a total dose of 0.4 mg/kg.
   d. 5 mg by IV bolus. Repeat doses may be given at 10 mg by IV bolus.

2. Propranolol is a nonselective beta-adrenergic blocking agent. Its blocking action reduces the rate and force of heart contractions and blood pressure. Which is *not* an adverse reaction or side effect of propranolol?
   a. Coma.
   b. Weakness.
   c. Congestive heart failure.
   d. Bronchospasm, wheezing.

3. The initial dosage of bretylium for a patient in ventricular fibrillation is 5 mg/kg by IV bolus, to be followed by defibrillation. If a subsequent dose must be given, the dosage is
   a. ½ the original dose every 10 min during resuscitation.
   b. 1 mg/kg by IV bolus.
   c. 5 mg/kg by IV bolus.
   d. 10 mg/kg by IV bolus.

4. What are the therapeutic benefits of giving epinephrine by IV bolus?
   a. Increase in rate, contractility, and automaticity of the heart.
   b. Increase in systemic vascular resistance and arterial blood pressure.
   c. Bronchodilation.
   d. All of the above.

5. Which of the following is *not* a contraindication for giving lidocaine?
   a. Bradycardia.
   b. High-degree AV block.
   c. History of seizures.
   d. Wolff-Parkinson-White syndrome.
      (1) a and b.
      (2) a and c.
      (3) b and c.
      (4) b and d.

6. Digoxin:
   a. Is helpful in the treatment of incomplete heart block.
   b. Is used in the treatment of bradyarrhythmias.
   c. Controls rapid ventricular response caused by atrial fibrillation or atrial flutter.
   d. Is used in the treatment of ventricular tachycardia in patients with a pulse who do not respond to more conventional therapy.

7. Diazoxide is used for the emergency treatment of malignant hypertension. Side effects include all *except:*
   a. Dizziness.
   b. Hypotension.

   c. Bradycardia.

   d. Sodium and water retention.

8. Morphine is contraindicated in patients with:

   a. Acute cardiogenic pulmonary edema.

   b. Severe pain associated with myocardial ischemia.

   c. Abnormally rapid respirations.

   d. Hypotension.

9. Why is dopamine one of the drugs of choice for the treatment of hemodynamically significant hypotension in the absence of hypovolemia?

   a. Dopamine increases blood pressure and cardiac output.

   b. Dopamine causes a decrease in preload.

   c. Dopamine improves blood flow to the kidneys.

   d. Dopamine may decrease oxygen demand on the heart.

     (1) b and c.

     (2) b and d.

     (3) a and b.

     (4) a, c, and d.

10. If isoproterenol is infused too rapidly, _____ could result.

   a. Bradycardia.

   b. Bronchospasm.

   c. Pulmonary edema.

   d. Ventricular fibrillation.

11. Adverse reactions or side effects of norepinephrine generally include all of the following *except:*

   a. Hypertension.

   b. Hypotension.

   c. Arrhythmias.

   d. Necrosis at the IV site.

12. What are the therapeutic benefits of nitroglycerin?

   a. It decreases the heart's ventricular work load

   b. It reduces the heart's oxygen demands

   c. It increases coronary blood flow

   d. It acts as an antagonist against vasospasm

     (1) a and b only.

     (2) b and c only.

     (3) b and d only.

     (4) All of the above.

13. Verapamil is used for the treatment of:

   a. Supraventricular tachyarrhythmias.

   b. Severe AV heart blocks.

   c. Ventricular tachycardia.

   d. Bradycardia.

14. You have been ordered to give a lidocaine bolus of 1 mg/kg to your 180-lb patient. The correct dosage is:

a. 180 mg.
b. 100 mg.
c. 82 mg.
d. 50 mg.

15. In the situation described in question 14, after the IV bolus of lidocaine the physician orders you to begin a lidocaine IV infusion at 2.0 mg/min. You have 2 gm of lidocaine and 500 mL of D₅W. What will the drug concentration be when the lidocaine is added to the D₅W? At what rate should the IV infusion run if you use a microdrip set?
a. 2 mg/mL—30 μgtts/min.
b. 4 mg/mL—30 μgtts/min.
c. 6 mg/mL—15 μgtts/min.
d. 8 mg/mL—15 μgtts/min

CASE STUDIES

1. Your patient is a 52-year-old man who says, "My heart feels like it is racing." The ECG monitor shows ventricular tachycardia (Fig. 7–3). At the present time the patient is hemodynamically stable. In this situation the prehospital drug of choice is:
a. Bretylium.
b. Verapamil.
c. Lidocaine.
d. Atropine.

2. You respond to a 46-year-old man who complains of severe substernal chest pain that radiates to his left shoulder, arm, and hand. He is short of breath and very apprehensive. The ECG monitor shows a sinus tachycardia at a regular rate of 120 beats/min (Fig. 7–4). After assessing vital signs, you note that they are within normal limits. Initial treatment should include oxygen, reassurance, and:
a. Nitroglycerin.
b. Lidocaine.
c. Bretylium.
d. Morphine.

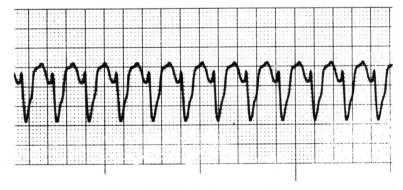

Figure 7–3. Ventricular tachycardia.

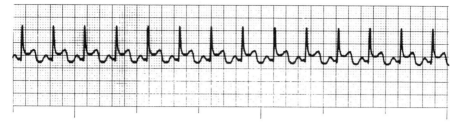

Figure 7–4. Sinus tachycardia. Rate: 120 beats/min.

3. You are called to a 67-year-old-woman who says that her heart feels like it is "fluttering." Your ECG monitor indicates the patient is experiencing paroxysmal supraventricular tachycardia at a regular rate of 180 beats/min (Fig. 7–5). Vital signs are currently within normal limits and she is tolerating the rhythm fairly well. Which is the drug of choice to treat stable paroxysmal supraventricular tachycardia?
   a. Isoproterenol.
   b. Procainamide.
   c. Adenosine.
   d. Verapamil.

EXTENDED CASE STUDY: Ventricular Ectopy

Response

You respond to a complaint of chest pain and shortness of breath. When you arrive, you find a 53-year-old man lying on the living room sofa complaining of substernal chest pain that radiates to his left shoulder and jaw. The patient says that he was watching television when the pain began, about an hour ago. He had passed the pain off as indigestion until it began radiating into his shoulder and jaw. He weighs 250 lb, has no previous cardiac history, and is not taking any medications. Your initial examination reveals the following:

- *Level of consciousness:* Alert and oriented.
- *Respirations:* 30/min.
- *Breath sounds:* Clear bilaterally.

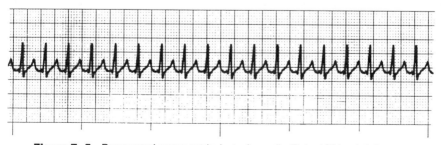

Figure 7–5. Paroxysmal supraventricular tachycardia. Rate: 100 beats/min.

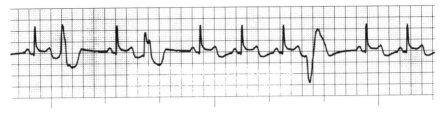

Figure 7–6. Sinus rhythm with multifocal premature ventricular contractions (PVCs).

- *Blood pressure:* 160/96.
- *Skin condition:* Cool, clammy.

ECG Interpretation

After connecting the patient to your ECG monitor, you see a rhythm like the one shown in Figure 7–6. You interpret the rhythm as a sinus rhythm with multifocal premature ventricular contractions (PVCs). Multifocal PVCs should be treated immediately. These PVCs are considered malignant, because the ectopic activity causing them originates from more than one area of the ventricles. The chances are high that multifocal PVCs will deteriorate to ventricular fibrillation, placing the patient in cardiopulmonary arrest.

Other malignant PVCs include:

- Unifocal PVCs that occur more than six times/min.
- Closely coupled PVCs.
- PVCs that occur in short bursts of three or more in succession (salvos).
- PVCs that occur on the preceding T wave (R-on-T phenomenon).

Management

After initial evaluation, the first step is reassurance. Next, place the patient on high-flow, humidified oxygen (100%) using a nonrebreather mask. Oxygen by itself may aid in controlling PVCs. Since the patient is short of breath, if may be appropriate to place him in a comfortable position such as sitting or semisitting.

Notify medical control as to the patient's condition and request an order for an IV of NS at a keep-open rate. Once the IV has been established, medical control should order you to administer a lidocaine bolus followed by an IV infusion of lidocaine.

Lidocaine is the drug of choice for the management of ventricular ectopy in the presence of an acute MI. Lidocaine suppresses ventricular ectopic activity and increases the ventricular fibrillation threshold, preventing PVCs from causing ventricular fibrillation.

The initial adult dose for lidocaine in this situation is 0.5 mg/kg by IV bolus. Since the patient weighs 250 lb, the initial bolus dose is 57 mg (250 lb ÷ 2.2 kg = 113.6 kg or 114 kg × 0.5 mg/kg = 57 mg). If this dose does not suppress the PVCs, administer additional boluses of lidocaine at 0.5 mg/kg every 2–5 min to a total dose of 2.0 mg/kg until the PVCs have been suppressed. Once the PVCs have been suppressed, start a lidocaine IV infusion running at 2–4 mg/min.

If you cannot use lidocaine with this patient, procainamide can be effective in the suppression of PVCs. Administer procainamide at 20–30 mg/min until the PVCs are suppressed, to a total dose of 17 mg/kg.

It is vital to make the best possible use of treatment time. Establish the IV lifeline and start drug therapy at the scene. Then, however, the patient should be moved to the ambulance for transport to the appropriate emergency facility. All other treatment and monitoring should be done en route. American Heart Association treatment algorithms begin on page 146.

VARIATION: Ventricular Ectopy Progresses to Ventricular Fibrillation

The initial response, ECG interpretation, and treatment remain the same. However, before you administer lidocaine bolus, the patient becomes unconscious and the monitor shows an ECG like that in Figure 7–7. The patient is now unresponsive, pulseless, and has no respirations. You interpret the above ECG rhythm as ventricular fibrillation.

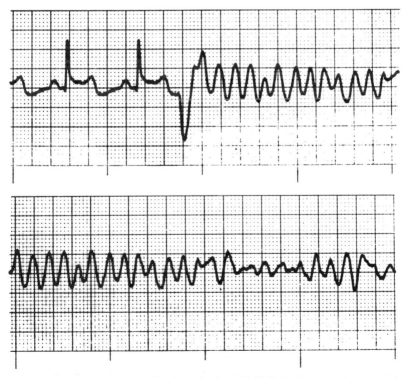

Figure 7–7. From a continuous strip: sinus rhythm with PVC *(top)* progressing to ventricular fibrillation *(bottom)*.

Management

As soon as it has been determined that the patient has no pulse or respirations, you administer a precordial thump. A precordial thump delivers approximately 2–3 J of energy, which may be enough to convert the ventricular fibrillation. If the precordial thump fails to convert the ventricular fibrillation, start CPR. The precordial thump is considered a Class IIb action in the witnessed arrest situation.

In this case the monitor/defibrillator is already connected to the patient. Therefore, the next step is immediate defibrillation, using 200 J. If, after defibrillation, the patient remains pulseless and ventricular fibrillation persists, make a second attempt at defi-

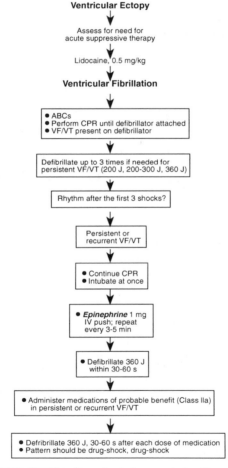

Figure 7–8. Treatment algorithm for extended case study. (Reproduced with permission. Adapted from Textbook of Advanced Cardiac Life Support, © American Heart Association; and from Guidelines for Cardiopulmonary Resuscitation and Emergency Care, 1992, copyright American Heart Association.)

brillation using 200–300 J. If the second defibrillation is also unsuccessful, attempt a third defibrillation using 360 J. Check the patient's pulse before and after each defibrillation attempt.

Maintain ventilations, using oxygen at a concentration of 100%. Thereafter, intubation assumes primary importance (remember, the IV lifeline is already in place).

Medical control should now direct you to administer 1 mg of a 1:10,000 solution of epinephrine by IV bolus. This should be repeated every 3–5 min during resuscitative efforts. If need be, a dose of 2–2.5 mg of epinephrine can be administered down the ET tube. After the epinephrine has had a chance to circulate, reattempt defibrillation using 360 J.

Epinephrine is a catecholamine with alpha-adrenergic and beta-adrenergic effects. It is a proven first-line drug used during resuscitative efforts for cardiac arrest. Epinephrine used during resuscitation can result in increased:

- Heart rate.
- Automaticity.
- Arterial blood pressure.
- Myocardial contraction.
- Systemic vascular resistance.
- Coronary and cerebral blood flow.
- Myocardial oxygen requirements.

Since epinephrine does cause the heart to require more oxygen, it is extremely important to maintain a patent airway and to ventilate the patient properly, using 100% oxygen.

The alpha-adrenergic effect of epinephrine may make ventricular fibrillation more susceptible to defibrillation. However, the $beta_1$-adrenergic effect may increase the heart's tendency to arrhythmia.

If the treatment just outlined is unsuccessful, begin therapy using an antiarrhythmic drug. Lidocaine is the recommended first drug of choice in this situation. Administer lidocaine by IV bolus of 1.5 mg/kg, followed by a repeat defibrillation attempt at 360 J. Subsequent treatment may include repeat doses of lidocaine at 0.5 mg/kg or an initial dose of 5 mg/kg of bretylium followed by subsequent doses of 10 mg/kg. Continue CPR for 1–2 min after each drug dose to allow the drug to reach the central circulation before defibrillation. Figure 7–8 illustrates the algorithm for this entire case.

Note: During the course of an actual prehospital emergency such as this, different circumstances and additional information may indicate treatment other than that outlined in this case study. Always follow local protocols and the direction of medical control.

Chapter 7 Appendix

American Heart Association Treatment Algorithms

ADULT ALGORITHMS (Figures 1 through 9)

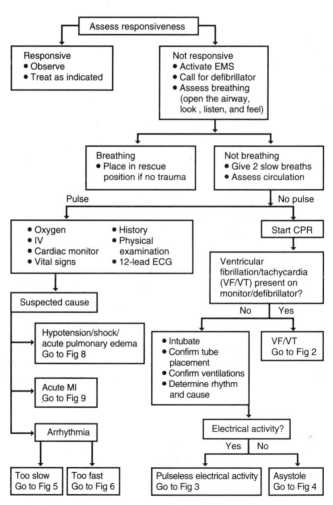

Figure 7A–1. Universal algorithm for adult emergency cardiac care (ECC). (Reproduced with permission from Guidelines for Cardiopulmonary Resuscitation and Emergency Care, 1992, copyright American Heart Association.)

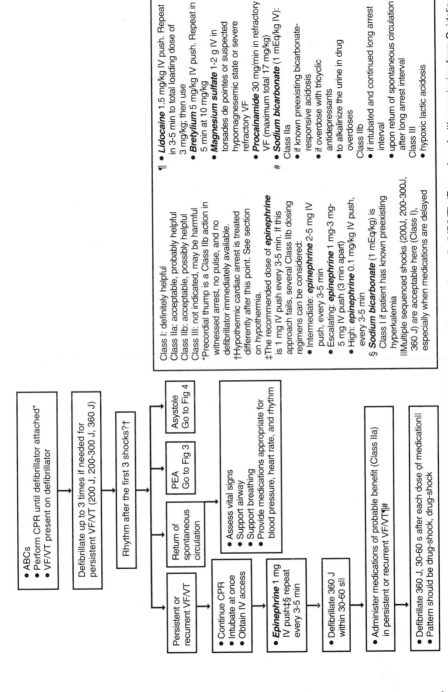

¶ • *Lidocaine* 1.5 mg/kg IV push. Repeat in 3-5 min to total loading dose of 3 mg/kg; then use
• *Bretylium* 5 mg/kg IV push. Repeat in 5 min at 10 mg/kg
• *Magnesium sulfate* 1-2 g IV in torsades de pointes or suspected hypomagnesemic state or severe refractory VF
• *Procainamide* 30 mg/min in refractory VF (maximum total 17 mg/kg)
• *Sodium bicarbonate* (1 mEq/kg IV):

Class IIa
• if known preexisting bicarbonate-responsive acidosis
• if overdose with tricyclic antidepressants
• to alkalinize the urine in drug overdoses

Class IIb
• if intubated and continued long arrest interval
• upon return of spontaneous circulation after long arrest interval

Class III
• hypoxic lactic acidosis

Class I: definitely helpful
Class IIa: acceptable, probably helpful
Class IIb: acceptable, possibly helpful
Class III: not indicated, may be harmful

*Precordial thump is a Class IIb action in witnessed arrest, no pulse, and no defibrillator immediately available.

†Hypothermic cardiac arrest is treated differently after this point. See section on hypothermia.

‡The recommended dose of *epinephrine* is 1 mg IV push every 3-5 min. If this approach fails, several Class IIb dosing regimens can be considered:
• Intermediate: *epinephrine* 2-5 mg IV push, every 3-5 min
• Escalating: *epinephrine* 1 mg-3 mg-5 mg IV push (3 min apart)
• High: *epinephrine* 0.1 mg/kg IV push, every 3-5 min

§ *Sodium bicarbonate* (1 mEq/kg) is Class I if patient has known preexisting hyperkalemia

‖Multiple sequenced shocks (200J, 200-300J, 360 J) are acceptable here (Class I), especially when medications are delayed

• ABCs
• Perform CPR until defibrillator attached*
• VF/VT present on defibrillator

Defibrillate up to 3 times if needed for persistent VF/VT (200 J, 200-300 J, 360 J)

Rhythm after the first 3 shocks?†

Asystole
Go to Fig 4

PEA
Go to Fig 3

Return of spontaneous circulation

• Assess vital signs
• Support airway
• Support breathing
• Provide medications appropriate for blood pressure, heart rate, and rhythm

Persistent or recurrent VF/VT

• Continue CPR
• Intubate at once
• Obtain IV access

• *Epinephrine* 1 mg IV push‡§ repeat every 3-5 min

• Defibrillate 360 J within 30-60 s‖

• Administer medications of probable benefit (Class IIa) in persistent or recurrent VF/VT¶#

• Defibrillate 360 J, 30-60 s after each dose of medication‖
• Pattern should be drug-shock, drug-shock

Figure 7A-2. Algorithm for ventricular fibrillation and pulseless ventricular tachycardia (VF/VT). (Reproduced with permission from Guidelines for Cardiopulmonary Resuscitation and Emergency Care, 1992, copyright American Heart Association.)

147

PEA includes   • Electromechanical dissociation (EMD)
                    • Pseudo-EMD
                    • Idioventricular rhythms
                    • Ventricular escape rhythms
                    • Bradyasystolic rhythms
                    • Postdefibrillation idioventricular rhythms

---

| • Continue CPR | • Obtain IV access |
| • Intubate at once | • Assess blood flow using Doppler ultrasound |

↓

Consider possible causes
(Parentheses=possible therapies and treatments)
• Hypovolemia (volume infusion)
• Hypoxia (ventilation)
• Cardiac tamponade (pericardiocentesis)
• Tension pneumothorax (needle decompression)
• Hypothermia (see hypothermia algorithm, Section IV)
• Massive pulmonary embolism (surgery, **thrombolytics**)
• Drug overdoses such as tricyclics, digitalis, β-blockers, calcium channel blockers
• Hyperkalemia*
• Acidosis†
• Massive acute myocardial infarction (go to Fig 9)

↓

• **Epinephrine** 1 mg IV push, *‡ repeat every 3-5 min

↓

• If absolute bradycardia (<60 beats/min) or relative bradycardia, give **atropine** 1 mg IV
• Repeat every 3-5 min up to a total of 0.04 mg/kg§

Class I: definitely helpful
Class IIa: acceptable, probably helpful
Class IIb: acceptable, possibly helpful
Class III: not indicated, may be harmful
***Sodium bicarbonate** 1 mEq/kg is Class I if patient has known preexisting hyperkalemia.
†**Sodium bicarbonate** 1 mEq/kg:
  Class IIa
  • if known preexisting bicarbonate-responsive acidosis
  • if overdose with tricyclic antidepressants
  • to alkalinize the urine in drug overdoses
  Class IIb
  • if intubated and long arrest interval
  • upon return of spontaneous circulation after long arrest interval
  Class III
  • hypoxic lactic acidosis
‡The recommended dose of **epinephrine** is 1 mg IV push every 3-5 min. If this approach fails, several Class IIb dosing regimens can be considered.
  • Intermediate: **epinephrine** 2-5 mg IV push, every 3-5 min
  • Escalating: **epinephrine** 1 mg-3 mg-5 mg IV push (3 min apart)
  • High: **epinephrine** 0.1 mg/kg IV push, every 3-5 min
§ Shorter **atropine** dosing intervals are possibly helpful in cardiac arrest (Class IIb).

Figure 7A–3. Algorithm for pulseless electrical activity (PEA) (electromechanical dissociation [EMD]). (Reproduced with permission from Guidelines for Cardiopulmonary Resuscitation and Emergency Care, 1992, copyright American Heart Association.)

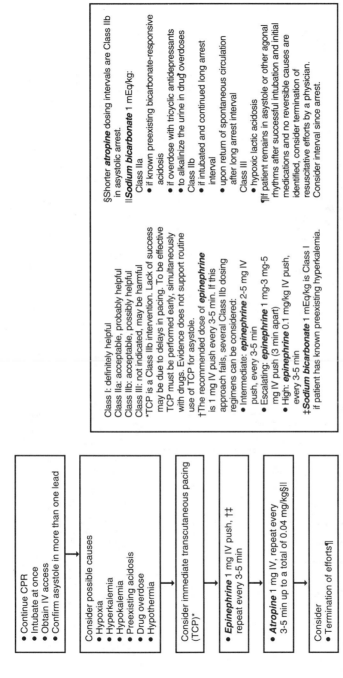

Figure 7A–4. Asystole treatment algorithm. (Reproduced with permission from Guidelines for Cardiopulmonary Resuscitation and Emergency Care, 1992, copyright American Heart Association.)

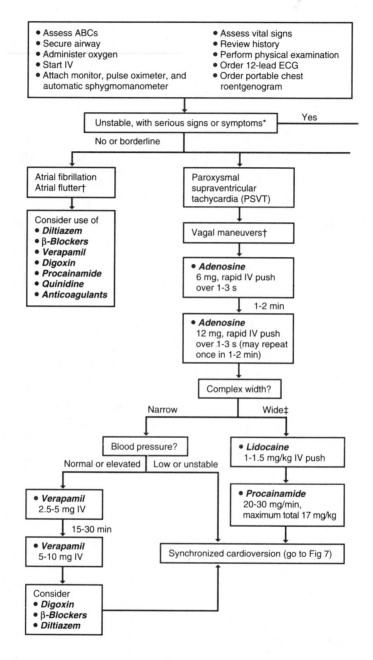

Figure 7A–5. Tachycardia algorithm. (Reproduced with permission from Guidelines for Cardio pulmonary Resuscitation and Emergency Care, 1992, copyright American Heart Association.)

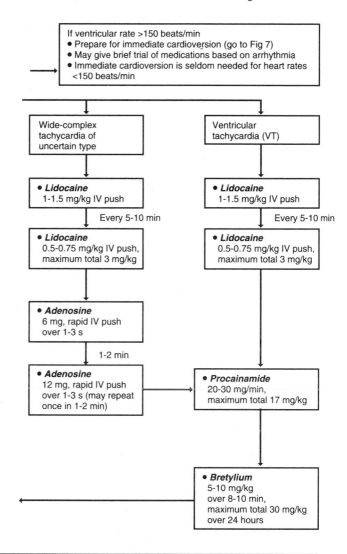

If ventricular rate >150 beats/min
- Prepare for immediate cardioversion (go to Fig 7)
- May give brief trial of medications based on arrhythmia
- Immediate cardioversion is seldom needed for heart rates <150 beats/min

| Wide-complex tachycardia of uncertain type | Ventricular tachycardia (VT) |

- *Lidocaine* 1-1.5 mg/kg IV push

Every 5-10 min

- *Lidocaine* 0.5-0.75 mg/kg IV push, maximum total 3 mg/kg

- *Lidocaine* 1-1.5 mg/kg IV push

Every 5-10 min

- *Lidocaine* 0.5-0.75 mg/kg IV push, maximum total 3 mg/kg

- *Adenosine* 6 mg, rapid IV push over 1-3 s

1-2 min

- *Adenosine* 12 mg, rapid IV push over 1-3 s (may repeat once in 1-2 min)

- *Procainamide* 20-30 mg/min, maximum total 17 mg/kg

- *Bretylium* 5-10 mg/kg over 8-10 min, maximum total 30 mg/kg over 24 hours

*Unstable condition must be related to the tachycardia. Signs and symptoms may include chest pain, shortness of breath, decreased level of consciousness, low blood pressure (BP), shock, pulmonary congestion, congestive heart failure, acute myocardial infarction.
†Carotid sinus pressure is contraindicated in patients with carotid bruits; avoid ice water immersion in patients with ischemic heart disease.
‡If the wide-complex tachycardia is known with certainty to be PSVT and BP is normal/elevated, sequence can include **verapamil**.

Figure 7A–5. Continued.

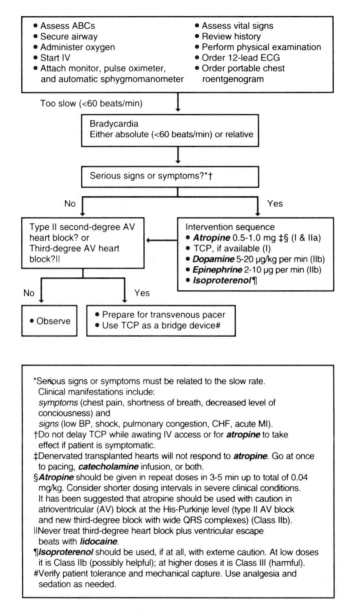

Figure 7A–6. Bradycardia algorithm (with the patient not in cardiac arrest). (Reproduced with permission from Guidelines for Cardiopulmonary Resuscitation and Emergency Care, 1992, copyright American Heart Association.)

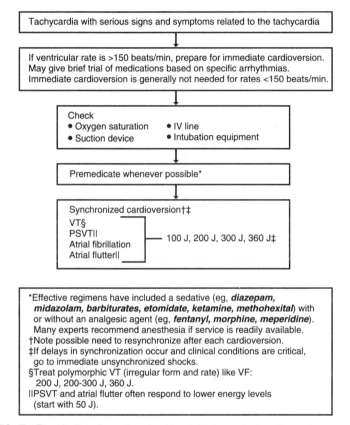

Tachycardia with serious signs and symptoms related to the tachycardia

If ventricular rate is >150 beats/min, prepare for immediate cardioversion.
May give brief trial of medications based on specific arrhythmias.
Immediate cardioversion is generally not needed for rates <150 beats/min.

Check
- Oxygen saturation   • IV line
- Suction device   • Intubation equipment

Premedicate whenever possible*

Synchronized cardioversion†‡
VT§
PSVT|| 100 J, 200 J, 300 J, 360 J‡
Atrial fibrillation
Atrial flutter||

*Effective regimens have included a sedative (eg, *diazepam, midazolam, barbiturates, etomidate, ketamine, methohexital*) with or without an analgesic agent (eg, *fentanyl, morphine, meperidine*).
Many experts recommend anesthesia if service is readily available.
†Note possible need to resynchronize after each cardioversion.
‡If delays in synchronization occur and clinical conditions are critical, go to immediate unsynchronized shocks.
§Treat polymorphic VT (irregular form and rate) like VF:
200 J, 200-300 J, 360 J.
||PSVT and atrial flutter often respond to lower energy levels
(start with 50 J).

Figure 7A–7. Electrical cardioversion algorithm (with the patient not in cardiac arrest). (Reproduced with permission from Guidelines for Cardiopulmonary Resuscitation and Emergency Care, 1992, copyright American Heart Association.)

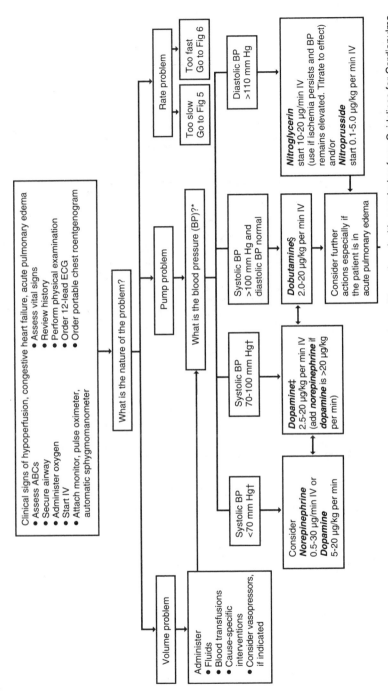

Clinical signs of hypoperfusion, congestive heart failure, acute pulmonary edema
- Assess ABCs
- Secure airway
- Administer oxygen
- Start IV
- Attach monitor, pulse oximeter, automatic sphygmomanometer
- Assess vital signs
- Review history
- Perform physical examination
- Order 12-lead ECG
- Order portable chest roentgenogram

What is the nature of the problem?

Volume problem

Administer
- Fluids
- Blood transfusions
- Cause-specific interventions
- Consider vasopressors, if indicated

Pump problem

What is the blood pressure (BP)?*

Systolic BP <70 mm Hg†

Consider
Norepinephrine
0.5-30 µg/min IV or
Dopamine
5-20 µg/kg per min

Systolic BP 70-100 mm Hg†

Dopamine‡
2.5-20 µg/kg per min IV
(add ***norepinephrine*** if ***dopamine*** is >20 µg/kg per min)

Systolic BP >100 mm Hg and diastolic BP normal

Dobutamine§
2.0-20 µg/kg per min IV

Consider further actions especially if the patient is in acute pulmonary edema

Rate problem

Too slow
Go to Fig 5

Too fast
Go to Fig 6

Diastolic BP >110 mm Hg

Nitroglycerin
start 10-20 µg/min IV
(use if ischemia persists and BP remains elevated. Titrate to effect)
and/or
Nitroprusside
start 0.1-5.0 µg/kg per min IV

Figure 7A–8. Algorithm for hypotension, shock, and acute pulmonary edema. (Reproduced with permission from Guidelines for Cardiopulmonary Resuscitation and Emergency Care, 1992, copyright American Heart Association.)

154

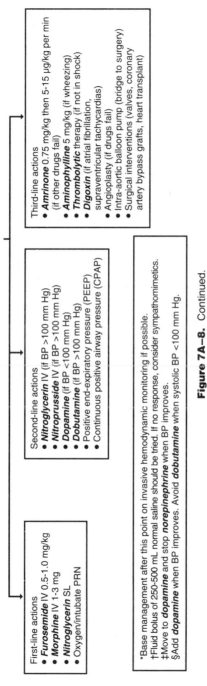

First-line actions
• **Furosemide** IV 0.5-1.0 mg/kg
• **Morphine** IV 1-3 mg
• **Nitroglycerin** SL
• Oxygen/intubate PRN

Second-line actions
• **Nitroglycerin** IV (if BP >100 mm Hg)
• **Nitroprusside** IV (if BP >100 mm Hg)
• **Dopamine** (if BP <100 mm Hg)
• **Dobutamine** (if BP >100 mm Hg)
• Positive end-expiratory pressure (PEEP)
• Continuous positive airway pressure (CPAP)

Third-line actions
• **Amrinone** 0.75 mg/kg then 5-15 µg/kg per min (if other drugs fail)
• **Aminophylline** 5 mg/kg (if wheezing)
• **Thrombolytic** therapy (if not in shock)
• **Digoxin** (if atrial fibrillation, supraventricular tachycardias)
• Angioplasty (if drugs fail)
• Intra-aortic balloon pump (bridge to surgery)
• Surgical interventions (valves, coronary artery bypass grafts, heart transplant)

*Base management after this point on invasive hemodynamic monitoring if possible.
†Fluid bolus of 250-500 mL normal saline should be tried. If no response, consider sympathomimetics.
‡Move to **dopamine** and stop **norepinephrine** when BP improves.
§Add **dopamine** when BP improves. Avoid **dobutamine** when systolic BP <100 mm Hg.

Figure 7A–8. Continued.

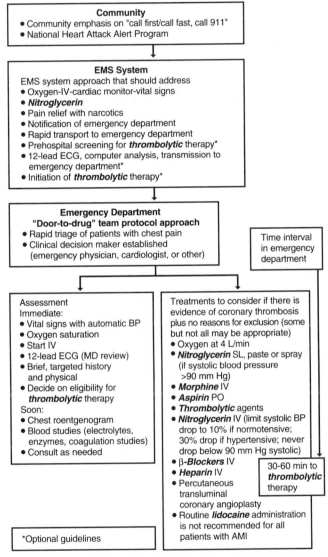

Figure 7A–9. Acute myocardial infraction (AMI) algorithm. Recommendations for early treatment of patients with chest pain and possible AMI. (Reproduced with permission from Guidelines for Cardiopulmonary Resuscitation and Emergency Care, 1992, copyright American Heart Association.)

PEDIATRIC ALGORITHMS (Figures 1 and 2)

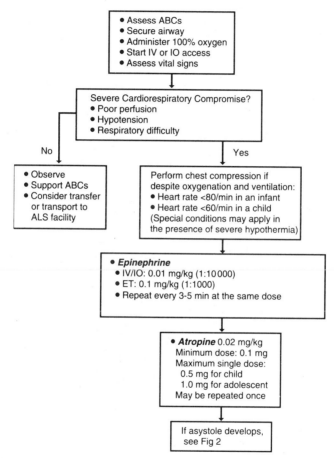

Figure 7P–1. Bradycardia decision tree. ABCs indicates airway, breathing, and circulation; ALS, advanced life support; ET, endotracheal; IO, intraosseous; and IV, intravenous. (Reproduced with permission from Guidelines for Cardiopulmonary Resuscitation and Emergency Care, 1992, copyright American Heart Association.)

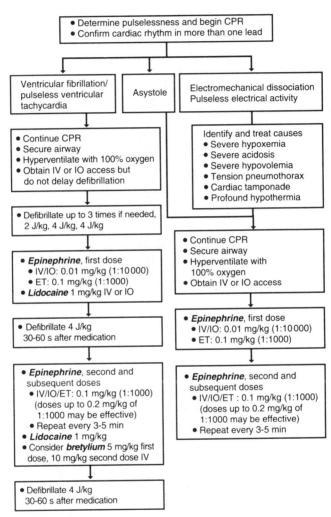

Figure 7P–2. Asystole and pulseless arrest decision tree. CPR indicates cardiopulmonary resuscitation; ET, endotracheal; IO, intraosseous; and IV, intravenous. (Reproduced with permission from Guidelines for Cardiopulmonary Resuscitation and Emergency Care, 1992, copyright American Heart Association.)

Chapter 8

Respiratory Emergencies

THERAPEUTIC CLASSIFICATIONS OF DRUGS USED FOR RESPIRATORY EMERGENCIES

BRONCHODILATORS
Albuterol
Aminophylline
Epinephrine (1:1000 solution)
Racemic epinephrine
Isoetharine
Metaproterenol
Terbutaline

CARDIAC STIMULATOR
Epinephrine

MEDICINAL GAS
Oxygen

PERIPHERAL VASOCONSTRICTOR
Epinephrine

Responding to a respiratory emergency is a common occurrence for prehospital emergency care professionals. A familiar scenario consists of a patient in a sitting position, leaning forward, and fighting to breathe, using accessory muscles. Wheezing is usually present, but may become fainter as the patient's condition becomes more severe. The problem—an acute asthma attack.

Fighting for breath can be a terrifying experience. The EMS professional must be able to act quickly and accurately when treating respiratory emergencies. In many respiratory emergencies, a calm EMS professional and 100%

159

humidified oxygen are all that is required to provide the patient with relief. However, if needed, several drugs are effective in relieving respiratory distress.

Except for oxygen, all of the drugs presented in this chapter are classified therapeutically as bronchodilators. A bronchodilator acts by relaxing the smooth muscles of the bronchial airways and pulmonary blood vessels, making it easier for the patient to breathe.

With the exception of aminophylline, all of the bronchodilators in this chapter are classified pharmacologically as adrenergic drugs. Adrenergic drugs primarily act on beta$_2$ receptors, relaxing bronchial smooth muscles. When beta$_2$ receptors are stimulated, however, beta$_1$ receptors are also stimulated, to a lesser extent. Beta$_1$ stimulation causes the heart to increase in both rate and contractile force.

Aminophylline is pharmacologically classified as a xanthine derivative. Xanthine is a compound that occurs naturally in muscle tissue. Aminophylline relaxes bronchial smooth muscles. Two common xanthines are caffeine and theophylline.

ALBUTEROL
Proventil, Ventolin

CLASSIFICATIONS
Pharmacologic: Adrenergic
Therapeutic: Bronchodilator

MECHANISM OF ACTION: Albuterol is a beta$_2$-adrenergic (pulmonary) agonist. It causes bronchodilation and stimulates the central nervous system (CNS) and the heart.

THERAPEUTIC BENEFIT: Albuterol relaxes bronchial smooth muscles, reducing airway resistance.

INDICATIONS FOR PREHOSPITAL USE: Albuterol is used to treat reversible airway obstruction caused by asthma or chronic obstructive pulmonary disease (COPD).

CONTRAINDICATIONS: Albuterol should not be given to patients who are hypersensitive to adrenergic amine drugs.

PRECAUTIONS: ■ Because of its cardiac effects, use caution in administering albuterol to patients with: ■ Heart disease. ■ Hypertension. ■ Diabetes.

ROUTE AND DOSAGE

Adult: 2 inhalations every 4–6 h (90 μg/spray).

Pediatric: Same as adult. Do not administer albuterol to children under 12.

ADVERSE REACTIONS AND SIDE EFFECTS

- *CNS:* Nervousness, tremor, headache.
- *Cardiovascular:* Hypertension, arrhythmias, chest pain.
- *Gastrointestinal:* Nausea, vomiting.

PARAMEDIC IMPLICATIONS: ▪ Because elderly patients are more prone to develop adverse reactions and side effects, local protocols may require lower dosages of albuterol. ▪ Monitor patient vital signs closely: high dosages increase the possibility of side effects.

DRUG INTERACTIONS: ▪ Additive adrenergic effects may occur if albuterol is used with other adrenergic drugs. ▪ Beta-blocking drugs may block the therapeutic effects of albuterol.

AMINOPHYLLINE
Aminophyllin, Somophyllin

CLASSIFICATIONS
Pharmacologic: Xanthine
derivative
Therapeutic: Bronchodilator

MECHANISM OF ACTION: Aminophylline relaxes bronchial smooth muscles. It also stimulates the heart and the respiratory center in the brain. In addition, aminophylline acts as a diuretic.

THERAPEUTIC BENEFIT: Therapeutic benefits of aminophylline include improved breathing as a result of bronchodilation and improved cardiac output as a result of increased heart rate.

INDICATIONS FOR PREHOSPITAL USE: Aminophylline is used to treat respiratory problems caused by asthma, COPD, pulmonary edema, and congestive heart failure (CHF).

CONTRAINDICATIONS: ▪ Do not administer aminophylline to patients with: ▪ Hypersensitivity to the drug. ▪ Uncontrolled cardiac arrhythmias.

PRECAUTIONS: ▪ Use caution in administering aminophylline to: ▪ Patients over 60. ▪ Patients with congestive heart failure. Consult medical control or local protocols for reduced dosages for these patients.

ROUTE AND DOSAGE

Adult: 250–500 mg (5–6 mg/kg) by IV infusion over 20–30 min.

Pediatric: 6 mg/kg by IV infusion over 20–30 min.
NOTE: Ideally, in patients who are currently receiving theophylline/aminophylline preparation, the loading dose should be deferred until the serum theophylline concentration is determined. However, when there is sufficient respiratory distress in these patients to warrant a small risk, half the usual loading dose (2.5–3 mg/kg) may be administered if no laboratory confirmation of serum theophylline levels is available.
To prepare infusion, add 250–500 mg of aminophylline to 50–100 mL of D_5W.

ADVERSE REACTIONS AND SIDE EFFECTS

- *CNS:* Nervousness, anxiety, headache, seizures.
- *Cardiovascular:* Arrhythmias, tachycardia, palpitations.
- *Gastrointestinal:* Nausea, vomiting.

PARAMEDIC IMPLICATIONS: ▪ Rapid administration of aminophylline (>25 mg/min) can cause ventricular fibrillation. Assess patient vital signs and ECG status continuously.

DRUG INTERACTIONS: ▪ Use with adrenergic drugs may cause additive CNS and cardiovascular side effects. ▪ Use with erythromycin and beta-blocking drugs may cause toxicity.

EPINEPHRINE (1:1000 SOLUTION)
Adrenalin

CLASSIFICATIONS
Pharmacologic: Beta-adrenergic agonist
Therapeutic: Bronchodilator, cardiac stimulator, peripheral vasoconstrictor

---

MECHANISM OF ACTION: Epinephrine is a catecholamine that stimulates both alpha-adrenergic and beta-adrenergic receptors in the sympathetic nervous system. Stimulation of cardiac beta$_1$-receptors increases the rate and force of contractions, resulting in an increase in cardiac output. Stimulation of beta$_2$ receptors relaxes the bronchial smooth muscles, thereby increasing vital lung capacity. Epinephrine's stimulation of alpha receptors causes the arterioles of the bronchioles to constrict, which can help reduce edema. Alpha-adrenergic stimulation also produces peripheral vasoconstriction, which aids in raising arterial blood pressure.

THERAPEUTIC BENEFIT: The therapeutic benefits of epinephrine include:
- Increased heart rate
- Increased contractility of the heart
- Increased automaticity of the heart
- Bronchodilation
- Increased arterial blood pressure
- Increased systemic vascular resistance

INDICATIONS FOR PREHOSPITAL USE: Epinephrine is used to treat bronchial asthma.

CONTRAINDICATIONS: ▪ Do not administer epinephrine to patients: ▪ In shock other than anaphylactic shock. ▪ With cardiac arrhythmias.

PRECAUTIONS: ▪ Use caution in administering epinephrine to patients with: ▪ Heart disease. ▪ Diabetes. ▪ Hypertension.

ROUTE AND DOSAGE

Adult: 0.3–0.5 mg (0.3–0.5 mL) SC of a 1:1000 solution.

Pediatric: 0.01 mg/kg (0.01 mL/kg) SC of a 1:1000 solution. Single doses should not exceed 0.5 mg.

ADVERSE REACTIONS AND SIDE EFFECTS

- *CNS:* Headache, nervousness, tremor.
- *Cardiovascular:* Arrhythmias, hypertension, chest pain.
- *Gastrointestinal:* Nausea, vomiting.

PARAMEDIC IMPLICATIONS: ■ Monitor patient closely; pay special attention to blood pressure, pulse, and ECG status. ■ Assess lungs before and after epinephrine administration. ■ An IV bolus injection of a 1:1000 solution of epinephrine may cause sudden hypertension or cerebral edema.

DRUG INTERACTIONS: ■ Beta-adrenergic blockers may block the therapeutic response to epinephrine. ■ The use of epinephrine with oxytocics or tricyclic antidepressants may cause severe hypertension. ■ Epinephrine in combination with other beta-adrenergic agonists can cause severe arrhythmias.

RACEMIC EPINEPHRINE
MicroNEFRIN

CLASSIFICATIONS:
Pharmacologic: Adrenergic
Therapeutic: Bronchodilator

MECHANISM OF ACTION: Racemic epinephrine stimulates both alpha-adrenergic and beta-adrenergic receptors. It is usually administered to pediatric patients for its beta$_2$ effects, which cause bronchial smooth muscle relaxation.

THERAPEUTIC BENEFIT: Racemic epinephrine causes bronchodilation, which relieves dyspnea.

INDICATIONS FOR PREHOSPITAL USE: Racemic epinephrine is used to treat **laryngotracheobronchitis** (croup), and patients with severe **dyspnea** during long transport times.

CONTRAINDICATIONS: ■ Do not administer racemic epinephrine to patients with: ■ **Epiglottitis.** ■ Severe tachycardia.

PRECAUTIONS: Excessive use of racemic epinephrine may cause bronchospasm, probably by rebound effect.

ROUTE AND DOSAGE

Adult: Not usually indicated for prehospital use.

Pediatric (<20 kg): 0.25 mL/kg by inhalation.

Pediatric (20–40 kg): 0.5 mL/kg by inhalation.

To administer, add 0.25–0.5 mL of a 2.25% epinephrine solution (1:1000 solution) to 2–3 mL of normal saline and administer via a nebulizer.

ADVERSE REACTIONS AND SIDE EFFECTS

- *CNS:* Headache, anxiety, fear, nervousness.
- *Cardiovascular:* Palpitations, tachycardia, arrhythmias.
- *Respiratory:* Respiratory weakness.
- *Gastrointestinal:* Nausea, vomiting.

PARAMEDIC IMPLICATIONS: Assess patient vital signs frequently, because adverse reactions and side effects can develop rapidly.

DRUG INTERACTIONS: ▪ Drugs classified as beta-adrenergic blockers may block the therapeutic response of racemic epinephrine. ▪ Additive effects may occur if racemic epinephrine is used with decongestants.

ISOETHARINE
Arm-a-Med, Beta-2, Bisorine, Bronkosol, Dey-Dose, Dey-Lute, Dispose-a-Med

CLASSIFICATIONS
Pharmacologic: Adrenergic
Therapeutic: Bronchodilator

MECHANISM OF ACTION: Isoetharine is a beta-adrenergic agonist, having a strong effect on beta$_2$-adrenergic (pulmonary) receptors.

THERAPEUTIC BENEFIT: Isoetharine relaxes bronchial smooth muscles, causing an increase in vital lung capacity and a decrease in airway resistance.

INDICATIONS FOR PREHOSPITAL USE: Isoetharine is used to relieve dyspnea caused by asthma or COPD.

CONTRAINDICATIONS: Do not administer isoetharine to patients who are hypersensitive to adrenergic amine drugs.

PRECAUTIONS: ▪ Use caution in administering isoetharine to patients with: ▪ Hypertension ▪ Hyperthyroidism. ▪ Acute coronary disease. ▪ Chest pain. ▪ Cardiac asthma.

Isoetharine can worsen any of these conditions.

ROUTE AND DOSAGE

Adult (Inhalation): One to two inhalations (340 μg/spray).

Adult (Oxygen Aerosol): 0.25–0.5 mL of a 1% solution diluted 1:3. For other concentrations:

- 2–4 mL of .125%
- 2.5 mL of 0.2%
- 2 mL of .25%

Adult (Nebulization): Four inhalations of a 0.5%–1% solution.

Pediatric: Not recommended for prehospital use.

ADVERSE REACTIONS AND SIDE EFFECTS

- *CNS:* Nervousness, tremor, headache, dizziness.
- *Cardiovascular:* Hypertension, arrhythmias, chest pain.
- *Gastrointestinal:* Nausea, vomiting.

PARAMEDIC IMPLICATIONS: ▪ Excessive use of inhalers can result in tolerance or paradoxic bronchospasm. ▪ Assess patient blood pressure, pulse rate, respirations, and lung sounds before and after administering isoetharine.

DRUG INTERACTIONS: ▪ Additive adrenergic effects may result if isoetharine is used with other adrenergic drugs. ▪ Beta-blocking drugs may block the therapeutic effects of isoetharine.

METAPROTERENOL
Alupent, Metaprel

CLASSIFICATIONS
Pharmacologic: Adrenergic
Therapeutic: Bronchodilator

MECHANISM OF ACTION: Metaproterenol is a beta-adrenergic agonist, having a strong effect on beta$_2$ (pulmonary) receptors. Its beta$_1$ effects produce CNS and cardiac stimulation.

THERAPEUTIC BENEFIT: Metaproterenol relaxes bronchial smooth muscles, resulting in an increase in lung capacity and a decrease in airway resistance.

INDICATIONS FOR PREHOSPITAL USE: Metaproterenol is used to treat dyspnea caused by asthma or COPD.

CONTRAINDICATIONS: ▪ Do not administer metaproterenol to patients with: ▪ Hypersensitivity to adrenergic amine drugs. ▪ Preexisting cardiac arrhythmias associated with tachycardia.

PRECAUTIONS: ▪ Use caution in administering metaproterenol to elderly patients. ▪ Use caution with patients with: ▪ Hypertension. ▪ Coronary artery disease. ▪ Congestive heart failure. ▪ Diabetes.

ROUTE AND DOSAGE

Adult (Inhalation): Two to three inhalations every 3–4 h by metered-dose inhaler (650 μg/spray).

Adult (Nebulization): Five to fifteen inhalations of an undiluted 5% solution three to four times per day. Also: 0.2–0.3 mL of a 5% solution diluted to 2.5 mL with normal saline.

Adult (Intermittent Positive Pressure Breathing [IPPB]): 0.2–0.3 mL of a 5% solution diluted in 2.5 mL of normal saline three to four times per day.

Pediatric: Same as adult. Not recommended for prehospital use in children under 12.

ADVERSE REACTIONS AND SIDE EFFECTS

- *CNS:* Nervousness, tremor, headache.
- *Cardiovascular:* Hypertension, arrhythmias, chest pain.
- *Gastrointestinal:* Nausea, vomiting.

PARAMEDIC IMPLICATIONS: ▪ Excessive use of inhalers can result in tolerance and paradoxical bronchospasm. ▪ Assess patient blood pressure, pulse rate, respirations, and lung sounds before and after administering metaproterenol.

DRUG INTERACTIONS: ▪ Additive adrenergic effects may result if metaproterenol is used with other adrenergic drugs. ▪ Beta-blocking drugs may block the therapeutic effects of metaproterenol.

OXYGEN

CLASSIFICATIONS
Pharmacologic: Medicinal gas
Therapeutic: Medicinal gas

MECHANISM OF ACTION: Oxygen is required to enable the cells to break down glucose into a usable energy form. Oxygen is a colorless, odorless, tasteless gas, essential to respiration. At sea level, oxygen makes up approximately 10%–16% of venous blood and 17%–21% of arterial blood. Oxygen is carried from the lungs to the body's tissues by hemoglobin in the red blood cells.

THERAPEUTIC BENEFIT: The administration of oxygen increases arterial oxygen tension (PaO_2) and hemoglobin saturation. This improves tissue oxygenation when circulation is adequately maintained.

INDICATIONS FOR PREHOSPITAL USE: Oxygen is used:

1. To treat severe chest pain that may be due to cardiac ischemia.
2. To treat hypoxemia from any cause.
3. In the treatment of cardiac arrest.

CONTRAINDICATIONS: None, for emergency use.

PRECAUTIONS: If the patient has a history of COPD, begin oxygen administration at low flow rates, increasing flow rates as necessary.

ROUTE AND DOSAGE

Adult: (Inhalation).   Several devices are used to administer oxygen, including masks, nasal cannulas, positive pressure devices, and volume-regulated ventilators. Some of the more commonly used oxygen devices and their delivery capacities include:

- *Nasal cannula:* O_2 concentrations of 24%–44% at flow rates of 1–6 L/min.
- *Face mask:* O_2 concentrations of 40%–60% at flow rates of 8–10 L/min.
- Face mask with oxygen reservoir: O_2 concentration of 60% at a flow rate of 6 L/min. An O_2 concentration of almost 100% can be achieved with a flow rate of 10 L/min.

- Venturi mask: O_2 concentrations:
  - 24% at 4 L/min
  - 28% at 4 L/min
  - 35% at 8 L/min
  - 40% at 8 L/min
- Mouth-to-mask: With supplemental O_2 at 10 L/min, O_2 concentrations can reach 50%. Without supplemental O_2, concentration reaches only approximately 17%.

Pediatric: Same as the adult.

ADVERSE REACTIONS AND SIDE EFFECTS

- *Respiratory:* In some cases of COPD oxygen administration may reduce respiratory drive. This is not a reason to withhold oxygen, but be prepared to assist ventilations.
- Miscellaneous: Oxygen that is not humidified may dry out or be irritating to mucous membranes.

PARAMEDIC IMPLICATIONS: ▪ Use humidified oxygen whenever possible. Nonhumidified oxygen may dry and irritate mucous membranes. ▪ Oxygen therapy may reduce respiratory drive in patients with COPD. If this should happen, it may be necessary to assist ventilations. If it is indicated, oxygen therapy should never be withheld. ▪ Reassure patients who are anxious about face masks but who require high concentrations of oxygen.

DRUG INTERACTIONS: A 50:50 nitrous oxide–oxygen mixture combination is an analgesic medicinal gas for use in the prehospital setting for pain relief.

TERBUTALINE
Brethaire, Brethine, Bricanyl

CLASSIFICATIONS
Pharmacologic: Adrenergic
Therapeutic: Bronchodilator

MECHANISM OF ACTION: Terbutaline is a beta-adrenergic agonist, having strong effects on beta$_2$ (pulmonary) receptors. High doses of terbutaline may cause CNS and cardiac stimulation.

THERAPEUTIC BENEFIT: Terbutaline relaxes bronchial smooth muscles, resulting in an increase in lung capacity and a decrease in airway resistance.

INDICATIONS FOR PREHOSPITAL USE: Terbutaline is used to treat dyspnea caused by asthma and COPD.

CONTRAINDICATIONS: Do not administer terbutaline to patients who are hypersensitive to adrenergic amine drugs.

PRECAUTIONS: ▪ Use caution in administering terbutaline to elderly patients. Use caution with patients with: ▪ Cardiac disease. ▪ Hyperthyroidism. ▪ Diabetes.

ROUTE AND DOSAGE

Adult (SC): 0.25 mg. Repeated in 15–30 min, if necessary. Terbutaline given parenterally may lose its beta$_2$ (pulmonary) selectiveness, but it will still be effective.

Adult (Inhalation): Two inhalations every 4–6 h (200 μg/spray).

Pediatric (Inhalation): Same as adult. Not recommended for prehospital use in children under 12.

ADVERSE REACTIONS AND SIDE EFFECTS

- *CNS:* Nervousness, tremor, headache.
- *Cardiovascular:* Hypertension, arrhythmias, chest pain.
- *Gastrointestinal:* Nausea, vomiting.

PARAMEDIC IMPLICATIONS: ▪ Assess patient blood pressure, pulse rate, respirations, and lung sounds before and after administering terbutaline. ▪ Cardiovascular effects may be increased if terbutaline is given parenterally.

DRUG INTERACTIONS: ▪ Additive adrenergic effects may result if terbutaline is used with other adrenergic drugs. ▪ Beta-blocking drugs may block the therapeutic effects of terbutaline.

CONCLUSION

Having to fight for each breath can be very frightening for a patient. Rapid assessment and proper recognition of presenting signs and symptoms by the EMS professional can be life-saving.

The most important drug used during a respiratory emergency is oxygen. However, conditions such as reversible airway obstruction caused by asthma or COPD may require appropriate drug therapy.

STUDY QUESTIONS

1. Bronchodilators are used to treat reversible airway obstruction. They work by:
   a. Decreasing edema.
   b. Reducing carbon dioxide content.
   c. Relaxing the bronchial smooth muscle.
   d. Increasing breathing by stimulation of the CNS.

2. To administer albuterol to a 13-year-old patient, the dosage needed is:
   a. One half the adult dose.
   b. One inhalation (90 μg). Repeated as necessary.
   c. Two inhalations every 4–6 h (90 μg/spray).
   d. Three inhalations every 4–6 h (90 μg/spray).

3. Aminophylline is contraindicated in patients:
   a. Who suffer from uncontrolled cardiac arrhythmias.
   b. With congestive heart failure.
   c. Over 60.
   d. With hypertension.

4. The adult dosage for epinephrine to treat bronchial asthma is:
   a. 0.3–0.5 mg by IV bolus of a 1:10,000 solution.
   b. 0.3–0.5 mg SC of a 1:1000 solution.
   c. 3–5 mg SC of a 1:1000 solution.
   d. 0.01 mg/kg SC of a 1:1000 solution.

5. The recommended initial dose for oxygen when treating a patient with COPD is:
   a. 15 L/min.
   b. 10 L/min.
   c. 4–6 L/min.
   d. 2–3 L/min.

6. Terbutaline is used to treat asthma and COPD by relaxing bronchial smooth muscles. The initial adult dose when given SC is:
   a. 0.25 mg.
   b. 25 mg.
   c. 0.5 mg.
   d. 50 mg.

7. The terbutaline dosage for an 8-year-old patient is:
   a. 0.25 mg.
   b. 0.5 mg.
   c. 1.0 mg.
   d. Not recommended.

CASE STUDIES

1. You respond to a 30-lb, 3-year-old patient in respiratory distress. She is hoarse, has a high-pitched harsh stridor, and a barking cough. You observe that the patient is using accessory muscles to breathe and her nostrils are flaring. After a careful assessment, you determine this patient has croup. The drug of choice for the treatment of croup is
   a. Epinephrine.
   b. Racemic epinephrine.
   c. Isoetharine.
   d. Metaproterenol.

2. You respond to a 28-year-old male patient having an acute asthma attack. The patient is sitting up, but leaning forward as he fights to breathe. He is coughing, and you can hear wheezing without your stethoscope. You also note that the patient is using his accessory muscles to help him breathe. You are giving humidified oxygen using an IPPB device. What other two drugs might medical control order to treat this patient?
   a. Epinephrine, 1:1000 solution and aminophylline.
   b. Epinephrine, 1:1000 solution and racemic epinephrine.
   c. Epinephrine, 1:10,000 solution and aminophylline.
   d. Epinephrine, 1:10,000 solution and terbutaline.

EXTENDED CASE STUDY: COPD versus CHF

Initial Response

You respond to the home of a 60-year-old man complaining of difficulty breathing. The patient is leaning forward in his chair, taking deep breaths. He tells you that he has been having this problem since late last night. As you take the patient's history, he tells you that he has no cardiac problems and is not taking any medications, but he does smoke about two packs of cigarettes per day. Initial assessment reveals the following:

- *Level of consciousness:* Alert, apprehensive.
- *Respirations:* 34/min, labored, pursed lips on exhalation.
- *Lung sounds:* Decreased breath sounds, expiratory wheezing with bilateral rales at the base of each lung, hyperresonant to percussion.
- *Pulse:* 124 beats/min, irregular.
- *Blood pressure:* 164/92.
- *Skin:* Pale, warm, moist.

Figure 8–1 illustrates the patient's ECG.

Management

You identify the rhythm in Figure 8–1 as sinus tachycardia with PACs. Place the patient on humidified oxygen at 4 L/min. This should be sufficient, since the patient is not clinically hypoxic. You should also start an IV lifeline, infusing D_5W at a keep-open rate.

Although it is difficult to determine in the prehospital setting, this patient is most likely suffering from either pulmonary edema or COPD. Frequent assessment of lung sounds reveals that the patient's wheezing is becoming more severe; his respiratory rate increases to 42/min. Wheezing is generally a distinguishing trait of bronchospasm, found in both COPD patients and patients suffering from CHF.

The prehospital drug of choice in this case should be aminophylline. Aminophylline is a bronchodilator used for treating bronchospasm in the management of both pulmonary edema associated with CHF and COPD. Administer 250–500 mg of aminophylline by IV infusion over 20–30 min.

While the aminophylline is being given, you notice the patient's level of consciousness begins to deteriorate; he is beginning to act confused. You also notice a change in the ECG monitor (Fig. 8–2).

You identify the new rhythm as sinus bradycardia. Reassessment of the patient reveals the following:

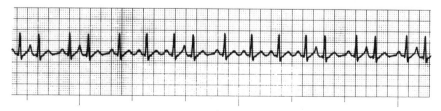

Figure 8–1. Sinus tachycardia with premature atrial contractions (PACs). Rate: 124 beats per minute.

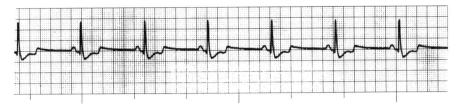

Figure 8–2. Sinus bradycardia. Rate: 120 beats per minute.

- *Level of consciousness:* Confused, anxious.
- *Respirations:* 10/min, labored.
- *Lung sounds:* Wheezing and rales.
- *Pulse:* 50 beats/min.
- *Blood pressure:* 110/60.
- *Skin:* Cool, diaphoretic.

This patient requires immediate assistance with his respirations and pharmacologic management to increase his heart rate and cardiac output. The drug of choice in this situation is atropine, 0.5–1 mg by IV bolus. Atropine is a parasympathetic blocker. It blocks the action of acetylcholine, and results in an increased heart rate.

If the first dose of atropine is ineffective, repeat doses can be given up to a total dose of 2 mg. If further treatment is necessary, use external pacing. If pacing is unavailable, administer 2–10 µg/min of isoproterenol by IV infusion (see page 148 for the AHA treatment algorithm for bradycardia). Isoproterenol is used for the immediate but temporary control of hemodynamically significant bradycardia that does not respond to atropine.

If you suspect COPD, use low flow rates of oxygen. High-flow oxygen administration can cause increasing acidosis in patients who rely on a hypoxic drive to breathe. As seen with this patient, an oxygen flow rate as low as 4 L/min can cause a patient to deteriorate rapidly.

Chapter 9

Metabolic Emergencies

THERAPEUTIC CLASSIFICATIONS
OF DRUGS USED FOR
METABOLIC EMERGENCIES

Dextrose 50% in Water ($D_{50}W$)   Insulin
Glucagon   Thiamine (Vitamin B_1)

CASE STUDIES

THERAPEUTIC CLASSIFICATIONS OF DRUGS USED FOR METABOLIC EMERGENCIES

ANTIDIABETIC   **HYPERGLYCEMIC**
Insulin   Dextrose 50% in water

ANTIHYPOGLYCEMIC   **VITAMIN**
Glucagon   Thiamine

Insulin shock (*hypo*glycemia) and diabetic coma or diabetic **ketoacidosis** (*hyper*glycemia) are two emergencies connected with metabolic disease that are commonly encountered by EMS professionals in the prehospital setting. The metabolic disease is diabetes mellitus, a disorder of carbohydrate metabolism that results from inadequate production or use of insulin.

When the condition is a result of the lack of insulin, it is called *insulin-dependent,* or *type I,* diabetes mellitus. When the condition is a result of the body's inability to use insulin that is present at normal levels, it is called *non-insulin-dependent,* or *type II,* diabetes mellitus. The symptoms are usually more serious in individuals with type I diabetes. In most cases, type II diabetes occurs in individuals over 40. Obesity is often times a factor.

Insulin is a hormone secreted by beta cells in the islets of Langerhans, which are clusters of specialized cells in the pancreas. In normal individuals, insulin enables the body's cells to take in and oxidize (metabolize) glucose. When there is no insulin in the bloodstream or when the individual cannot properly use insulin that is present, the level of glucose in the blood rises above normal (hyperglycemia). The level of sugar in the urine also rises above normal *(glycosuria).*

Hypoglycemia can occur in an insulin-dependent diabetic as a result of taking too much insulin or not eating enough food, or a combination of both. The brain requires glucose for metabolism. If hypoglycemia develops, the glucose shortage reduces brain metabolism and causes neurologic and psychiatric

172

symptoms. If hypoglycemia is not corrected, permanent brain damage may occur.

Hypoglycemia can develop very rapidly. Signs and symptoms of hypoglycemia include a weak, rapid pulse; cold, clammy skin; weakness; headache; and irritable or bizarre behavior. Hypoglycemic patients may appear intoxicated. In severe cases, patients may develop seizures and coma.

Hyperglycemia occurs when the circulating blood sugar becomes too high. This happens because the person with diabetes has taken an inadequate amount of insulin or has not taken insulin at all. As the blood sugar level increases, the patient excretes more urine. This, together with vomiting, causes dehydration and, in severe cases, shock. Without insulin, the body cannot use glucose. Therefore, the body changes over to metabolizing fat for energy. Fat metabolism generates acids and **ketones** as waste. Unlike hypoglycemia, hyperglycemia progresses slowly, usually taking 12–48 h. Signs and symptoms of hyperglycemia include excessive urination, excessive thirst, nausea and vomiting, tachycardia, **Kussmaul respirations,** fruity odor on the breath, and hypotension. Table 9-1 compares hyperglycemia and hypoglycemia.

This chapter presents three drugs that are used to treat diabetes mellitus: insulin, glucagon, and a solution of 50% dextrose in water, called $D_{50}W$. Insulin is administered when the body cannot produce its own supplies. Glucagon and $D_{50}W$ are administered to increase the level of sugar in the bloodstream.

Another drug included in this chapter is the vitamin thiamine. Thiamine is necessary for the metabolism of carbohydrates and fats. Physicians or EMT-Ps administer thiamine to restore the body's supply when necessary.

DEXTROSE 50% IN WATER ($D_{50}W$)

CLASSIFICATIONS
Pharmacologic: Carbohydrate
Therapeutic: Hyperglycemic

MECHANISM OF ACTION: Dextrose 50% in water increases circulating blood sugar levels to normal. It also acts briefly as an **osmotic diuretic.**

THERAPEUTIC BENEFIT: Dextrose 50% in water restores circulating blood sugar levels to normal in hypoglycemic states.

INDICATIONS FOR PREHOSPITAL USE: Dextrose 50% in water is used to treat patients in coma due to hypoglycemia and patients in coma of an unknown cause. Patients with an altered level of consciousness whose reagent strip reading indicates less than 45 mg should also be given $D_{50}W$. Some EMS protocols also recommend giving $D_{50}W$ in certain cardiac arrest situations.

CONTRAINDICATIONS: Do not administer $D_{50}W$ to patients with intracranial hemorrhage.

PRECAUTIONS: ■ Use caution in administering $D_{50}W$ to patients: ■ With diabetes mellitus. ■ Who cannot tolerate carbohydrate agents.

Table 9–1. HYPOGLYCEMIA AND HYPERGLYCEMIA (KETOACIDOSIS)

	Hypoglycemia	Hyperglycemia
Definition	Abnormally low level of sugar in the blood	An abnormally high level of sugar in the blood
	Develops rapidly, usually within 30–60 min	Develops slowly, usually over 12–48 h
Precipitating factors	1. Insulin overdose	1. Low or nonexistent insulin level
	2. Fasting	2. Infection (respiratory, urinary, or gastroenteritis)
	3. Increased alcohol intake without increased carbohydrate intake	
	4. Excessive physical activity without sufficient intake of food	
Signs and Symptoms		
History	Recent insulin injection, inadequate food intake, excessive physical activity after insulin	Often acute infection in the diabetic, inadequate intake of insulin, perhaps no history of diabetes
Skin	Pale, sweating	Flushed, dry
Breath	Normal odor (acetone odor rare)	Acetone odor
Thirst	Absent	Intense
Respirations	Shallow	Deep, rapid (Kussmaul)
Pulse	Full, bounding	Rapid, weak
Blood pressure	Normal	Low
Abdominal pain	Absent	Often acute

ROUTE AND DOSAGE

Adult: 25 g by slow IV bolus. Repeat if needed.

Pediatric: Dilute 1:1 with sterile water to make a 25% solution ($D_{25}W$) (0.25 mg/mL). 0.5–1.0 g/kg by slow IV bolus.

ADVERSE REACTIONS AND SIDE EFFECTS

- *Central nervous system (CNS):* May cause neurologic symptoms in the alcoholic patient.
- *Cardiovascular:* May aggravate hypertension and congestive heart failure in susceptible patients.
- *Skin:* May cause tissue necrosis at the injection site.

PARAMEDIC IMPLICATIONS: ■ Before establishing an IV line, take a blood sample for glucose analysis. ■ Establish the IV line in the largest vein possible and run it wide open during slow administration of the $D_{50}W$. ■ Thiamine should be administered before the $D_{50}W$ in the comatose patient. Thiamine is necessary for carbohydrate metabolism. Administering dextrose to an alcohol-dependent patient who is deficient in thiamine can cause Wernicke's encephalopathy or Korsakoff's syndrome (see Thiamine, page 169). Remember, it is vital to administer thiamine before dextrose to an alcohol-dependent patient or a patient in coma of unknown cause that may be alcohol related.

DRUG INTERACTIONS: None, concerning prehospital use.

GLUCAGON

CLASSIFICATIONS
Pharmacologic: Antihypoglycemic
Therapeutic: Antihypoglycemic

MECHANISM OF ACTION: Glucagon is a hormone excreted by the alpha cells of the pancreas. When released, glucagon increases the level of circulating blood sugar by stimulating the release of **glycogen** from the liver. The glycogen is quickly broken down to become glucose.

THERAPEUTIC BENEFIT: Glucagon causes an increase in the plasma glucose levels of the circulating blood, causes smooth muscle relaxation, and has positive **inotropic** and **chronotropic** effects on the heart.

INDICATIONS FOR PREHOSPITAL USE: Glucagon is given to treat hypoglycemia in the unconscious patient, in the combative patient, or in a patient in which an IV cannot be started.

CONTRAINDICATIONS: Do not administer glucagon to a patient who is hypersensitive to the drug.

PRECAUTIONS: Use caution in administering glucagon to patients with pheochromocytoma. A pheochromocytoma is a catecholamine-secreting tumor that may cause hypertension. Glucagon stimulates the release of catecholamines, which could further increase blood pressure.

ROUTE AND DOSAGE

Adult: 0.5–1 U IM, SC, or IV. If the patient does not respond in about 20 min, administer up to 2 more doses. Glucagon comes in vials that contain 1 U of powder and 1 mL of diluting solution. Glucagon must be reconstituted before use.

Pediatric: Not usually administered in the prehospital setting.

ADVERSE REACTIONS AND SIDE EFFECTS

- *CNS:* Dizziness.
- *Cardiovascular:* Possible hypotension.
- *Gastrointestinal:* Nausea, vomiting.

PARAMEDIC IMPLICATIONS: ■ In emergency situations, $D_{50}W$ is the drug of choice. Use glucagon only if you cannot start an IV and administer glucose. ■ Before administering glucagon, draw a blood sample for glucose determination.

DRUG INTERACTIONS: A precipitate will form if glucagon is mixed with chloride solutions.

INSULIN (ANIMAL-DERIVED OR BIOSYNTHETIC)
Humulin, Novolin, Iletin

CLASSIFICATIONS
Pharmacologic: Pancreatic hormone
Therapeutic: Antidiabetic

MECHANISM OF ACTION: Insulin lowers blood glucose levels and promotes the conversion of glucose to glycogen. Glycogen is the form in which carbohydrates are stored until they are converted into sugar.

THERAPEUTIC BENEFITS: Insulin helps to control blood sugar levels in patients with diabetes.

INDICATIONS FOR PREHOSPITAL USE: Insulin is used to treat patients with diabetic ketoacidosis (severe hyperglycemia).

CONTRAINDICATIONS: Certain individuals are hypersensitive to beef or pork. Do not administer insulin products derived from these sources to these patients. Another animal-derived insulin to which the patient is not hypersensitive or a biosynthetic insulin should be used in these cases.

PRECAUTIONS: Use caution in administering insulin, because the effects of a dosage can vary greatly depending on such factors as diet, exercise, stress, and work patterns.

ROUTE AND DOSAGE

Adult (IV): 2–10 U (0.1 U/kg) loading dose, followed by 2–10 U (0.1 U/kg/h) by continuous IV infusion.

To prepare the infusion, add 100 U of regular insulin to 1000 mL of normal saline; this yields a concentration of 0.1 U/mL.

Adult (IV, SC): 25–150 U by IV bolus initially. Administer additional doses every h based on blood glucose levels.

or

50–100 U by IV bolus plus 50–100 U SC initially. Administer additional SC doses every 2–6 h as needed.

Pediatric (IV): 0.1 U/kg by IV bolus followed by a continuous IV infusion of 0.1 U/kg/h.

Pediatric (IV, SC): 0.5–1 U divided into 2; administer ½ dose by IV bolus and ½ dose SC.

ADVERSE REACTIONS AND SIDE EFFECTS

- *Local reactions:* Itching, swelling, redness.
- *Endocrine:* Hypoglycemia.
- *Miscellaneous:* Allergic reactions, usually to traces of beef or pork protein in the preparation.

PARAMEDIC IMPLICATIONS: ▪ Only regular insulin can be administered IV. ▪ When administering insulin by IV bolus, administer each 50 U over 1 min. ▪ Assess patient constantly for signs of hypoglycemia. Keep glucose available.

DRUG INTERACTIONS: ▪ Some of the signs and symptoms of hypoglycemia (such as tachycardia) may be masked by beta-adrenergic blocking drugs. ▪ Corticosteroids and thiazide diuretics can cause increases in the insulin required.

Table 9–2 compares some of the common insulin preparations.

THIAMINE (VITAMIN B₁)
Betalin S

CLASSIFICATIONS
*Pharmacologic: Water-soluble
   vitamin*
Therapeutic: B-complex vitamin

MECHANISM OF ACTION: Thiamine is required for the metabolism of carbohydrates and fats. It is necessary for the freeing of energy and the oxidation of pyruvic acid. Without enough thiamine, the cells of the body cannot use most of the energy usually available in glucose. The organ most sensitive to thiamine deficiency is the brain.

THERAPEUTIC BENEFIT: Administering thiamine when deficiency exists restores the body's supply of the vitamin.

INDICATIONS FOR PREHOSPITAL USE: Thiamine is used to treat patients in a coma of unknown origin, patients in coma due to alcohol, and patients suffering from delerium tremens.

Table 9–2. COMPARISON OF COMMON INSULIN
PREPARATIONS

Insulin	Onset	Peak	Duration
Rapid Acting			
Regular			
Regular Iletin	½–1 h	2–4 h	6–8 h
Humulin R*	½–1 h	2–4 h	6–8 h
Novolin R	½ h	2½–5 h	8 h
Prompt Zinc Suspension			
Semilente	1½ h	5–10 h	16 h
Semilente Ilentin I	1–3 h	3–8 h	10–16 h
Intermediate Acting			
Isophane Suspension			
NPH Ilentin	1–4 h	6–12 h	18–26 h
Humulin N*	1–2 h	6–12 h	18–24 h
Insulatard NPH	1½ h	4–12 h	24 h
Novolin N	1½ h	4–12 h	24 h
Zinc Suspension			
Lente Ilentin	2–4 h	6–12 h	18–26 h
Humulin L*	1–3 h	6–12 h	18–21 h
Novolin L	2½ h	7–15 h	22 h
Long Acting			
Protamine Zinc Suspension			
Protamine Zinc Iletin	4–8 h	14–24 h	28–36 h
Extended Zinc Suspension			
Ultralente	4 h	10–30 h	36 h

* Humulin insulins have a slightly more rapid onset and a shorter duration of action than animal-derived insulins.

CONTRAINDICATIONS: None.

PRECAUTIONS: Thiamine deficiency can cause Wernicke's encephalopathy and Korsakoff's syndrome in the alcohol-dependent patient.

- *Wernicke's encephalopathy:* Wernicke's encephalopathy is an acute and reversible disorder associated with chronic alcoholism. It is characterized by poor voluntary muscle coordination, eye muscle weakness, and mental derangement.
- *Korsakoff's syndrome:* Korsakoff's syndrome is a frequent result of chronic alcoholism. It is characterized by disorientation, illusions, hallucinations, and painful extremities; in addition, the patient may have bilateral foot drop.

ROUTE AND DOSAGE

Adult: Before Administering D$_{50}$W:

1. Dilute 100 mg of thiamine in 50–100 mL of normal saline or D$_5$W and infuse over 15–20 min.

2. Administer 50 mg by slow IV bolus and 50 mg IM.

NOTE: Too-rapid administration of thiamine may cause hypotension.

Pediatric: Not recommended for prehospital use.

ADVERSE REACTIONS AND SIDE EFFECTS

- *Cardiovascular:* Rapid administration of thiamine may cause vasodilation and hypotension.
- *Respiratory:* Excessive administration of thiamine may cause dyspnea or respiratory failure.

PARAMEDIC IMPLICATIONS: Thiamine is necessary for carbohydrate metabolism. The administration of dextrose to an alcohol-dependent patient who is deficient in thiamine may cause Wernicke's encephalopathy or Korsakoff's syndrome. Therefore, it is important to administer thiamine before administering dextrose to an alcohol-dependent patient.

DRUG INTERACTIONS: N/A.

Patients suffering from metabolic disorders can exhibit many different signs and symptoms. Treatment for the diabetic patient depends on accurately assessing the patient. Correct, timely treatment is vital. For example, the brain relies on glucose for its metabolism. If a patient becomes severely hypoglycemic, the brain cannot function properly. If the hypoglycemia is left untreated for an extended period, permanent brain damage could result.

A patient found in a coma needs a rapid, accurate assessment. Drug treatment for these patients are diagnostic in nature as well as being potentially life-saving. Treatment can include thiamine, glucose, and naloxone (see Chapter 12).

STUDY QUESTIONS

1. Dextrose 50% in water is indicated for
   a. Reagent strip reading <45 mg with an altered LOC.
   b. Coma of unknown cause.
   c. Medical cardiac arrest.
   d. All of the above.

2. The pediatric dosage for $D_{50}W$ is
   a. 25 g by slow IV bolus.
   b. 0.05–0.1 g/kg by slow IV bolus.
   c. 0.5–1.0 g/kg by slow IV bolus.
   d. 5–10 g/kg by slow IV bolus.

3. Before giving glucose to your patient, you should first
   a. Take a blood sample.
   b. Monitor cardiac rhythm.
   c. Start an IV of D_5W.
   d. Dilute 1:1 with sterile distilled water.

4. Insulin is indicated for the treatment of
   a. Hypoglycemia.
   b. Hyperglycemia.

   c. Coma of unknown cause.
   d. Metabolic acidosis.

5. Glucagon causes an increase in the plasma glucose levels of the circulating blood. The adult dose of glucagon in the prehospital setting is
   a. 0.25–0.5 U.
   b. 0.5–1 U.
   c. 1–1.5 U.
   d. 1.5–2.5 U.

6. The organ most sensitive to the effects of thiamine deficiency is the
   a. Heart.
   b. Liver.
   c. Brain.
   d. Kidney.

7. Thiamine is used as a diagnostic tool in the patient in a coma of unknown cause. The adult dosage of thiamine is
   a. 50 mg.
   b. 75 mg.
   c. 100 mg.
   d. 1 mg/kg.

8. The pancreas is responsible for the production of insulin. Without insulin,
   a. Hypoglycemia will result.
   b. A buildup of carbon dioxide produces acidosis.
   c. Starches cannot be metabolized into glucose.
   d. Glucose cannot pass into the body's cells.

CASE STUDIES

1. You respond to an unconscious, unresponsive man who was found lying in his car. There is nothing to indicate that trauma has occurred. The patient has a patent airway, vital signs are within normal limits, and there are no apparent physical injuries. You notice several empty beer cans on the floor of the car. What is the first drug that medical control might order after you complete your assessment?
   a. $D_{50}W$.
   b. Insulin.
   c. Thiamine.
   d. Glucagon.

2. You respond to the home of an unconscious, unresponsive female patient. Your assessment finds the patient presenting with Kussmaul respirations at 40/min. The ECG monitor shows sinus tachycardia at a rate of 120 beats/min (Figure 9–1). Skin is warm and dry and the patient has a fruity odor on her breath. Her blood pressure is low. This patient is presenting with classic signs and symptoms of
   a. Insulin overdose.
   b. Ketoacidosis.
   c. Metabolic acidosis.
   d. Respiratory acidosis.

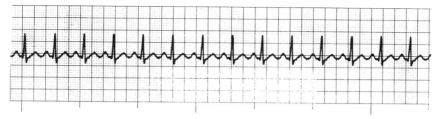

Figure 9–1. Sinus tachycardia. Rate: 120 beats/min.

3. After your initial assessment, treatment for the patient in question 2 should include
   a. IV for volume replacement and insulin.
   b. IV and D₅₀W.
   c. IV, thiamine, and D₅₀W.
   d. IV, D₅₀W, and insulin.

EXTENDED CASE STUDY: Diabetic Emergency—Diabetic Ketoacidosis

Initial Response

You respond to the residence of an unconscious woman. On arrival you find a female patient, about 30, lying on the bedroom floor. A rapid assessment reveals that the patient's breathing is deep and rapid; she has a weak, rapid pulse and responds only to painful stimuli. While placing the patient on oxygen and connecting the ECG monitor, you notice a Medic-Alert bracelet that indicates she has diabetes. There is no evidence of alcohol or drug use. Additional assessment reveals the following:

- *Level of consciousness:* Unconscious, responds only to pain.
- *Respirations:* Kussmaul, at a rate of 40/min.
- *Pulse:* 120 beats/min and weak. ECG shows sinus tachycardia (Figure 9–2).
- *Blood pressure:* 112/82.
- *Skin:* Warm and dry—dehydrated.

Management

Differentiating between diabetic ketoacidosis and hypoglycemia can be difficult in the prehospital setting. Therefore, management of the unconscious diabetic patient is

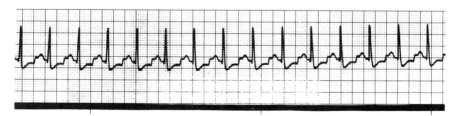

Figure 9–2. Sinus tachycardia. Rate: 120 beats/min.

generally directed toward treating hypoglycemia, which is the more severe condition. Prehospital management of this patient should proceed as follows:

- Maintain a patent airway; be prepared to intubate and to assist ventilation if necessary.
- Attempt to draw a blood sample for glucose analysis at the hospital.
- Measure glucose level using a glucose reagent strip. However, this may not be accurate. A reading of <45 mg indicates a need for further treatment.
- Begin an IV of D_5W at a keep-open rate.
- Administer 25 g of $D_{50}W$ by slow IV bolus. $D_{50}W$ is a hyperglycemic drug that increases circulating blood sugar levels in the hypoglycemic patient.
- If you cannot establish an IV line, administer 0.5–1 mg of glucagon IM. Glucagon elevates blood sugar levels by stimulating the release of glycogen from the liver. Glucagon does not produce results as quickly as $D_{50}W$. $D_{50}W$ shows immediate results, while glucagon may take as long as 20 min.
- Monitor vital signs and cardiac rhythm closely.
- Transport to the nearest appropriate hospital.

Depending on the circumstances at the scene, management can usually take place while the patient is being transported. In this case, the patient's condition does not change during transport. The patient is trying to compensate for metabolic acidosis by creating respiratory alkalosis through the Kussmaul respirations. Diabetic ketoacidosis starves red blood cells of glucose as well as producing a low pH. After arrival at the hospital, treatment will include decreasing serum glucose levels with insulin.

How would you manage this patient if she were in a coma of unknown cause with no available previous history? After the airway has been appropriately managed, blood drawn, and an IV started, the following treatment should take place:

- If the patient is suspected of being alcohol dependent, administer 100 mg of thiamine by slow IV bolus.
- Administer 25 g of $D_{50}W$ by slow IV bolus.
- If the above treatment is not successful, consider giving naloxone. Naloxone is a narcotic antagonist sometimes used in comas of unknown cause if narcotic drugs are suspected or to rule out narcotic drugs. Chapter 12 has a detailed discussion of naloxone.
- Transport to the nearest appropriate hospital. Depending on the circumstances at the scene, management can usually take place while the patient is being transported.

Chapter 10

Neurologic Emergencies

THERAPEUTIC CLASSIFICATIONS
OF DRUGS USED FOR
NEUROLOGIC EMERGENCIES

Dexamethasone   Methylprednisolone
Diazepam   Phenobarbital
Mannitol   Phenytoin

CASE STUDIES

THERAPEUTIC CLASSIFICATIONS OF DRUGS USED FOR NEUROLOGIC EMERGENCIES

ANTIANXIETY AGENT
Diazepam

DIURETIC
Mannitol

ANTICONVULSANTS
Diazepam
Phenobarbital
Phenytoin

SEDATIVE-HYPNOTIC
Phenobarbital

SKELETAL MUSCLE RELAXANT
Diazepam

ANTI-INFLAMMATORIES
Dexamethasone
Methylprednisolone

Neurologic emergencies are often very difficult to manage. Frequently, patients experiencing a neurologic emergency show signs and symptoms that are very subtle, ranging from a headache to coma. This makes for difficulty in diagnosis, which can greatly complicate prehospital treatment.

Most pharmacologic agents for neurologic emergencies are for nontraumatic problems, such as major motor seizures or **status epilepticus.** Emergencies such as these can be managed with anticonvulsant drugs such as diazepam or phenobarbital. Anticonvulsants depress abnormal neuron discharges in the central nervous system (CNS) that may result in seizure activity.

Neurologic emergencies commonly seen in the prehospital setting are cerebrovascular accidents (CVA/strokes). A CVA generally occurs due to a clot or hemorrhage in the brain, causing weakness, paralysis, speech impairment, confusion, and coma. Some signs and symptoms of CVA can mimic those of hypoglycemia and drug or alcohol abuse, which can make diagnosis difficult. Table 10–1 compares the signs and symptoms of CVA, hypoglycemia, and alcohol/drug abuse.

183

Table 10-1. SIGNS AND SYMPTOMS OF CEREBROVASCULAR
ACCIDENT (CVA), HYPOGLYCEMIA, AND ALCOHOL/DRUG ABUSE*

CVA	Hypoglycemia	Alcohol/Drug Intoxication
Headache	Headache	Headache
Confusion	Abnormal behavior—may	Confusion
Paralysis (usually one side of	appear intoxicated	Profuse perspiration
the body)	Confusion	Abnormal behavior
Facial flacidity, drooling	Convulsions	Elevated or normal blood
Impaired speech	Arrhythmias	pressure
Impaired vision	Profuse perspiration	Arrhythmias
Elevated or normal blood	Drooling	Convulsions
pressure	Normal blood pressure	Coma
Arrhythmias	Coma	
Convulsions		
Coma		

* Some of the signs and symptoms of hypoglycemia often mimic those of CVA or alcohol or drug intoxication.

Treatment for neurologic trauma is mainly supportive, with rapid transport. For example, the primary concerns for patients with traumatic head injury are head and neck stabilization, airway maintenance, and treatment of other injuries as needed. By the time trauma patients are stabilized, they are generally at or very close to the receiving emergency facility. However, there are drugs appropriate for prehospital treatment for neurologic trauma, especially when transport times are long. For example, dexamethasone is an anti-inflammatory drug that has been used to aid in reducing brain edema. Mannitol is a diuretic that can be used to reduce intracranial pressure.

Methylprednisolone is a newly developed drug that may have use in improving muscle function and sensation caused by traumatic injury to the spinal cord. Methylprednisolone, currently under investigation, is an anti-inflammatory steroid that can be used to protect nerve fibers and to inhibit swelling, ischemia, nerve cell death, and electrolyte imbalance to the spinal cord caused by traumatic injury. If proven successful, methylprednisolone could be of great patient benefit in traumatic spinal cord injuries where the patient has lost sensation and/or muscle function.

Remember, however, that no matter what type of neurologic emergency a prehospital healthcare professional encounters, rapid assessment and appropriate treatment are essential.

DEXAMETHASONE
Decadron, Hexadrol

CLASSIFICATIONS
Pharmacologic: Glucocorticoid
Therapeutic: Anti-inflammatory

MECHANISM OF ACTION: Dexamethasone is a long-acting **steroid** that suppresses inflammation and normal immune response.

THERAPEUTIC BENEFIT: Dexamethasone suppresses allergic tissue response and improves circulatory status in shock.

INDICATIONS FOR PREHOSPITAL USE: Dexamethasone is used to treat shock, acute cerebral edema, and severe allergic reactions.

CONTRAINDICATIONS: There are no contraindications for a single prehospital dose of dexamethasone.

PRECAUTIONS: ▪ Use caution in administering dexamethasone to patients with: ▪ Hypertension. ▪ Diabetes mellitus. ▪ Seizures. ▪ Congestive heart failure. ▪ Glaucoma. ▪ Dexamethasone may cause CNS excitement.

ROUTE AND DOSAGE

Adult (shock):   100 mg (1–6 mg/kg) by slow IV bolus.

Adult (cerebral edema):   10 mg by slow IV bolus.

Adult (severe allergic reactions):   4 mg by slow IV bolus.

Pediatric: Not recommended for prehospital use.

ADVERSE REACTIONS AND SIDE EFFECTS

- *CNS:* Headache, depression, restlessness.
- *Cardiovascular:* Hypertension.
- *Eyes:* Increased intracranial pressure.
- *Fluids and electrolytes:* Fluid retention, hypokalemia.
- *Gastrointestinal:* Nausea, vomiting.

PARAMEDIC IMPLICATIONS: ▪ Dexamethasone is sensitive to temperature extremes, so these conditions should be avoided. ▪ Dexamethasone is incompatible with other drugs.

DRUG INTERACTIONS: ▪ Simultaneous use of dexamethasone and diuretics may cause additive hypokalemia, which increases the risk of digitalis glycoside toxicity. ▪ Barbiturates and phenytoin may decrease the effectiveness of dexamethasone.

DIAZEPAM
Valium, Valrelease

CONTROLLED SUBSTANCE—
SCHEDULE IV
CLASSIFICATIONS
Pharmacologic: Benzodiazepine
Therapeutic: Antianxiety agent,
anticonvulsant, skeletal muscle
relaxant

MECHANISM OF ACTION: Diazepam causes CNS depression. It blocks spinal cord interneuronal transmission, causing relaxation of skeletal muscles.

Diazepam freely crosses the blood-brain barrier, but its actual mechanism of action is unknown.

THERAPEUTIC BENEFIT: In prehospital emergency care, diazepam is mainly used to control convulsions and to decrease anxiety. It is also used in orthopedic emergencies as a skeletal muscle relaxant.

INDICATIONS FOR PREHOSPITAL USE: Diazepam is used to treat status epilepticus and major motor seizures. It can also be used as a skeletal muscle relaxant in treating orthopedic injuries.

CONTRAINDICATIONS: ■ Do not administer diazepam to patients with: ■ Hypersensitivity to the drug. ■ Preexisting CNS depression. ■ Acute **narrow-angle glaucoma.**

PRECAUTIONS: ■ Use caution in administering diazepam to patients with a history of psychosis or drug addiction. ■ Administer lower than adult doses of diazepam to elderly patient, because they are usually more sensitive to the drug's CNS effects.

ROUTE AND DOSAGE

Adult (seizures/muscle relaxant): 2–5 mg by slow IV bolus. Repeat if needed, but do not exceed a total dose of 10 mg.

Adult (status epilepticus): 5–10 mg by slow IV bolus. Repeat every 10–15 min if needed, to a maximal dose of 30 mg.

Pediatric (seizures/skeletal muscle relaxant): 0.2–0.5 mg/kg by slow IV bolus over 3 min. Maximal doses:

- <*5 y:* 5 mg.
- >*5 y:* 10 mg.

Pediatric (status epilepticus)

- <*5 y:* 0.2–0.5 mg by slow IV bolus or IM every 2–5 min to a total dose of 5 mg.
- >*5 y:* 1 mg every 2–5 min by slow IV bolus or IM to a total dose of 10 mg.

ADVERSE REACTIONS AND SIDE EFFECTS:

- *CNS:* Dizziness, drowsiness, mental depression, headache.
- *Cardiovascular:* Hypotension.
- *Respiratory:* Respiratory depression.
- *Eyes:* Blurred vision, increased intraocular pressure in patients with narrow-angle glaucoma.

PARAMEDIC IMPLICATIONS: ■ Diazepam may cause respiratory arrest if administered too rapidly or in excess. ■ Do not mix diazepam with any other drug—diazepam may even react with the IV tubing. To minimize such reactions, administer diazepam at the IV site, not higher in the tubing. Thoroughly flush the IV line before administering diazepam if other drugs have already been administered. ■ Assess the patient's vital signs continuously.

DRUG INTERACTIONS: Additive CNS depression may occur if diazepam is administered with other CNS depressants, such as antihistamines, tricyclic antidepressants, alcohol, narcotics, or other sedatives or hypnotics.

MANNITOL
Osmitrol

CLASSIFICATIONS
Pharmacologic: Osmotic diuretic
Therapeutic: Diuretic

MECHANISM OF ACTION: Mannitol increases osmotic pressure in the **glomerular filtrate.** This inhibits the reabsorption of water and electrolytes, which causes their excretion in the urine.

THERAPEUTIC BENEFIT: The diuretic action of mannitol causes a dehydrating effect on the brain.

INDICATION FOR PREHOSPITAL USE: Mannitol is used to relieve excessive intracranial pressure.

CONTRAINDICATIONS: ■ Do not administer mannitol to patients with: ■ Hypersensitivity to the drug. ■ Preexisting dehydration. ■ Active intracranial bleeding.

PRECAUTIONS: Use caution in administering mannitol to patients who show a tendency to congestive heart failure, because mannitol may cause a sudden expansion of extracellular fluid, which could bring on congestive heart failure.

ROUTE AND DOSAGE

Adult: 1.5–2 g/kg of a 20% solution by IV infusion, using an in-line IV filter. Mannitol comes in a 5, 10, 15, or 20% 500-mL solution.

Pediatric: Not recommended for prehospital use.

ADVERSE REACTIONS AND SIDE EFFECTS

- *CNS:* Headache, confusion.
- *Cardiovascular:* Tachycardia, chest pain, congestive heart failure, pulmonary edema.
- *Eyes:* Blurred vision.
- *Fluids and electrolytes:* Dehydration.
- *Gastrointestinal:* Nausea, vomiting, thirst.

PARAMEDIC IMPLICATIONS: ■ Monitor the patients closely for any signs of dehydration, which include: ■ Fever. ■ Thirst. ■ Decreased skin turgor. ■ Dry skin and mucous membranes. ■ Mannitol has a tendency to crystalize at temperatures below 45°F. Use an in-line filter when administering mannitol to filter any crystals out of the solution.

DRUG INTERACTIONS: ■ Additive CNS depression can result if mannitol is administered with other CNS depressants. ■ Mannitol can also cause additive adrenergic effects and anticholinergic effects when used with CNS depressants.

METHYLPREDNISOLONE
A-methapred, Medrol, Solu-
Medrol

CLASSIFICATIONS
Pharmacologic: Glucocorticoid
Therapeutic: Anti-inflammatory

MECHANISM OF ACTION: Methylprednisolone suppresses inflammation of tissue. It is believed to protect nerve fibers and inhibit swelling, ischemia, nerve cell death, and electrolyte imbalance to the spinal cord caused by traumatic injury.

THERAPEUTIC BENEFIT: Methylprednisolone is believed to improve muscle and sensory function following traumatic injury to the spinal cord.

INDICATIONS FOR PREHOSPITAL USE: Methylprednisolone is sometimes used in the prehospital treatment of patients who have sustained traumatic spinal cord injury and demonstrate a loss of motor function or sensation.

CONTRAINDICATIONS: None, during emergency use.

PRECAUTIONS: ■ Use caution in administering methylprednisolone to patients with: ■ Hypertension. ■ Diabetes. ■ Congestive heart failure.

ROUTE AND DOSAGE

Adult: 30 mg/kg by IV bolus, followed by an IV infusion of 5.4 mg/kg/h.

Pediatric: The pediatric dosage for traumatic spinal cord injury has not yet been established.

ADVERSE REACTIONS AND SIDE EFFECTS

- *Cardiovascular:* Hypertension.
- *Fluids and electrolytes:* Hypokalemia, fluid retention.
- *Gastrointestinal:* Nausea, vomiting.

PARAMEDIC IMPLICATIONS: ■ For methylprednisolone to be effective, treatment should begin as soon as possible. According to recent studies, this means that treatment must begin within 8 h of the injury for methylprednisolone to be effective. ■ Doses <30 mg/kg are considered ineffective.

DRUG INTERACTIONS: Additive hypokalemia may result if methylprednisolone is used with diuretics. Hypokalemia increases the risk of digitalis toxicity.

PHENOBARBITAL
Luminal

CONTROLLED SUBSTANCE—
SCHEDULE IV
CLASSIFICATIONS
Pharmacologic: Barbiturate

---

*Therapeutic: Anticonvulsant,
sedative hypnotic*

MECHANISM OF ACTION: Phenobarbital causes depression of the CNS and respiratory system and lowers heart rate and blood pressure.

THERAPEUTIC BENEFIT: Phenobarbital's actions inhibit the transmission of signals within the CNS. This inhibition raises the seizure threshold, suppressing the spread of seizure activity.

INDICATIONS FOR PREHOSPITAL USE: In the prehospital setting phenobarbital is most often used to treat grand mal, partial, and febrile seizures in children.

CONTRAINDICATIONS: ■ Do not administer phenobarbital to patients with: ■ Hypersensitivity to barbiturates. ■ CNS depression. ■ Respiratory system depression.

PRECAUTIONS: ■ Use caution in administering phenobarbital to patients: ■ With severe liver or kidney dysfunction. ■ Who may be drug-dependent. ■ Because elderly patients are more likely to experience the side effects of phenobarbital, they should receive reduced doses (⅔–¾ the normal adult dose).

ROUTE AND DOSAGE

Adult (anticonvulsant): 100–300 mg by slow IV bolus.

Pediatric (anticonvulsant): 10–20 mg/kg by slow IV bolus.

Adult (status epilepticus): 10–20 mg/kg by slow IV bolus.

Pediatric (status epilepticus): 15–20 mg/kg by slow IV bolus.

ADVERSE REACTIONS AND SIDE EFFECTS

- *CNS:* Drowsiness, headache, vertigo, possibly paradoxical excitement.
- *Respiratory:* Bronchospasm, laryngospasm, respiratory depression.
- *Cardiovascular:* Hypotension.
- *Gastrointestinal:* Nausea, vomiting.
- *Skin:* Rash, allergic reaction.

PARAMEDIC IMPLICATIONS: ■ Assess patients frequently for respiratory status, pulse, and blood pressure. ■ Advanced airway resuscitation equipment should be readily available in case severe respiratory depression develops during phenobarbital use.

DRUG INTERACTIONS: ■ Phenobarbital may cause added CNS depression if used with other CNS depressants including: ■ Alcohol. ■ Antidepressants. ■ Antihistamines. ■ Narcotics. ■ Sedatives/hypnotics.

PHENYTOIN
Dilantin

CLASSIFICATIONS
*Pharmacologic: Hydantoin
derivative*
Therapeutic: Anticonvulsant

MECHANISM OF ACTION: Phenytoin causes an increase in the transport of sodium out of motor cortex cell neurons. This increase helps to limit cell depolarization, thus preventing the spread of seizure activity.

THERAPEUTIC BENEFIT: Phenytoin's action controls or prevents **grand mal (tonic-clonic) seizures** and **partial seizures.**

INDICATIONS FOR PREHOSPITAL USE: Phenytoin is used to prevent or treat grand mal seizures and partial seizures.

CONTRAINDICATIONS: ■ Do not administer phenytoin to patients who are hypersensitive to the drug. ■ Because of its effect on AV conduction, do not administer phenytoin to patients with bradycardia or heart block.

PRECAUTIONS: ■ Use caution in administering phenytoin to: ■ Elderly patients. ■ Patients with severe cardiac or respiratory problems.

ROUTE AND DOSAGE

Adult: 150–250 mg by slow IV bolus. Repeat with a dose of 100–150 mg after 30 min if needed. Some medical controls prefer a loading dose of 15–18 mg/kg by slow IV bolus, not to exceed an administration rate of 25–50 mg/min.

Pediatric: 10–15 mg/kg by slow IV bolus, at a rate of 0.5–1.5 mg/kg/min.

ADVERSE REACTIONS AND SIDE EFFECTS

- *CNS:* Double vision, dizziness, headache, nervousness.
- *Cardiovascular:* Hypotension, ventricular fibrillation, cardiac depression.
- *Fluids and electrolytes:* Hypocalcemia.
- *Skin:* Rashes.
- *Gastrointestinal:* Nausea, vomiting.

PARAMEDIC IMPLICATIONS: ■ Slow administration of phenytoin helps prevent toxicity. ■ Elderly patients may develop toxic effects more rapidly than younger patients. ■ Monitor the patients closely for developing hypotension and respiratory and cardiac problems. ■ Administer phenytoin through an IV established in a large vein. Do not use veins in the hands.

DRUG INTERACTIONS: ■ Phenytoin may cause additive CNS depression if administered with other CNS depressants, including alcohol, antidepressants, antihistamines, narcotics, and other sedative/hypnotics. ■ Phenytoin is not compatible with dextrose solutions; a precipitate will form.

The drugs presented in this chapter are effective, but they should not be used until basic treatment has been given. For example, the primary treatment for patients having a seizure is to maintain an adequate airway and to keep the patient from injuring himself or herself. Immediate treatment for the patient who has sustained a head injury includes stabilization of the head and neck while simultaneously maintaining an adequate airway. Once basic treatment has been given, then the use of drugs can proceed, if indicated.

A drug which appears to be making new advances in treating traumatic spinal cord injury is methylprednisolone. Current research shows that methylprednisolone inhibits spinal cord swelling, ischemia, nerve cell death, and electrolyte imbalance. However, current information also indicates that immediate methylprednisolone therapy is not necessary, but can wait as long as 8 h before administration. Immediate treatment for patients suspected of sustaining traumatic spinal cord injury is stabilization of the head and neck while simultaneously maintaining an adequate airway.

STUDY QUESTIONS

1. The initial recommended adult dosage of diazepam for the patient experiencing status epilepticus is
   a. 2–5 mg by slow IV bolus.
   b. 5–10 mg by slow IV bolus.
   c. 10–20 mg by slow IV bolus.
   d. 20–30 mg by slow IV bolus.

2. A potentially life-threatening side effect of diazepam is
   a. Cardiac arrhythmia.
   b. Hypotension.
   c. Respiratory arrest.
   d. Anaphylaxis.

3. Dexamethasone is a steroid that suppresses allergic tissue response and improves circulatory status in shock. The dosage for dexamethasone for severe allergic reactions is
   a. 4 mg by slow IV bolus.
   b. 10 mg by slow IV bolus.
   c. 50 mg by slow IV bolus.
   d. 100 mg by slow IV bolus.

4. Which of the following situations demands caution in the use of mannitol?
   a. Active intracranial bleeding.
   b. Preexisting dehydration.
   c. Hypersensitivity.
   d. Tendency to develop congestive heart failure.

5. Methylprednisolone may improve muscle function and sensation following traumatic injury to the spinal cord. A patient estimated to weigh 180 lb should receive __mg of methylprednisolone by IV bolus, followed by an IV infusion of __mg/h.
   a. 5400 mg; 972 mg.
   b. 2700 mg; 486 mg.
   c. 2460 mg; 443 mg.
   d. 1230 mg; 222 mg.

6. A contraindication for the use of phenobarbital sodium is
   a. Kidney dysfunction.
   b. Elderly patient.
   c. Pediatric patient.
   d. Hypersensitivity to barbiturates.

7. The pediatric dose of phenytoin for the treatment of a grand mal seizure is
   a. 0.5–1.5 mg/kg.
   b. 10–15 mg/kg.
   c. 20–30 mg/kg.
   d. 150–250 mg.

8. A contraindication for the use of phenytoin is
   a. Heart block.
   b. Elderly patient.
   c. Respiratory problem.
   d. Headache.

CASE STUDIES

1. You respond to the home of a woman "unable to walk and speak." On arrival you find a 70-year-old woman sitting in a chair at the kitchen table. She is conscious and her eyes follow movements in the room, which indicates she is aware of her surroundings. However, she cannot stand to walk and she cannot speak. Your initial assessment reveals the following:
   - *Level of consciousness:* Conscious, apparently aware of surroundings, but unable to communicate.
   - *Respirations:* 16 breaths/min.
   - *Pulse:* 90 beats/min, irregular. ECG shows atrial fibrillation (Fig. 10–1).
   - *Blood pressure:* 152/112.
   - *Skin:* Normal, slight drooling.
   - *Pupils:* Equal and reactive.
   - Paralysis affecting only the left side of the patient's body.

   The patient's husband states that his wife is currently being treated for high blood pressure, and she has a history of heart disease. His wife appeared normal about 1 h ago. Immediate treatment for this patient should include:
   a. IV line of D_5W, verapamil, rapid transport.
   b. IV line of D_5W, rapid transport.
   c. Humidified oxygen, rapid transport.
   d. Humidified oxygen, precautionary IV line, rapid transport.

2. You respond to an alley where you find a man, approximately 50, passed out. There are several empty beer cans and wine bottles in the area. There is no indication that trauma is a factor. Your assessment reveals the following:
   - *Level of consciousness:* Unconscious, responds to pain.
   - *Respirations:* 20 breaths/min, no respiratory difficulty, breath smells of alcohol.
   - *Pulse:* 50 beats/min, irregular. ECG monitor shows a second-degree heart block, Type II (Fig. 10–2).
   - *Blood pressure:* 196/94.
   - *Skin:* Cool, clammy.

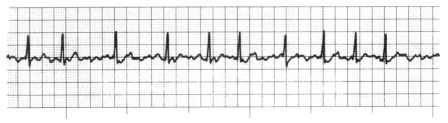

Figure 10–1. Atrial fibrillation. Rate: 90 beats/min.

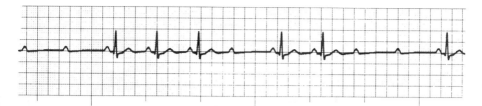

Figure 10–2. Second-degree heart block, Type II. Rate: 50 beats/min.

There is no medical identification on the patient.

Medical control orders an IV of normal saline started at a keep-open rate. As soon as the IV is established, the patient begins to experience active seizures. The drug of choice to control this seizure activity is

a. Phenytoin.
b. Diazepam.
c. Methylprednisolone.
d. Dexamethasone.

EXTENDED CASE STUDY: Status Epilepticus

Initial Response

You respond to the home of a man "having a seizure." On arrival, you find a man, who appears to be approximately 40, experiencing active seizures. His extremities are outstretched, his jaw is clenched, and he is drooling. As you approach, seizure activity appears to be slowing down. However, just as you begin to place the patient on oxygen, seizures begin again. Family members state he has been going from one seizure to another.

This patient is experiencing status epilepticus. Status epilepticus is considered a major emergency because the patient may aspirate, become extremely hypoxic, fracture long bones including the spinal column, or sustain myocardial damage due to cardiac ischemia. Hyperthermia and exhaustion can result from prolonged seizures and cause death.

Management

Patients experiencing status epilepticus are very difficult to manage. This is a life-threatening situation, however, so rapid treatment is essential.

Maintain the patient's airway with the administration of high flow rates of high concentrations of oxygen. Assist ventilations if necessary. Monitor cardiac function. It may be difficult to keep ECG leads attached or to record an accurate strip because of seizure activity. If possible, establish an IV line of normal saline at a keep-open rate. Normal saline is the fluid of choice in case phenytoin is administered. Phenytoin is not compatible with D_5W, because a precipitate forms when phenytoin comes in contact with dextrose. Phenytoin causes an increase in the transport of sodium out of motor cortex cell neurons to limit cell depolarization, thus preventing the spread of seizure activity. The suggested route and dosage of phenytoin is 150–250 mg by slow IV bolus.

Once an IV has been established, there are two prehospital agents of choice: diazepam and $D_{50}W$. Diazepam is a CNS depressant with anticonvulsant properties. The suggested route and dosage for diazepam in this case is 5–10 mg by slow IV bolus initially, repeated if necessary, but not to exceed a total dose of 30 mg. Dextrose 50% in water increases circulating blood sugar levels to normal in hypoglycemic states. Hypoglycemia may be a factor in treating status epilepticus. The suggested route and dosage of $D_{50}W$ for an adult is 25 g by slow IV bolus, repeated as necessary.

Status epilepticus is a true emergency. Rapid transport to the nearest appropriate emergency facility is essential.

Chapter 11

Obstetric and Gynecologic Emergencies

THERAPEUTIC CLASSIFICATIONS
OF DRUGS USED FOR
OBSTETRIC AND
GYNECOLOGIC EMERGENCIES
Diazepam
Magnesium Sulfate
Oxytocin

CASE STUDIES

THERAPEUTIC CLASSIFICATIONS OF DRUGS USED IN OBSTETRIC AND GYNECOLOGIC EMERGENCIES

ANTIANXIETY AGENT
Diazepam

SKELETAL MUSCLE RELAXANT
Diazepam

ANTICONVULSANTS
Diazepam
Magnesium Sulfate

OXYTOCIC
Oxytocin

For most prehospital emergency care professionals, the opportunity to assist in the delivery of a new life into the world is one of the most exciting and fulfilling events in their careers. Most prehospital deliveries occur without complications. During and after delivery, prehospital treatment for both the mother and infant is usually supportive.

In some cases, however, prehospital emergency care providers face one of two potentially fatal obstetric and gynecologic emergencies: **postpartum hemorrhage** and **toxemia of pregnancy** or **eclampsia**.

Postpartum hemorrhage is the loss (by the mother) of more than 500 mL of blood within 24 h after delivery. Because it may be difficult to estimate how much blood the patient has lost at the scene or during transport, it is important to assess frequently the patient's clinical appearance and vital signs in order to determine blood loss.

The initial treatment for severe postpartum hemorrhage is the same as for anyone experiencing hypovolemia due to hemorrhage. This treatment includes maintaining an adequate airway, using supplemental oxygen, and administering intravenous volume expanders. Some EMS systems may use the pneumatic antishock garment (PASG) when treating severe postpartum hemorrhage. Controversy exists as to the actual benefit from using the PASG. Follow local pro-

195

tocols. If prehospital pharmacologic therapy is needed, the drug of choice in treating postpartum hemorrhage is oxytocin. If treatment of postpartum hemorrhage is delayed, a life-threatening situation could rapidly develop.

Eclampsia generally occurs during the last trimester of pregnancy. The cause of eclampsia is unknown. However, it is associated with preexisting hypertension (blood pressure exceeding 140/90), renal disease, and diabetes; it is more prevalant in women experiencing their first pregnancy. Eclampsia is characterized by hypertension and diffuse edema. It develops in approximately 1 out of 200 patients and is usually fatal if untreated. The drugs used for the prehospital treatment of eclampsia are diazepam and a solution of 10% magnesium sulfate.

Preeclampsia is a toxemia of pregnancy characterized by increasing blood pressure, headaches, and edema of the lower extremities. If left untreated, preeclampsia may develop into true eclampsia.

DIAZEPAM
Valium, Valrelease

CONTROLLED SUBSTANCE—
SCHEDULE IV
CLASSIFICATIONS
Pharmacologic: Benzodiazepine
Therapeutic: Antianxiety agent,
anticonvulsant, skeletal muscle
relaxant

MECHANISM: Diazepam causes central nervous system (CNS) depression. It blocks spinal cord interneuronal transmission, causing relaxation of skeletal muscles. Diazepam freely crosses the blood-brain barrier, but its actual mechanism of action is unknown.

THERAPEUTIC BENEFIT: In prehospital emergency care, diazepam is mainly used to control convulsions and to decrease anxiety. It is also used in orthopedic emergencies as a skeletal muscle relaxant.

INDICATIONS FOR PREHOSPITAL USE: Diazepam is used to treat status epilepticus and major motor seizures. It can also be used as a skeletal muscle relaxant in treating orthopedic injuries.

CONTRAINDICATIONS: Do not administer diazepam to patients with:

■ Hypersensitivity to the drug. ■ Preexisting CNS depression. ■ Acute narrow-angle glaucoma.

PRECAUTIONS: ■ Use caution in administering diazepam to patients with a history of psychoses or drug addiction. ■ Administer lower than adult doses of diazepam to elderly patients, because they are usually more sensitive to the drug's CNS effects.

ROUTE AND DOSAGE

Adult (seizures/muscle relaxant): 2–5 mg by slow IV bolus. Repeat if needed, but do not exceed a total dose of 10 mg.

Adult (status epilepticus): 5–10 mg by slow IV bolus. Repeat every 10–15 min if needed, to a maximal dose of 30 mg.

Adult (eclampsia): 5–10 mg by slow IV bolus.

Pediatric (seizures/skeletal muscle relaxant): 0.2–0.5 mg/kg by slow IV bolus over 3 min. Maximal doses:

- $<5y$: 5 mg.
- $>5y$: 10 mg.

Pediatric (status epilepticus):

- $<5y$: 0.2–0.5 mg by slow IV bolus or IM every 2–5 min to a total dose of 5 mg.
- $>5y$: 1 mg every 2–5 min by slow IV bolus or IM to a total dose of 10 mg.

ADVERSE REACTIONS AND SIDE EFFECTS

- *CNS:* Dizziness, drowsiness, mental depression, headache.
- *Cardiovascular:* Hypotension.
- *Respiratory:* Respiratory depression.
- *Eyes:* Blurred vision, increased intraocular pressure in patients with narrow-angle glaucoma.

PARAMEDIC IMPLICATIONS: ■ Diazepam may cause respiratory arrest if administered too rapidly or in excess. ■ Do not mix diazepam with any other drug—it may even react with the IV tubing. To minimize such reactions, administer diazepam at the IV site, not higher in the tubing. Thoroughly flush the IV line before introducing diazepam if other drugs have already been administered. ■ Assess the patient's vital signs continuously.

DRUG INTERACTIONS: Additive CNS depression may result from using diazepam with other CNS depressants, such as antihistamines, tricyclic antidepressants, alcohol, narcotics, or other sedatives or hypnotics.

MAGNESIUM SULFATE

CLASSIFICATIONS
Pharmacologic: Electrolyte
Therapeutic: Anticonvulsant

MECHANISM OF ACTION: Magnesium sulfate affects neuromuscular transmission, depressing the CNS, which in turn can depress respirations. It also acts as a peripheral vasodilator. High doses of magnesium sulfate can cause hypotension.

THERAPEUTIC BENEFIT: Magnesium sulfate resolves convulsive seizures associated with toxemia of pregnancy (eclampsia).

INDICATIONS FOR PREHOSPITAL USE: Magnesium sulfate is used as an anticonvulsant in the prevention or control of seizures in preeclampsia or eclampsia.

CONTRAINDICATIONS: ■ Do not administer magnesium sulfate to patients with: ■ Heart block. ■ Heart damage. ■ Respiratory depression.

PRECAUTIONS: Use caution in administering magnesium sulfate to patients with decreased renal function.

ROUTE AND DOSAGE

Adult: 2–4 g of a 10% solution by IV bolus over 3 min. This drug concentration yields the following drug amounts:

- *2 g:* 20 mL.
- *3 g:* 30 mL.
- *4 g:* 40 mL.

Follow the IV bolus dose with an IV infusion of 1–2 g/h.

Pediatric: Magnesium sulfate is not used in pediatric patients.

ADVERSE REACTIONS AND SIDE EFFECTS

- *CNS:* Drowsiness.
- *Respiratory:* Respiratory depression.
- *Cardiovascular:* Bradycardia, arrhythmias, hypotension.
- *Gastrointestinal:* Nausea, vomiting.
- *Skin:* Rash

PARAMEDIC IMPLICATIONS: ▪ Rapid IV injection of magnesium sulfate may cause respiratory or cardiac arrest. Before administering magnesium sulfate, be sure that the patient's respiratory rate is at least 16 breaths/min. ▪ An overdose of magnesium sulfate may cause respiratory depression and heart block. To reverse these effects, hyperventilate the patient using 100% oxygen and administer an IV bolus of 10% calcium gluconate at 5–10 mEq (10–20 mL). ▪ Constant monitoring of the patient's blood pressure is extremely important. The patient's blood pressure must not fall below 130/80. If maternal blood pressure falls below that level, the uterus may not remain adequately perfused, which could result in damage to the fetus.

DRUG INTERACTIONS: ▪ Additive CNS effects may result when magnesium sulfate is administered with: ▪ Alcohol. ▪ Narcotics. ▪ Barbiturates. ▪ Antidepressants. ▪ Hypnotics. ▪ Antipsychotics. ▪ Cardiac conduction changes may occur if magnesium sulfate is administered with cardiac glycosides.

OXYTOCIN
Pitocin, Syntocinon

CLASSIFICATIONS
Pharmacologic: Hormone
Therapeutic: Oxytocic

MECHANISM OF ACTION: Oxytocin is a pituitary hormone that stimulates uterine muscle contraction. Oxytocin also has vasopressor and antidiuretic effects, but these effects are much less pronounced.

THERAPEUTIC BENEFIT: Oxytocin contracts uterine blood vessels, which reduces postpartum bleeding.

INDICATIONS FOR PREHOSPITAL USE: Oxytocin is used to control postpartum hemorrhage.

CONTRAINDICATIONS: Do not administer oxytocin to patients who are hypersensitive to the drug.

PRECAUTIONS: Do not administer oxytocin until the mother has delivered both the baby and placenta.

ROUTE AND DOSAGE

Adult (IV infusion): 10–20 U added to 1000 mL of lactated Ringer's or normal saline, titrated to severity of hemorrhage.

Adult (IM): 3–10 U.

Pediatric: Oxytocin is not administered to children.

ADVERSE REACTIONS AND SIDE EFFECTS

In the hospital, oxytocin is administered to induce labor at term or to facilitate uterine contractions at term. In those cases, of course, the drug enters the fetal bloodstream. Because it is possible that you will be required to administer oxytocin before delivery, you should learn adverse reactions and side effects for both mother and fetus:

Mother

- *CNS:* Seizures, coma.
- *Cardiovascular:* Hypotension, arrhythmias, increased heart rate and cardiac output.
- *Fluids and electrolytes:* Water intoxication.
- *Gastrointestinal:* Nausea, vomiting.

Fetal

- *CNS:* Intracranial hemorrhage.
- *Respiratory:* Hypoxia, asphyxia.
- *Cardiovascular:* Arrhythmias, PVCs, bradycardia.

PARAMEDIC IMPLICATIONS: ■ If possible, place the newborn at the mother's breast. The baby's sucking action promotes the secretion of oxytocin, which will also aid in controlling postpartum hemorrhage. ■ Oxytocin overdose can cause uterine rupture. Because of this risk, monitor the patient's vital signs frequently.

DRUG INTERACTIONS: Using oxytocin with vasoconstrictors may cause severe hypertension.

Most prehospital OB/GYN emergencies do not require pharmacologic intervention. The prehospital professional can manage the majority of these emergencies by maintaining an adequate airway, using supplemental oxygen, and administering intravenous volume expanders, if needed. If prehospital pharmacologic intervention is needed in severe cases of postpartum hemorrhage, the drug of choice is oxytocin. If prehospital pharmacologic intervention is needed to treat preeclampsia, the drug of choice is magnesium sulfate. If prehospital pharmacologic intervention is needed to treat seizures caused by eclampsia, the drugs used should be diazepam and magnesium sulfate.

In treating prehospital OB/GYN emergencies, medical control may order other drugs in place of or in addition to the drugs presented in this chapter. For example, the physician may elect to order an antihypertensive drug to treat malignant hypertension associated with the OB/GYN patient. Other OB/GYN prehospital emergencies will call for other kinds of flexibility in treatment. It is important that EMS professionals be knowledgeable about local protocols so that they are ready to carry out treatment orders from medical control.

STUDY QUESTIONS

1. The prehospital indication for oxytocin is for the
   a. Control of seizures.
   b. Treatment of hypertension.
   c. Control of postpartum hemorrhage.
   d. Treatment of severe bronchospasm.

2. Oxytocin can be administered both by IV infusion or IM. The IV infusion dosage is __, and the IM dosage is __.
   a. 10–20 U IV; 3–10 U IM.
   b. 3–10 U IV; 10–20 U IM.
   c. 10–20 mEq IV, 3–10 U IM.
   d. 2–5 mg IV, 0.5–2 mg IM.

3. A major concern in a patient with eclampsia is seizures. The prehospital drug of choice in the treatment of severe eclampsia is
   a. Oxytocin.
   b. Magnesium sulfate.
   c. Diazepam.
   d. Labetalol.

4. The prehospital dosage for magnesium sulfate is
   a. 3–10 U IV.
   b. 1 mg/kg IV.
   c. 2–5 mg IV.
   d. 2–4 g IV.

5. The dose of diazepam for a patient having seizures caused by eclampsia is
   a. 2–5 mg.
   b. 5–10 mg.
   c. 10–20 mg.
   d. 30 mg.

CASE STUDIES

1. You are dispatched to the home of a "woman having chest pain." On arrival you find a 24-year-old patient who says that she is 8 mon pregnant. She also reports that she has had a headache for the past 2 days, and today has developed chest pain. Further history and physical examination identify the chest pain as epigastric pain. Initial assessment reveals the following:
   • *Level of consciousness:* Alert, oriented.
   • *Respirations:* 18 breaths/min, lungs clear bilaterally.
   • *Pulse:* 96 beats/min, regular.

- *Blood pressure:* 164/110.
- *Skin:* pale, edematous.

The patient says that this is her first pregnancy. She has no history of high blood pressure or any other illness.

All signs and symptoms indicate this patient is preeclamptic. Preeclampsia can lead to true eclampsia. Do not delay transport to the emergency department. Headache and epigastric pain in this situation could be signs of impending seizure activity.

The drug of choice for the prevention of seizure activity in the preeclamptic patient is

a. Diazepam.
b. Oxytocin.
c. Mannitol.
d. Magnesium sulfate.

2. You are called to the home of a woman "having seizures." On arrival you find a woman in her late 20s experiencing active seizures. The patient's mother says that her daughter is 7 mon pregnant. She also reports this is her daughter's second seizure since she called for help. Earlier in the day the patient had complained of severe headache, dizziness, nausea, chest pain, and spots before her eyes. Seizure control for this patient should begin with:

a. Diazepam.
b. Calcium gluconate.
c. Magnesium sulfate.
d. Oxytocin.

EXTENDED CASE STUDY: OB/GYN Emergency

Initial Response

Your ambulance is dispatched to a "woman in labor." On arrival, you find a 32-year-old patient who is experiencing strong uterine contractions every 2 min, each lasting approximately 1 min. The patient tells you that this is her second child, but it is not due for another 3 wk. On visual examination, you notice that the baby's buttocks are visible, which indicates that delivery is imminent. Preparations for delivery are quickly made.

Place the mother on 100% oxygen. If delivery complications arise, it is important to increase oxygen content and oxygen delivery to the tissues.

As the baby emerges, the buttocks and legs come out smoothly but the head remains in the birth canal. In this situation, an adequate airway must be provided, because the baby may attempt to begin spontaneous respirations. You form an airway at the bottom of the birth canal*, but there is no evidence of respirations. After approximately 2 min, the baby's head delivers. Initial assessment of the baby reveals the following:

- *Level of consciousness:* Unconscious.
- *Respirations:* None.
- *Pulse:* None.

---

* While wearing gloves, fingers are inserted into the birth canal to form a space, making a temporary airway for the baby.

Management

Immediately use suction to clear the baby's airway and ventilate, with 100% oxygen using a bag-valve mask and chest compressions. There is a risk that 100% oxygen will have toxic effects on the baby's lungs and eyes, but oxygen should never be withheld from an infant during an emergency.

Assessment of ventilations reveals good breath sounds over the chest and gastric area. It is now a good idea to place an ET tube in the baby for airway protection and administration of emergency drugs if necessary. Vascular access in a newborn is difficult at best, so in most cases ET access for drug administration is preferable. The ECG monitor shows asystole.

Once the ET is in place and adequate ventilations are achieved, administer approximately 0.1 mg (0.04 mL) epinephrine in a 1:1000 solution down the ET tube. The dosage of epinephrine is 0.01 mg/kg IV of a 1:10,000 solution or 0.1 mg/kg of a 1:1000 solution via the ET tube. (The average normal birthweight of a newborn is 4–5 kg.) When administering epinephrine ET, it is best to dilute the drug with normal saline solution.

Epinephrine is a natural catecholamine that stimulates both alpha-adrenergic and beta-adrenergic receptors. It elevates perfusion pressure during cardiac compressions, improves cardiac contractions, and stimulates spontaneous contractions in asystole. (See Chapter 7.) In this case, the newborn responds to the epinephrine and ventilations with a heart rate beginning at 40 beats/min and gradually increasing to a normal sinus rhythm. In the newborn, a heart rate less than 80 beats/min is considered bradycardia, and it does not produce adequate perfusion. Therefore, chest compressions are necessary until the epinephrine and ventilation gradually increase the newborn's heart rate to normal.

The key to successful resuscitation of a newborn is adequate airway maintenance and ventilation using supplemental oxygen. Medical control may call for medications if the patient does not respond to ventilation and chest compressions. In this case the newborn now has a sinus rhythm at a rate of 144 beats/min, with a good pulse and adequate respirations.

While attention was focused on the baby, another member of your team began having problems with the mother. She complained of severe abdominal pain after delivery of the placenta and soon began hemorrhaging.

Hemorrhage after delivery calls for several prehospital management techniques. Immediately one of the ALS team begins massaging the patient's fundus while another team member starts an IV lifeline of lactated Ringer's or normal saline. The patient should remain on high-flow 100% oxygen. If massaging the fundus does not control the hemorrhage, the drug of choice used for prehospital hemorrhage control is oxytocin. Oxytocin is a hormone secreted by the pituitary gland that stimulates uterine contractions. In this prehospital emergency, oxytocin is used to contract uterine blood vessels, thus reducing postpartum hemorrhage. If possible, the newborn should be placed at the mother's breast. The sucking action of the baby will promote the secretion of oxytocin, also aiding in controlling hemorrhage. However, in this case the baby should be closely monitored while enroute to the emergency department due to its potentially unstable condition. The oxytocin dosage is 10–20 U added to lactated Ringer's or normal saline at a rate adjusted to the severity of the hemorrhage.

Chapter 12

Anaphylactic Emergencies

THERAPEUTIC CLASSIFICATIONS
OF DRUGS USED IN
ANAPHYLACTIC EMERGENCIES

Diphenhydramine	Hydrocortisone
Epinephrine (1:1000 and 1:10,000 Solutions)	Methylprednisolone

CASE STUDIES

THERAPEUTIC CLASSIFICATIONS OF DRUGS USED FOR ANAPHYLACTIC EMERGENCIES

ANTIHISTAMINE
Diphenhydramine

BRONCHODILATOR
Epinephrine

ANTI-INFLAMMATORIES
Hydrocortisone
Methylprednisolone

IMMUNOSUPPRESSANTS
Hydrocortisone
Methylprednisolone

Anaphylaxis is an acute allergic hypersensitive reaction of the body to an **antigen**. An antigen is a foreign particle or substance (usually a protein) whose presence in the body causes the body's immune system to produce an antibody. Antibodies are also proteins, of a special class of serum proteins called *immunoglobins*. Each antibody is produced in response to the presence of a specific antigen, and it reacts only with that antigen. The antigen-antibody interaction is the basis of the cell-mediated immune response in normal individuals.

Allergies occur when a substance, such as a drug or food, that does not normally stimulate an immune response does so. Such substances are called *allergens*. The person is said to be hypersensitive to the substance. For some reason, the hypersensitive person's body contains antibodies to the allergen. The antibodies may have been produced in response to previous exposures to the allergen or they may be naturally occurring. In either case, these antibodies, if present in sufficient quantities, cause the allergic reaction when the allergen enters the body.

Smooth muscle cells, such as those in the respiratory tract, have two kinds of **histamine** receptors, H_1 and H_2. Most of the effects of histamine in allergic reactions are due to the stimulation of H_1 receptors. Stimulation of H_1 receptors causes bronchoconstriction, making it difficult to breathe. The treatment most frequently used to block the stimulation of H_1 receptors is the administration of an H_1-receptor antagonist, such as diphenhydramine.

203

There are two types of allergic hypersensitive reactions: the delayed and the immediate. Anaphylaxis is the immediate hypersensitive reaction. This reaction causes contraction of the smooth muscles and increased loss of fluid from capillaries into tissue spaces. Severe anaphylaxis, which is called anaphylactic shock, is a severe allergic reaction that may cause respiratory and/or circulatory failure and death. Anaphylactic shock may develop within seconds after the exposure. Individual signs and symptoms depend on the severity of the anaphylactic reaction. Common signs of anaphylactic shock include hives, flushing, and edema. If the condition is not corrected, laryngeal edema, constriction of the bronchial tree, and hypotension can rapidly develop and lead to death. The first and most important prehospital response to anaphylactic emergencies is to alleviate the bronchial constriction.

DIPHENHYDRAMINE
Benadryl, Benylin

CLASSIFICATIONS
Pharmacologic: Antihistamine
Therapeutic: Antihistamine (H₁-receptor antagonist)

MECHANISM OF ACTION: Diphenhydramine competes with histamine for H_1 receptor sites. It is a strong central nervous system (CNS) depressant; in addition, diphenhydramine has significant anticholinergic properties. Diphenhydramine blocks the effects of histamine, including: vasodilation, increased gastrointestinal tract secretions, increased heart rate, and hypotension.

THERAPEUTIC BENEFIT: Diphenhydramine blocks the effects of histamine release on H_1 receptor sites. By blocking these effects, diphenhydramine relieves symptoms associated with allergic reactions.

INDICATIONS FOR PREHOSPITAL USE: Diphenhydramine is used in addition to epinephrine for the symptomatic relief of allergic symptoms caused by histamine release.

CONTRAINDICATIONS: ▪ Do not administer diphenhydramine to patients who are hypersensitive to the drug. ▪ Do not administer to patients experiencing acute asthma attacks, because diphenhydramine thickens bronchial secretions.

PRECAUTIONS: ▪ Administer diphenhydramine with caution to patients with: ▪ Narrow-angle glaucoma. ▪ Cardiovascular disease. ▪ Hypertension.

ROUTE AND DOSAGE

Adult: 10–50 mg by slow IV bolus or deep IM injection at a rate of approximately 1 mL/min. Some patients may need up to 100 mg.

Pediatric: 2–5 mg/kg by slow IV bolus or deep IM injection. The usual dosage is 10–30 mg.

ADVERSE REACTIONS AND SIDE EFFECTS

- *CNS:* Drowsiness, dizziness, headache, and (possibly) paradoxic excitement in children.
- *Respiratory:* Wheezing, thickening of bronchial secretions, tightness of the chest.
- *Cardiovascular:* Palpitations, hypotension.
- *Eyes:* Blurred vision.
- *Gastrointestinal:* Dry mouth, anorexia, nausea, vomiting, diarrhea.

PARAMEDIC IMPLICATIONS: Assess the patient's lung sounds, respiratory function, and airway patency frequently.

DRUG INTERACTIONS: ▪ Additive CNS depression may result if diphenhydramine is used with: ▪ Other antihistamines. ▪ Alcohol. ▪ Narcotics. ▪ Sedatives/hypnotics.

EPINEPHRINE (1:1000 AND 1:10,000 SOLUTIONS)
Adrenalin

CLASSIFICATIONS
Pharmacologic: Adrenergic
Therapeutic: Bronchodilator

MECHANISM OF ACTION: Epinephrine stimulates both alpha-adrenergic and beta-adrenergic receptors. Alpha-adrenergic receptors, located in smooth muscle cells of the veins and arteries, control vasoconstriction. Beta-adrenergic receptors, located in the heart, bronchioles, and peripheral vessels, control heart rate, myocardial contractions, and dilation of the bronchioles of the peripheral vessels. Epinephrine constricts dilated blood vessels, raises the heart rate, improves myocardial contractions, and dilates the bronchioles. Epinephrine also prevents the release of histamines, which helps to reverse histamine-caused bronchoconstriction, vasodilation, and edema.

THERAPEUTIC BENEFIT: Epinephrine causes bronchodilation and cardiac stimulation in cases of anaphylaxis.

INDICATIONS FOR PREHOSPITAL USE: Epinephrine is used as the primary drug in treating anaphylaxis.

CONTRAINDICATIONS: ▪ Do not administer epinephrine to patients with: ▪ Hypersensitivity to the drug. ▪ Heart disease. ▪ Arrhythmias. ▪ Narrow-angle glaucoma.

PRECAUTIONS: ▪ Use caution in administering epinephrine to: ▪ Elderly patients. Use caution in administering the drug to patients with: ▪ Hypertension. ▪ Hyperthyroidism. ▪ Diabetes.

ROUTE AND DOSAGE:

Adult (mild/moderate anaphylaxis): 0.3–0.5 mg (0.3–0.5 mL) of a 1:1000 solution SC.

Adult (severe anaphylaxis): 0.3–0.5 mg slow IV bolus (3–5 mL of a 1:10,000 solution). In addition to the IV bolus, an IV infusion may be necessary at 1 µg/min but not to exceed 4 µg/min.
To prepare the infusion add 2 mg. of a 1:1000 solution to 500 mL of D₅W, making a concentration of 4 µg/mL.

Pediatric (mild/moderate anaphylaxis): 0.01 mL/kg of a 1:1000 solution SC.

Pediatric (severe anaphylaxis): 0.1 ml/kg of a 1:10,000 solution by IV bolus.

ADVERSE REACTIONS AND SIDE EFFECTS

- *CNS:* Nervousness, restlessness, tremor, headache.
- *Endocrine:* Hyperglycemia.
- *Gastrointestinal:* Nausea, vomiting.

PARAMEDIC IMPLICATIONS: ▪ Assess the patient's condition frequently, especially blood pressure, pulse, and ECG changes. ▪ Assess lung sounds before and during treatment. ▪ Inadvertent IV injection of a 1:1000 solution instead of a 1:10,000 solution may result in sudden hypertension or cerebral hemorrhage.

DRUG INTERACTIONS: ▪ Beta-adrenergic blocking drugs may block the therapeutic response to epinephrine. ▪ Administering epinephrine with other adrenergic drugs may produce additive effects.

HYDROCORTISONE
Cortef, Cortisol,
   Hydrocortone, Solu-Cortef

CLASSIFICATIONS:
Pharmacologic: Glucocorticoid
Therapeutic: Anti-inflammatory

MECHANISM OF ACTION: Hydrocortisone is the pharmaceutical name of the hormone cortisol, which is produced in the adrenal cortex. The drug is used to replace the naturally occurring hormone in deficient states.

THERAPEUTIC BENEFIT: Hydrocortisone is used in the replacement of cortisol in deficiency states. It is used for the short-term management of inflammatory and allergic reactions.

CONTRAINDICATIONS: There are no contraindications for the use of hydrocortisone for severe anaphylaxis.

PRECAUTIONS: ▪ Use caution in administering hydrocortisone to patients with: ▪ Renal disease. ▪ Hypertension. ▪ Diabetes. ▪ Seizures. ▪ Congestive heart failure.

ROUTE AND DOSAGE

Adult: 100–500 mg by IV bolus or IM. Dilute IV bolus dosages >100 mg in 50–100 mL of D_5W or normal saline solution. Hydrocortisone comes in powdered form, which must be reconstituted before use.

Pediatric: 0.16–1.0 mg/kg by IV bolus or IM.

ADVERSE REACTIONS AND SIDE EFFECTS

- *CNS:* Depression, euphoria.
- *Eyes:* Increased intraocular pressure.
- *Fluids and electrolytes:* Sodium retention, hypokalemia.
- *Gastrointestinal:* Nausea, vomiting.

PARAMEDIC IMPLICATIONS: Assess patient frequently for peripheral edema, rales, or dyspnea.

DRUG INTERACTIONS: ▪ Phenytoin and phenobarbital may decrease the effectiveness of hydrocortisone. ▪ Digitalis glycoside toxicity may develop if the patient becomes hypokalemic (decreased serum potassium level).

METHYLPREDNISOLONE
A-methaPred, Medrol, Solu-Medrol

CLASSIFICATIONS
Pharmacologic: Glucocorticoid
Therapeutic: Anti-inflammatory, immunosuppressant

MECHANISM OF ACTION: Methylprednisolone decreases the body's inflammatory response as well as suppressing the body's immune system.

THERAPEUTIC BENEFIT: Methylprednisolone suppresses the body's inflammatory response and modifies the body's normal immune response.

INDICATIONS FOR PREHOSPITAL USE: Methylprednisolone is used in the treatment of severe anaphylaxis.

CONTRAINDICATIONS: Do not administer methylprednisolone to patients who are hypersensitive to adrenocorticoid preparations.

PRECAUTIONS: ▪ Use caution in administering methylprednisolone to patients with: ▪ Renal disease. ▪ Hypertension. ▪ Diabetes. ▪ Seizures. ▪ Congestive heart failure.

ROUTE AND DOSAGE

Adult: 100–200 mg by IV bolus or IM. Methylprednisolone comes in powdered form and must be reconstituted before use. It may be further diluted in D_5W or normal saline solution.

Pediatric: Methylprednisolone is not recommended for prehospital use.

ADVERSE REACTIONS AND SIDE EFFECTS:

- *CNS:* Depression, euphoria, restlessness, headache.
- *Cardiovascular:* Hypertension.
- *Eyes:* Increased intraocular pressure.
- *Endocrine:* Hyperglycemia.
- *Fluids and electrolytes:* Hypokalemia, fluid retention.
- *Gastrointestinal:* Nausea, vomiting.

PARAMEDIC IMPLICATIONS: Assess the patient frequently for signs of peripheral edema, rales, or dyspnea.

DRUG INTERACTIONS: Methylprednisolone used with diuretics may cause additive hypokalemia, which in turn may increase the risk of digitalis glycoside toxicity.

Anaphylactic reactions are common prehospital emergencies. Many anaphylactic reactions occur suddenly and therefore must be managed aggressively. In severe cases of anaphylaxis, death usually occurs from spasm of the bronchial smooth muscles.

Generally, prehospital drug therapy for anaphylactic reactions should include epinephrine, diphenhydramine, and in severe cases hydrocortisone and methylprednisolone. In some situations, medical control may order aminophylline. However, aminophylline is generally not administered in cases of severe anaphylaxis because of its side effects, which include hypotension (see Chapter 8).

The body's response to the invasion of antigens is very complex. The patient's response can be an uncomfortable but not serious reaction, or it can quickly develop into a life-threatening emergency. When anaphylaxis is suspected, it is important to monitor the patient closely. If symptoms develop, it is vital to treat the patient aggressively.

Remember that anaphylactic shock can be treated with a variety of drugs. It the responsibility of each EMS professional to keep current with local treatment protocols.

STUDY QUESTIONS

1. Diphenhydramine acts in the treatment of allergic reactions by
   a. Competing with histamine for H_1-receptor sites to prevent further reaction.
   b. Releasing catecholamines, preventing further reaction.
   c. Dilating bronchial passages to relieve airway obstruction.
   d. Reversing the chemical actions of histamine.

2. The usual pediatric dosage of diphenhydramine is
   a. 100 mg.
   b. 10–50 mg.
   c. 10–30 mg.
   d. 2–5 mg.

3. Epinephrine is the prehospital drug of choice in cases of anaphylaxis because it
   a. Binds to both H_1- and H_2-receptor sites.
   b. Reverses the chemical actions of histamine.

   c. Decreases the oxygen requirements of the heart.

   d. Constricts peripheral blood vessels and dilates the bronchioles.

4. In cases of severe anaphylaxis, the adult dose of epinephrine is
   a. 0.3–0.5 mg of a 1:1000 solution.
   b. 0.3–0.5 mg of a 1:10,000 solution.
   c. 0.1 mL/kg of a 1:10,000 solution.
   d. 3–5 mL of a 1:1000 solution.

5. Hydrocortisone acts in treating anaphylaxis by
   a. Neutralizing histamine.
   b. Blocking H_1- and H_2-receptor sites.
   c. Promoting dilation of the bronchioles.
   d. Overcoming insufficiencies of the naturally occurring hormone to suppress the immune reaction.

6. The adult dosage range of hydrocortisone for an allergic reaction is
   a. 100–500 mg.
   b. 50–100 mg.
   c. 30–50 mg.
   d. 5 mg/kg.

7. After giving methylprednisolone, the paramedic should frequently assess the patient for
   a. Tachyarrhythmias.
   b. Peripheral edema.
   c. Hypoglycemia.
   d. Hypotension.

8. The pediatric dosage of methylprednisolone for allergic reactions is
   a. 10–50 mg.
   b. 0.1 mL/kg.
   c. 0.16–1 mg/kg.
   d. Not recommended.

CASE STUDIES

1. You are called to a picnic area where you find a 10-year-old female patient having difficulty breathing. Initial patient assessment reveals that she has severe headache, abdominal cramps, and a rapid pulse and shows slight facial swelling. The patient says that just before these signs and symptoms began she had been playing in a wooded area of the picnic grounds. This patient is most likely experiencing
   a. An asthma attack.
   b. An anaphylactic reaction.
   c. A diabetic emergency.
   d. Heat exhaustion.

2. In the situation described, you decide your patient has developed a moderate case of anaphylaxis. What are the drugs that medical control is likely to order first?
   a. Epinephrine and diphenhydramine.
   b. Epinephrine and dopamine.

c. Epinephrine and hydrocortisone.
d. Epinephrine and methylprednisolone.

EXTENDED CASE STUDY

Initial Response

You are dispatched to a man experiencing shortness of breath. On arrival you find a 36-year-old man sitting on his front steps. His wife states that he had been mowing the lawn when he suddenly became short of breath. The patient appears flushed and very anxious. He says that his throat feels like it is closing up, making it very hard to breathe. You notice hives on his back, chest, and upper abdomen. Initial assessment of the patient reveals the following:

- *Level of consciousness:* Alert, very anxious.
- *Respirations:* Rapid, shallow, bilateral wheezing on both inspiration and expiration.
- *Pulse:* Rapid and weak.
- *Blood pressure:* 92/60.
- *Skin:* Flushed, hives.

The patient says he has no history of cardiac problems or any other recent illness. All signs and symptoms of this patient strongly suggest anaphylaxis.

Management

After you contact medical control and completely assess the patient, it is decided to place the patient on high-flow oxygen, to start an IV of lactated Ringer's, to connect him to a cardiac monitor, and to administer 0.3 mg of a 1:1000 solution of epinephrine SC. After administering the epinephrine you are ordered to start an IV of lactated Ringer's at a keep-open rate, using a large-bore catheter. The ECG monitor shows a sinus tachycardia at a regular rate of 138/min.

Epinephrine is given to the anaphylactic patient because of its bronchodilating effects on the lower airways and its constricting action on the peripheral circulation. Once epinephrine is administered, keep track of its effects by frequent auscultation of the patient's lungs and monitoring of blood pressure. If you haven't already placed the patient in the ambulance and begun transport, do so now.

After the epinephrine has been given and the IV established, a reassessment of vital signs reveals the following:

- *Level of consciousness:* Conscious, anxious, confused.
- *Respirations:* 36/min, labored. Lung sounds unchanged.
- *Pulse:* 146/min, weak.
- *Blood pressure:* 70/52.

At this point, medical control orders you to administer another injection of 0.3 mg of epinephrine, to increase the IV rate to wide open, and to start a second IV of lactated Ringer's at a wide-open rate.

As anaphylaxis progresses, respiration becomes compromised due to developing edema and spasm of the upper airway and bronchii. Anaphylaxis can also cause hypovolemia due to peripheral vasodilation and the pooling of blood. In most cases of mild or moderate anaphylaxis, an SC injection of 0.3 mg of epinephrine is the appropriate initial treatment. However, if the patient's blood pressure continues to fall, the circulation fails to distribute the drug properly and the patient deteriorates. In this case, the initial blood pressure was 92/60 and quickly fell to 70/52. Therefore, in order for the epinephrine to be effective, you must take steps to correct the hypovolemia.

If this patient had been experiencing severe anaphylaxis when you first assessed him, 2 wide-open IVs of lactated Ringer's would have been indicated. The initial drug of choice would still have been epinephrine, but the dosage would have been 0.3–0.5 mg of a 1:10,000 solution by slow IV bolus. Medical control may have also ordered an epinephrine infusion.

Diphenhydramine can be used as an adjunct to epinephrine in cases of anaphylaxis. Diphenhydramine is used for the symptomatic relief of allergic reactions caused by histamine release. The initial adult dosage of diphenhydramine is 10–50 mg by slow IV bolus or deep IM.

Diphenhydramine has little effect, however, if the allergic reaction has had time to fully develop. In such cases, one possible plan for correcting hypotension is to administer a dopamine infusion. Add 800 mg of dopamine to 500 mL of D_5W, which yields a drug concentration of 1600 μg/mL. Dopamine is a catecholamine that corrects hypotension by increasing cardiac output without significantly affecting heart rate (see Chapter 7).

Chapter 13

Toxicologic Emergencies

THERAPEUTIC CLASSIFICATIONS
OF DRUGS USED FOR
TOXICOLOGIC EMERGENCIES

Activated Charcoal	Physostigmine
Amyl Nitrite	Pralidoxime
Atropine	Sodium Nitrite
Diazepam	Sodium Thiosulfate
Naloxone	Syrup of Ipecac

CASE STUDIES

THERAPEUTIC CLASSIFICATIONS OF DRUGS USED FOR TOXICOLOGIC EMERGENCIES

ANTICONVULSANT
Diazepam

ANTIDOTES
Activated charcoal
Atropine (to cholinesterase inhibitors)
Physostigmine (antimuscarinic)
Pralidoxime (to cholinesterase inhibitors)

CYANIDE POISONING ADJUNCTS
Amyl nitrite
Sodium nitrite
Sodium thiosulfate

EMETIC
Syrup of ipecac

NARCOTIC ANTAGONIST
Naloxone

Prehospital toxicologic emergencies include the management of poisonings and overdoses. A **poison** is any substance taken into the body that interferes with normal physiologic functions. As this definition implies, almost any substance is a potential poison. Prehospital management of poisoning emergencies includes identifying the poison, attempting to slow or stop the absorption process, and administering an antidote.

Overdose, too, is a common prehospital emergency. An overdose is the intake of a substance, usually a drug of abuse, in sufficient amount to cause an acute reaction in the body. Acute reactions range from excessive excitement to coma or even death.

Cyanide compounds are among the most common and most deadly poisons known. Cyanide poisoning can occur from exposure through the skin, inhalation, or by oral ingestion. Fortunately, cyanide poisoning is relatively rare. When the poison is inhaled, symptoms of cyanide poisoning usually occur within seconds to minutes. Cyanide inhibits cellular respirations, which cause cellular hypoxia and death. Symptoms generally begin with giddiness and progress rapidly to headache, palpitations, vomiting, unconsciousness, convulsions, and death. Cyanide poisoning may cause the patient's breath to smell like "bitter almonds." Do not, however, rely heavily on odor for diagnosis: many people do not know what bitter almonds smell like. Treatment for cyanide poisoning should be immediate. Drug therapy usually consists of a three-step protocol beginning with amyl nitrite, followed by sodium nitrite and sodium thiosulfate.

Organophosphates are a major component of many insecticides. Toxicity can occur by absorption through the skin or lungs or by ingestion. The manifestations of organophosphate poisoning include nausea, profuse sweating, epigastric and substernal tightness, abdominal cramps, and profuse salivation and muscle twitching. Severe cases of organophosphate poisoning may produce seizures and respiratory arrest. Pharmacologic treatment for severe cases of organophosphate poisoning includes the administration of atropine followed by pralidoxime.

Most overdoses affect the central nervous system (CNS), causing an altered level of consciousness and respiratory depression. Prehospital management of overdose emergencies is aimed at stabilizing the ABCs; in some cases treatment includes the administration of antidotes.

ACTIVATED CHARCOAL
Arm-a-char, Charcoaide, InstaChar

CLASSIFICATIONS
Pharmacologic: Adsorbent
Therapeutic: Antidote

MECHANISM OF ACTION: Activated charcoal binds to and adsorbs ingested poisons: this **adsorption** inhibits their absorption in the gastrointestinal tract.

THERAPEUTIC BENEFIT: Activated charcoal inhibits the absorption of many poisons in the gastrointestinal tract.

INDICATIONS FOR PREHOSPITAL USE: Activated charcoal is used in the treatment of certain cases of poisoning and overdoses in the alert patient after the stomach has been emptied.

CONTRAINDICATIONS: ▪ Do not administer charcoal to patients who have ingested: ▪ Cyanide. ▪ Mineral acids. ▪ Strong bases. ▪ Methanol. ▪ Ethanol.
Activated charcoal is ineffective with these substances.

PRECAUTIONS: Activated charcoal may cause vomiting. Be prepared to take appropriate action if vomiting should occur.

ROUTE AND DOSAGE:

Adult: 30–60 g (5–10 tbs) mixed in tap water to make a slurry.

Pediatric: 10–30 g (3–5 tbs) mixed in tap water to make a slurry.

ADVERSE REACTIONS AND SIDE EFFECTS

- *Gastrointestinal:* Constipation, diarrhea. Large doses of activated charcoal may cause vomiting.

PARAMEDIC IMPLICATIONS: Activated charcoal is most effective if it is administered within 30 min after ingestion of the toxic substance.

DRUG INTERACTIONS: ▪ Do not administer activated charcoal before or simultaneously with syrup of ipecac, because activated charcoal will absorb the ipecac and render it ineffective. Avoid milk products when using activated charcoal, because milk products decrease activated charcoal's effectiveness.

AMYL NITRITE

CLASSIFICATIONS
Pharmacologic: Nitrite/nitrate
Therapeutic: Cyanide poisoning
adjunct

MECHANISM OF ACTION: Amyl nitrite converts hemoglobin into methemoglobin. Methemoglobin reacts with cyanide and chemically binds it, which prevents it from having any toxic effect.

THERAPEUTIC BENEFIT: Amyl nitrite degrades cyanide in cases of cyanide poisoning.

INDICATION FOR PREHOSPITAL USE: Amyl nitrite is used for the immediate treatment of cyanide poisoning.

CONTRAINDICATIONS: None, in cases of cyanide poisoning.

PRECAUTIONS: ▪ Use caution in administering amyl nitrite to patients: ▪ Who are hypersensitive to the drug. ▪ Who have sustained head trauma or cerebral hemorrhage (amyl nitrite dilates meningeal blood vessels). ▪ Who are hypotensive. ▪ Who have glaucoma.

ROUTE AND DOSAGE

Adult: 1–2 ampules crushed and the volatile contents inhaled for 30 sec. Repeated as needed until the patient arrives at the emergency department. Each amyl nitrite ampule contains 0.3 mL of the drug.

Pediatric: 1 ampule crushed and the volatile contents inhaled for 30 sec. Repeated as needed until the patient arrives at the emergency department. Each amyl nitrite ampule contains 0.3 mL of the drug.

NOTE: Amyl nitrite administration is the first step in a 3-step treatment protocol for cyanide poisoning. After administering amyl nitrite, administer sodium nitrite, then sodium thiosulfate.

ADVERSE REACTIONS AND SIDE EFFECTS

- *CNS:* Severe headache, dizziness, weakness, muscle twitching.
- *Cardiovascular:* Orthostatic hypotension, tachycardia, fainting.
- *Gastrointestinal:* Nausea, vomiting.
- *Skin:* Flushing, cold sweats.

PARAMEDIC IMPLICATIONS: ■ Assess the patient frequently; be alert for signs of developing hypotension. ■ The patient should remain sitting or lying down while amyl nitrite is being given.

DRUG INTERACTIONS: ■ Additive hypotension may result if amyl nitrite is administered simultaneously with: ■ Phenothiazines. ■ Beta-blockers. ■ Antihypertensives.

ATROPINE
N/A

CLASSIFICATIONS
Pharmacologic: Anticholinergic
Therapeutic: **Anticholinesterase** *inhibitor (organophosphate poisoning antidote)*

MECHANISM OF ACTION: Atropine blocks the action of acetylcholine in the parasympathetic nervous system, aiding in the treatment of anticholinesterase poisoning from organophosphate pesticides. Table 13–1 lists some of the more common organophosphate pesticides with which an individual may come in contact.

THERAPEUTIC BENEFIT: Atropine reverses the adverse effects of organophosphate poisoning.

INDICATIONS FOR PREHOSPITAL USE: Atropine is used in the treatment of organophosphate poisoning.

Table 13–1. ORGANOPHOSPHATE PESTICIDES

High Toxicity	Moderate Toxicity	Mild Toxicity
Demeton	Coumaphos	Chlorthion
Disulfoton	Diazinon	Dimethoate
OMPA	Dichlorvos	Malathion
Parathion		
Phosdrin		
Schradon		
TEPP		

CONTRAINDICATIONS: There are no contraindications for atropine when used in severe cases of organophosphate poisoning.

PRECAUTIONS: ■ Very young and very old patients are more prone to experience adverse reactions to atropine. ■ Use caution in administering atropine to patients with: ■ Chronic renal disease. ■ Cardiac disease. ■ Pulmonary disease.

ROUTE AND DOSAGE

Adult: 1 mg by IV bolus initially. If there is no improvement, administer one additional dose of 2–5 mg by IV bolus. Medical control may order additional doses while you are en route.

Pediatric: 0.05 mg/kg by IV bolus. Repeat doses may be necessary.

ADVERSE REACTIONS AND SIDE EFFECTS

- *CNS:* Drowsiness, confusion, excitation.
- *Cardiovascular:* Tachycardia.
- *Eyes:* Dry eyes, blurred vision.
- *Gastrointestinal:* Dry mouth.

PARAMEDIC IMPLICATIONS: ■ Assess the patient frequently for any signs of developing adverse reactions and side effects. ■ Severe cases of organophosphate poisoning may require the administration of pralidoxime in addition to atropine.

DRUG INTERACTIONS: Administering atropine simultaneously with other anticholinergic drugs, including antihistamines, tricyclic antidepressants, and quinidine, may cause additive anticholinergic effects.

DIAZEPAM
Valium, Valrelease

CLASSIFICATIONS
Pharmacologic: Benzodiazepine
Therapeutic: Antianxiety agent,
anticonvulsant, skeletal muscle
relaxant

MECHANISM OF ACTION: Diazepam causes CNS depression. It blocks spinal cord interneuronal transmission, causing relaxation of skeletal muscles. Diazepam freely crosses the blood-brain barrier, but its actual mechanism of action is unknown.

THERAPEUTIC BENEFIT: In prehospital emergency care, diazepam is mainly used to control convulsions and to decrease anxiety. It is also beneficial in orthopedic emergencies as a skeletal muscle relaxant.

INDICATIONS FOR PREHOSPITAL USE: Diazepam has been shown to be effective in controlling advancing CNS overstimulation and seizures caused by cocaine overdose.

CONTRAINDICATIONS: ▪ Do not administer diazepam to patients with: ▪ Hypersensitivity to the drug. ▪ Preexisting CNS depression. ▪ Acute narrow-angle glaucoma.

PRECAUTIONS: ▪ Use caution in administering diazepam to patients with a history of psychosis or drug addiction because of the possible development of adverse reactions. ▪ Administer less than adult doses of diazepam to elderly patients, because they are usually more sensitive to the drug's CNS effects.

ROUTE AND DOSAGE

Adult (advancing CNS overstimulation): 2.5–5 mg by slow IV bolus.

Adult (active seizure activity): 5–10 mg by slow IV bolus over 2–3 min. Repeated every 10–15 min, as needed, to a maximum of 30 mg.

Pediatric: Not recommended for prehospital use for cocaine overdose.

ADVERSE REACTIONS AND SIDE EFFECTS

- *CNS:* Dizziness, drowsiness, mental depression, headache.
- *Cardiovascular:* Hypotension.
- *Respiratory:* Respiratory depression.
- *Eyes:* Blurred vision, increased intraocular pressure in patients with narrow-angle glaucoma.

PARAMEDIC IMPLICATIONS: ▪ Diazepam may cause respiratory arrest if administered too rapidly or in excess. ▪ Do not mix diazepam with any other drug—diazepam may even react with the IV tubing. To minimize these effects, administer diazepam at the IV site, not higher in the tubing. Thoroughly flush the IV line before administering diazepam if other drugs have already been administered. ▪ Assess the patient's vital signs continuously.

DRUG INTERACTIONS: Additive CNS depression may occur if diazepam is administered with other CNS depressants, such as antihistamines, tricyclic antidepressants, alcohol, narcotics, or other sedatives or hypnotics.

NALOXONE
Narcan

CLASSIFICATIONS
Pharmacologic: Narcotic
*   antagonist*
Therapeutic: Narcotic antagonist

MECHANISM OF ACTION: Naloxone's mechanism of action is not fully understood. It appears that naloxone competes with narcotic drugs opiate receptors in the CNS. This competitive action displaces narcotic analgesics from their receptor sites, blocking their effects, which include CNS depression and respiratory depression.

THERAPEUTIC BENEFIT: Naloxone reverses the effects of narcotics.

INDICATIONS FOR PREHOSPITAL USE: Naloxone is used to treat symptomatic narcotic overdose. It can also be administered as a diagnostic tool in a coma of unknown origin. If the patient is in a coma because of a narcotic overdose, the naloxone will produce improvement. If the coma is from another cause, the naloxone will not harm the patient.

CONTRAINDICATIONS: Do not administer naloxone to patients who are hypersensitive to the drug.

PRECAUTIONS: ■ Use caution in administering naloxone to patients with: ■ Supraventricular   arrhythmias. ■ Head   injury. ■ Increased   intracranial pressure. ■ Naloxone may cause seizures, so use caution in administering it to patients with convulsive disorders.

ROUTE AND DOSAGE

Adult: 0.4–2 mg by slow IV bolus. Repeat at intervals of 2–3 min if needed. If no response is seen after 10 mg has been administered, consider another cause.

Pediatric: 0.01 mg/kg by slow IV bolus. If no response, increase the dose to 0.1 mg/kg.

Neonate: 0.01 mg/kg by slow IV bolus or slowly through the umbilical vein. Repeated after 2–3 min if needed.

To prepare the solution, add 0.4 mg (1 mL) of naloxone to 9 mL of D_5W, making a drug concentration of 0.04 mg/mL. Give naloxone slowly while monitoring the rate and depth of the patient's respirations.

NOTE: If an IV line cannot be established, naloxone can be administered IM, SC, or, *with extreme care,* ET.

ADVERSE REACTIONS AND SIDE EFFECTS

- *Cardiovascular:* Ventricular tachycardia, ventricular fibrillation, hypotension, or hypertension.
- *Gastrointestinal:* Nausea, vomiting.

PARAMEDIC IMPLICATIONS: ■ Because the duration of action of naloxone is shorter than that of narcotics, repeated doses of naloxone may be necessary when treating the nonaddicted narcotic overdose patient. ■ Use caution in administering naloxone to the patient addicted to a narcotic, because naloxone may cause an acute withdrawal syndrome.

DRUG INTERACTIONS: Naloxone may cause withdrawal syndrome in the narcotic-dependent patient. **Withdrawal syndrome** is the partial collapse of an individual resulting from withdrawal of alcohol, stimulants, or some opiates. Individuals experiencing withdrawal syndrome may become very combative.

PHYSOSTIGMINE
Antilirium

CLASSIFICATIONS
Pharmacologic: Cholinergic,
cholinesterase inhibitor
Therapeutic: Antimuscarinic

MECHANISM OF ACTION: Physostigmine inhibits the breakdown of acetylcholine, resulting in the accumulation of acetylcholine at cholinergic synapses. This antagonizes anticholinergics and counteracts the anticholinergic side effects of tricyclic antidepressant overdose. Physostigmine produces generalized cholinergic responses, including bronchial constriction and bradycardia.

THERAPEUTIC BENEFIT: Physostigmine reverses the CNS effects of tricyclic antidepressant overdose and anticholinergic poisoning. These effects include delirium, hallucinations, and coma.

INDICATIONS FOR PREHOSPITAL USE: Physostigmine is used to treat tricyclic antidepressant overdose and anticholinergic poisoning.

CONTRAINDICATIONS: ■ Do not administer physostigmine to patients with: ■ Narrow-angle glaucoma. ■ Hypersensitivity to cholinesterase inhibitors.

PRECAUTIONS: ■ Use caution in administering physostigmine to patients with: ■ Diabetes. ■ Hypotension. ■ Bradycardia.

ROUTE AND DOSAGE:

Adult: 0.5–2 mg by slow IV bolus. If an IV cannot be started, administer IM.

Pediatric: 0.02 mg/kg by slow IV bolus. If an IV cannot be started, administer IM.

ADVERSE REACTIONS AND SIDE EFFECTS

- *CNS:* Restlessness, weakness, dizziness, hallucinations, seizures.
- *Cardiovascular:* Bradycardia, hypotension.
- *Respiratory:* Bronchospasm.
- *Eyes:* Pupillary constriction, tearing.
- *Gastrointestinal:* Nausea, vomiting, abdominal cramps, diarrhea.

PARAMEDIC IMPLICATIONS: ■ Assess patient vital signs frequently, especially neurologic status, heart rate, respiratory status, and blood pressure. ■ Ensure that atropine is readily available as an antidote. ■ Administer antidote if the patient shows signs of physostigmine overdose, which include:

bradycardia	stomach cramps
respiratory distress	diarrhea
seizures	diaphoresis
weakness	increased salivation/tearing
nausea/vomiting	

DRUG INTERACTIONS: Drugs with anticholinergic properties, such as atropine, antihistamines, antidepressants, haloperidol, phenothiazines, and quinidine, may antagonize the cholinergic effects of physostigmine.

PRALIDOXIME
Protopam

CLASSIFICATIONS
Pharmacologic: Quaternary
ammonium oxime
Therapeutic: Antidote—
anticholinesterase poisoning
inhibitor

MECHANISM OF ACTION: Pralidoxime reactivates cholinesterase that has been inactivated due to organophosphate pesticide poisoning.

THERAPEUTIC BENEFIT: Pralidoxime reverses respiratory paralysis and paralysis of skeletal muscles caused by organophosphate pesticide poisoning.

INDICATIONS FOR PREHOSPITAL USE: Pralidoxime is administered after atropine in severe cases of organophosphate pesticide poisoning.

CONTRAINDICATIONS: Do not administer pralidoxime to patients who have been poisoned by inorganic phosphates.

PRECAUTIONS: The dosage of pralidoxime may need to be reduced for patients with impaired renal function, because the drug may accumulate to unacceptable concentrations.

ROUTE AND DOSAGE

Adult: 1–2 g by IV infusion over 30–60 min; after the administration of atropine.

Pediatric: 20–40 mg/kg by IV infusion over 30–60 min.
Infusion Preparation: Add 1 g of pralidoxime to 500 mL of normal saline, making a drug concentration of 2 mg/mL.

ADVERSE REACTIONS AND SIDE EFFECTS

- *CNS:* Dizziness, headache.
- *Cardiovascular:* Tachycardia.
- *Eyes:* Blurred vision.
- *Gastrointestinal:* Nausea.

PARAMEDIC IMPLICATIONS: ■ Too-rapid administration may cause tachycardia, laryngospasm, or muscle rigidity. ■ Draw a blood sample for red blood cell and cholinesterase evaluation before giving pralidoxime.

DRUG INTERACTIONS: Patients who have sustained anticholinesterase poisoning should not receive morphine, theophylline, aminophylline, succinylcholine, phenothiazines, or other respiratory depressants while simultaneously receiving pralidoxime.

SODIUM NITRITE

CLASSIFICATIONS
Pharmacologic: Nitrite
Therapeutic: Cyanide poisoning
adjunct

MECHANISM OF ACTION: Sodium nitrite reacts with hemoglobin to form methemoglobin. Methemoglobin reacts with cyanide causing the cyanide to be chemically bound, which prevents it from having any toxic effect. Subsequent administration of sodium thiosulfate produces thiocyanate, which is excreted in the urine, thereby detoxifying the body.

THERAPEUTIC BENEFIT: Sodium nitrite degrades cyanide in cases of cyanide poisoning.

INDICATION FOR PREHOSPITAL USE: Sodium nitrite is the second of a 3-step treatment protocol for cyanide poisoning. It should be preceded by amyl nitrite and followed by sodium thiosulfate.

CONTRAINDICATIONS: None.

PRECAUTIONS: Sodium nitrite is a strong vasodilator. If administered too rapidly, it could cause significant hypotension.

ROUTE AND DOSAGE:

Adult: 300 mg (one 10-mL ampule of a 3% solution) after amyl nitrite inhalation. Administer either by slow IV bolus over 5 min or by diluting the 300 mg in 50–100 mL of normal saline and infusing slowly, monitoring blood pressure closely.

Pediatric: 0.15–0.33 mL/kg by slow IV bolus.

ADVERSE REACTIONS AND SIDE EFFECTS:

- *Cardiovascular:* Hypotension, tachycardia, fainting.
- *Gastrointestinal:* Nausea, vomiting.

PARAMEDIC IMPLICATIONS: ■ Monitor blood pressure during the administration of sodium nitrite. ■ Excessive doses of sodium nitrite may cause methemoglobinemia and death. **Methemoglobinemia** occurs when more than 1% of the hemoglobin in the blood has been oxidized to the ferric form. Oxidized hemoglobin is incapable of transporting oxygen. Signs of methemoglobinemia include cyanosis, vomiting, shock, and coma.

DRUG INTERACTIONS: Not applicable.

SODIUM THIOSULFATE

CLASSIFICATIONS
Pharmacologic: Thiosulfate
Therapeutic: Cyanide poisoning
* adjunct*

MECHANISM OF ACTION: Sodium thiosulfate converts cyanide to the less toxic thiocyanate. The thiocyanate is then excreted in the urine and the body is detoxified.

THERAPEUTIC BENEFIT: Sodium thiosulfate detoxifies the body in cases of cyanide poisoning.

INDICATION FOR PREHOSPITAL USE: Sodium thiosulfate is the third of a 3-step treatment protocol for cyanide poisoning. It should be preceded by amyl nitrite and sodium nitrite.

CONTRAINDICATIONS: None.

PRECAUTIONS: None.

ROUTE AND DOSAGE

Adult: 12.5 by slow IV bolus (one 50 mL ampule of a 25% solution).

Pediatric: 1.65 mL/kg of a 25% solution by slow IV bolus.

ADVERSE REACTIONS AND SIDE EFFECTS: None have been reported.

PARAMEDIC IMPLICATIONS: If the clinical response to treatment is inadequate, administer a second dose of both sodium nitrite and sodium thiosulfate at half the initial doses, 30 min after the initial doses.

DRUG INTERACTIONS: Not applicable.

SYRUP OF IPECAC

CLASSIFICATIONS
Pharmacologic: Alkaloid emetic
Therapeutic: Emetic

MECHANISM OF ACTION: Syrup of ipecac irritates the gastrointestinal mucosa and stimulates the emetic center in the brain, thus causing vomiting.

THERAPEUTIC BENEFIT: Syrup of ipecac causes vomiting to rid the stomach of ingested poisons.

INDICATIONS FOR PREHOSPITAL USE: Syrup of ipecac is used to induce vomiting in cases of poisoning or overdose in the alert patient.

CONTRAINDICATIONS: ■ Do not administer syrup of ipecac to patients who have a reduced level of consciousness, who have lost their gag reflex, or who are experiencing seizures. ▪ Do not administer syrup of ipecac to patients who have ingested caustic or petroleum products. ▪ Do not administer in cases of poisoning by ingestion of an antiemetic.

PRECAUTIONS: Use extreme caution in administering syrup of ipecac to patients with cardiac disease, because absorption or ingestion of an overdose can cause arrhythmias or myocarditis.

ROUTE AND DOSAGE

Adult: 15–30 mL PO, followed by several glasses of warm water. Repeated once after 20 min, if needed.

Pediatric (6 mo–1 y): 5–10 mL PO, followed by warm water.

Pediatric (>1 y): 15–25 mL PO, followed by warm water.

ADVERSE REACTIONS AND SIDE EFFECTS:

- *CNS:* Depression.
- *Cardiovascular:* Arrhythmias, hypotension.
- *Gastrointestinal:* Diarrhea.

PARAMEDIC IMPLICATIONS: Use carbonated sodas, fruit juice, or any other acceptable liquid the patient will drink if warm water is not available or not tolerated. However, avoid following syrup of ipecac with milk, because milk may delay the onset of action.

DRUG INTERACTIONS: ▪ Do not administer activated charcoal simultaneously with syrup of ipecac, because the charcoal will absorb the ipecac and render it ineffective. ▪ Take care not to confuse ipecac fluid extract with syrup of ipecac. Ipecac fluid extract is 14 times more concentrated and may be fatal if administered in the same volume as the syrup.

Toxicologic emergencies are becoming more and more common in prehospital emergency care. Patients who are experiencing either poisoning or overdose emergencies should be treated symptomatically. The initial prehospital management of toxicologic emergencies should include management of the ABCs, the administration of oxygen, the establishment of an IV line, and placing the patient on a cardiac monitor.

Management of poisoning emergencies includes identifying the poison, attempting to slow or stop the absorption process, and administrating an antidote. Management of overdose emergencies is aimed at stabilizing the ABCs, and in some cases antidotes.

STUDY QUESTIONS

1. Amyl nitrite is indicated in the treatment of
   a. Organophosphate poisoning.
   b. Cyanide poisoning.
   c. Narcotic overdose.
   d. Anticholinergic poisoning.

2. The initial adult dose for amyl nitrite is
   a. 1–2 mL.
   b. 0.5–1 mL.
   c. 0.3–0.6 mL.
   d. 0.1–0.3 mL.

3. Activated charcoal is used in the treatment of certain cases of poisoning and over-doses. The use of activated charcoal is contraindicated if the patient has taken
   a. Aspirin.
   b. Phenytoin.
   c. Strychnine.
   d. Cyanide.

4. The pediatric dosage for activated charcoal is
   a. 60–80 g.
   b. 30–60 g.
   c. 10–30 g.
   d. 5–10 g.

5. The two main uses for atropine in the prehospital setting are to treat symptomatic bradycardia and to treat
   a. Narcotic overdose.
   b. Organophosphate poisoning.
   c. Cyanide poisoning.
   d. Ethanol poisoning.

6. Medical control has ordered you to administer 1 mg of atropine by IV bolus to an adult patient suffering from organophosphate poisoning. If there is no improve-ment, the repeat dosage of atropine is
   a. ½ the original dose.
   b. 1 mg.
   c. 2–5 mg.
   d. 5–10 mg.

7. Naloxone is classified therapeutically as a(n)
   a. Emetic.
   b. Cyanide poisoning adjunct.
   c. Cholinesterase poisoning antidote.
   d. Narcotic antagonist.

8. The initial adult dose for naloxone to treat a patient in a coma of unknown cause is
   a. 10 mg.
   b. 2–4 mg.
   c. 0.4–2 mg.
   d. 0.4 mg/kg.

9. If a patient is overdosed with physostigmine during treatment, _____can be used as an antidote.
   a. Naloxone.
   b. Pralidoxime.
   c. Syrup of ipecac.
   d. Atropine.

10. Your pediatric patient is suffering from a severe case of organophosphate poisoning. Medical control instructs you to give the patient atropine. While you are en route to the emergency department, medical control instructs you to administer pralidoxime. How would you administer the pralidoxime?
    a. 1–2 g by IV infusion over 30–60 min.
    b. 20–40 mg/kg by IV infusion over 30–60 min.
    c. 1 mg by IV bolus. Repeat every 2–3 min as needed.
    d. 20–40 g/kg by IV infusion over 30–60 min.

11. The recommended dosage of syrup of ipecac for a 3-year-old is
    a. 5–10 mL.
    b. 15–25 mL.
    c. 15–30 mL.
    d. 30–40 mL.

CASE STUDIES

1. You are dispatched to a farm, where you are directed to a cotton field. On arrival, you find a male patient lying on the ground, shivering. The patient's son says that his father was spraying malathion on the cotton crop when he started "acting funny" just before he collapsed. Initial patient assessment reveals the following:
   - *Level of consciousness:* Depressed, responds to pain, in obvious distress.
   - *Respirations:* 36/min, shallow.
   - *Pulse:* 42/min, regular.
   - *Blood pressure:* 60 systolic.
   - *Skin:* Diaphoretic.
   - *Eyes:* Watering, constricted pupils.

   The patient is also salivating and has a watering nose. His shivering is caused by virtually all his skeletal muscles twitching simultaneously.
   A. This patient is probably suffering from
      (1) Cerebrovascular accident.
      (2) Organophosphate poisoning.
      (3) Cyanide poisoning.
      (4) Narcotic overdose.
   B. Pharmacologic treatment for this patient will probably include
      (1) Atropine and physostigmine.
      (2) Amyl nitrite and sodium nitrite.
      (3) Naloxone and pralidoxime.
      (4) Atropine and pralidoxime.

   Pralidoxime reactivates cholinesterase that has been inactivated due to organophosphate poisoning. It reverses respiratory paralysis as well as paralysis of skeletal muscles. Pralidoxmine should be given after the administration of atropine for it to be most effective. The dosage of pralidoxime is 1–2 g IV infusion over 30–60 min.

   Due to the urgency of this type of emergency, and barring no scene delays, the patient should be transported after the primary assessment and after washing has been completed. Pharmacologic therapy should ideally be done while transporting the patient to the emergency department.

2. You respond to the home of a known cocaine abuser. On arrival, you find the patient, a 21-year-old man, lying unresponsive in a closet. He has a pair of panty hose tied around his right upper arm. There are obvious "tracks" on both arms. The patient's roommate says the patient had been high on cocaine and suddenly became unconscious. Further assessment reveals:

- *Level of consciousness:* Unconscious: responds to painful stimuli by occasional tonic and clonic jerking movements and incoherent speech.
- *Respirations:* 28/min, shallow.
- *Pulse:* 124 beats/min, irregular.
- *Blood pressure:* 190/102.
- *Skin:* Warm and moist.
- *Pupils:* Dilated, slow to react.

Medical control instructs you to start an IV of normal saline at a keep-open rate. The first drug ordered in this case will probably be

a. Diazepam.
b. Naloxone.
c. Atropine.
d. Pralidoxime.

EXTENDED CASE STUDY: Overdose

Initial Response

Your ambulance is dispatched to a "possible overdose." On arrival, an anxious mother directs you to her 17-year-old son's room. You find the patient on the bedroom floor; his level of consciousness is depressed and he is unable to speak coherently. His mother says that she has not noticed anything unusual concerning her son lately. In a rapid survey of the patient's room, you notice 4 empty beer cans and an empty medication bottle labeled "Tofranil-PM, 50 mg. Take two tablets at bedtime." Initial assessment of the patient reveals the following:

- *Level of consciousness:* Conscious, disoriented, slurred speech.
- *Respirations:* 16/min, shallow.
- *Pulse:* 124 beats/min, regular.
- *Blood pressure:* 122/84.
- *Skin:* Warm, dry.
- *Pupils:* Equal, do not respond to light.

Tofranil-PM is a tricyclic antidepressant (TCA) prescribed for various forms of depression, often in conjunction with psychotherapy. It has significant anticholinergic properties and increases the effect of norepinephrine. Tofranil-PM is often used in suicide attempts. Adverse reactions and side effects of Tofranil-PM include sedation, drowsiness, confusion, hypotension, convulsions, life-threatening cardiac arrhythmias, and coma.

The evidence of alcohol ingestion in conjunction with a TCA overdose means that this is truly an emergency situation. It is necessary to maintain the patient's airway and to administer oxygen. Establish an IV line using D_5W at a keep-open rate.

Do not administer syrup of ipecac to any patient who has taken an overdose of tricyclic drugs, even an alert patient. An overdose of a TCA is sure to lead to a depressed level of consciousness, often very rapidly, even before the syrup of ipecac can have an effect.

Place the patient in the ambulance at this point, and continue treatment while en route to the emergency department.

On the way to the hospital, the patient develops seizure activity. You can administer the drug of choice in this situation, physostigmine, while en route.

Indications for physostigmine in a TCA overdose include anticholinergic seizures, severe anticholinergic delirium, and severe anticholinergic movement disorders. Physostigmine is a cholinesterase inhibitor that can reverse the toxic effects of anticholinergic and tricyclic drugs. It produces generalized cholinergic responses, including bronchial constriction and bradycardia. In this case, the adult dose of physostigmine is 0.5–2 mg by slow IV bolus. If you cannot establish an IV, administer the drug IM. If the patient shows signs of physostigmine toxicity, you can administer atropine as an antidote.

While you are en route to the emergency department, medical control orders 2 mg of physostigmine. The only noticeable result of this dose is a decrease in the patient's heart to 100 beats/min. The lack of improvement in the patient's condition could be due to his blood alcohol level, the possible ingestion of another drug, or hypoglycemia. It would not be inappropriate to administer 25 g (50 mL) of $D_{50}W$ to reverse possible hypoglycemia while still en route.

Prehospital treatment of TCA overdose is symptomatic. Toxic symptoms such as cardiac arrhythmias, seizures, and congestive failure can occur rapidly. The patient must be transported rapidly to the emergency department.

Chapter 14

Behavior Emergencies

THERAPEUTIC CLASSIFICATIONS
OF DRUGS USED FOR
BEHAVIOR EMERGENCIES
Chlorpromazine   Haloperidol
Diazepam   Hydroxyzine

CASE STUDIES

THERAPEUTIC CLASSIFICATIONS OF DRUGS USED FOR BEHAVIOR EMERGENCIES

ANTIANXIETY AGENTS
Diazepam
Hydroxyzine

ANTIPSYCHOTICS
Chlorpromazine
Haloperidol

SEDATIVE
Hydroxyzine

SEDATIVE/HYPNOTIC
Diazepam

Many prehospital emergency care professionals feel most uncomfortable and unprepared when treating patients in behavior emergencies. As a result, many EMS professionals are uncertain when faced with behavior emergencies. This uncertainty stems in part from the lack of behavior protocols for prehospital use and in part from the knowledge that the outcome of a behavior emergency is not as predictable as that of trauma or other medical emergencies. The behavioral emergency presents us with the most unpredictable scenarios and patient outcomes.

There are no definite presenting signs or symptoms for individuals with a behavior disorder. Basically, a behavior "emergency" call is a result of anxiety or panic on the part of the patient, the patient's family, or bystanders. The problem for the responder is that abnormal behavior may stem from mental illness or some other condition. For example, drug or alcohol abuse, cerebrovascular accident, infection, and metabolic disorders—each can cause symptoms that appear to indicate a behavior or mental problem.

These are the basic principles to follow when treating an individual who shows signs of psychologic or emotional disorder:

1. Clearly identify yourself, being as calm and direct as possible.
2. If possible, interview the patient alone, letting the individual tell his or her own story.

228

3. Provide honest reassurance, maintaining a nonjudgmental attitude.
4. Take a definite plan of action. This will help to relieve the patient's anxiety.
5. Never leave the patient alone, and never assume it is impossible to talk with the patient unless you have tried.

Currently, not even the most progressive EMS systems use pharmacologic interventions when treating behavior emergencies. Patient management is generally directed at supportive measures and the attempt to give the patient a feeling of friendly and secure surroundings.

There are, however, four drugs used in some prehospital emergency care systems to treat patients in behavior emergencies: chlorpromazine, diazepam, haloperidol, and hydroxyzine.

CHLORPROMAZINE
Promapar, Thorazine

CLASSIFICATIONS
Pharmacologic: Phenothiazine
Therapeutic: Antipsychotic

MECHANISM OF ACTION: Chlorpromazine inhibits by postsynaptic blockage the effects of dopamine in the central nervous system (CNS); this blockage has antipsychotic effects.

THERAPEUTIC BENEFIT: Chlorpromazine decreases the signs and symptoms of **psychosis.**

INDICATIONS FOR PREHOSPITAL USE: Chlorpromazine is used to treat acute psychotic episodes and mild alcoholic withdrawal.

CONTRAINDICATIONS: ■ Do not administer chlorpromazine to patients with: ■ Hypersensitivity to the drug. ■ CNS depression. ■ Circulatory compromise. ■ Do not administer to patients who have taken hallucinogens.

PRECAUTIONS: Because chlorpromazine may lower the seizure threshold, use caution when administering it to patients with seizure disorders.

ROUTE AND DOSAGE

Adult (psychosis): 25 mg IM.

Adult (alcohol withdrawal): 25 mg IM.

Pediatric (psychosis): 0.55 mg/kg IM.

ADVERSE REACTIONS AND SIDE EFFECTS

- *CNS:* Sedation, drowsiness, headache.
- *Cardiovascular:* Hypotension, tachycardia.
- *Eyes:* Dry eyes, blurred vision.
- *Gastrointestinal:* Dry mouth, constipation.

PARAMEDIC IMPLICATIONS: Frequently assess the patient's vital signs, especially mental status, orthostatic blood pressure, pulse, and respirations.

DRUG INTERACTIONS: ■ Additive hypotension may develop if chlorpromazine is used simultaneously with antihypertensives. ■ Additive depression may develop if chlorpromazine is used with other CNS depressants. ■ Additive anticholinergic effects may occur if chlorpromazine is used with other anticholinergic drugs.

DIAZEPAM
Valium, Valrelease

CLASSIFICATIONS:
Pharmacologic: Benzodiazepine
Therapeutic: Antianxiety agent,
*   anticonvulsant, skeletal muscle*
*   relaxant*

MECHANISM OF ACTION: Diazepam causes CNS depression. It blocks spinal cord interneuronal transmission, causing relaxation of skeletal muscles. Diazepam freely crosses the blood-brain barrier, but its actual mechanism of action is unknown.

THERAPEUTIC BENEFIT: In prehospital emergency care, diazepam is mainly used to control convulsions and decrease anxiety. It is also used in orthopedic emergencies as a skeletal muscle relaxant.

INDICATIONS FOR PREHOSPITAL USE: Diazepam is used to treat status epilepticus and major motor seizures. It can be used as a skeletal muscle relaxant for orthopedic injuries. Diazepam is used as a sedative for prehospital emergency treatment of severe anxiety.

CONTRAINDICATIONS: ■ Do not administer diazepam to patients with: ■ Hypersensitivity to the drug. ■ Preexisting CNS depression. ■ Acute narrow-angle glaucoma.

PRECAUTIONS: ■ Use caution in administering diazepam to patients with a history of psychosis or drug addiction. ■ Administer less than adult doses of diazepam to elderly patients, because they are usually more sensitive to the drug's CNS effects.

ROUTE AND DOSAGE

Adult (antianxiety/sedative):   2–10 mg by slow IV bolus or slow IM injection.

Adult (seizures/muscle relaxant):   2–5 mg by slow IV bolus. Repeat if needed, but do not exceed a total dose of 10 mg.

Adult (status epilepticus):   5–10 mg by slow IV bolus. Repeat every 10–15 min, if needed, to a maximal dose of 30 mg.

Pediatric (antianxiety/sedative):   Not recommended for prehospital use.

Pediatric (seizures/skeletal muscle relaxant):   0.2–0.5 mg/kg by slow IV bolus over 3 min. Maximal doses:
- *<5 y:* 5 mg.
- *>5 y:* 10 mg.

Pediatric (status epilepticus):

- $<5\,y$: 0.2–0.5 mg by slow IV or IM every 2–5 min, to a total dose of 5 mg.
- $>5\,y$: 1 mg every 2–5 min by slow IV or IM, to a total dose of 10 mg.

ADVERSE REACTIONS AND SIDE EFFECTS

- *CNS:* Dizziness, drowsiness, mental depression, headache.
- *Cardiovascular:* Hypotension.
- *Respiratory:* Respiratory depression.
- *Eyes:* Blurred vision, increased intraocular pressure in patients with narrow-angle glaucoma.

PARAMEDIC IMPLICATIONS: ▪ Diazepam may cause respiratory arrest if administered too rapidly or in excess. ▪ Do not mix diazepam with any other drug—diazepam may even react with the IV tubing. To minimize such reactions, administer diazepam at the IV site, not higher in the tubing. Flush the IV line before administering diazepam if other drugs have already been administered. ▪ Assess the patient's vital signs continuously.

DRUG INTERACTIONS: Additive CNS depression may occur if diazepam is administered with other CNS depressants, such as antihistamines, tricyclic antidepressants, alcohol, narcotics, or other sedatives or hypnotics.

HALOPERIDOL
Haldol

CLASSIFICATIONS
Pharmacologic: Butyrophenone
Therapeutic: Antipsychotic

MECHANISM OF ACTION: Haloperidol exerts antipsychotic effects by blocking the effects of dopamine in the CNS. It also has weak peripheral anticholinergic effects.

THERAPEUTIC BENEFIT: Haloperidol decreases the signs and symptoms of psychoses.

INDICATIONS FOR PREHOSPITAL USE: Haloperidol is used to treat acute and chronic psychoses.

CONTRAINDICATIONS: ▪ Do not administer haloperidol to patients with: ▪ Hypersensitivity to the drug. ▪ CNS depression. ▪ Circulatory compromises.

PRECAUTIONS: Use caution in administering haloperidol to patients with seizure disorders, because the drug may lower the seizure threshold.

ROUTE AND DOSAGE

Adult: 2–5 mg IM.

Pediatric: Haloperidol is not recommended for pediatric patients in the prehospital setting.

ADVERSE REACTIONS AND SIDE EFFECTS

- *CNS:* Sedation, confusion, restlessness, seizures.
- *Respiratory:* Respiratory depression.

- *Cardiovascular:* Hypotension, tachycardia.
- *Gastrointestinal:* Dry mouth, constipation.

PARAMEDIC IMPLICATIONS: Assess patient mental status, blood pressure, pulse, and respirations before and frequently after drug administration.

DRUG INTERACTIONS: ▪ Haloperidol use with antihypertensives or nitrates may produce additive hypotension. ▪ Use with other CNS depressants may cause additive CNS depression. ▪ Using haloperidol with anticholinergics may cause additive anticholinergic effects. ▪ Phenobarbital may decrease the effectiveness of haloperidol.

HYDROXYZINE
Atarax, Vistaril

CLASSIFICATIONS
Pharmacologic: Antihistamine
Therapeutic: Antianxiety agent,
  sedative

MECHANISM OF ACTION: Hydroxyzine acts as a CNS depressant through suppression of activity at the subcortical levels in the brain.

THERAPEUTIC BENEFIT: Hydroxyzine causes relief of anxiety and sedation.

INDICATIONS FOR PREHOSPITAL USE: Hydroxyzine is used in treatment of anxiety.

CONTRAINDICATIONS: Do not administer hydroxyzine to patients who are hypersensitive to the drug.

PRECAUTIONS: Use caution when administering hydroxyzine to elderly patients; use less than adult dosages.

ROUTE AND DOSAGE

Adult: 50–100 mg deep IM.

Pediatric: 1.0 mg/kg deep IM.

ADVERSE REACTIONS AND SIDE EFFECTS

- *CNS:* Drowsiness, dizziness, weakness, headache.
- *Respiratory:* Wheezing, chest tightness.
- *Gastrointestinal:* Dry mouth, nausea.

PARAMEDIC IMPLICATIONS: Administer hydroxyzine deep into well-developed muscle to prevent subcutaneous tissue infiltration. Inadvertent injection into the subcutaneous tissue may cause tissue damage.

DRUG INTERACTIONS: ▪ Additive CNS depression may occur if hydroxyzine is used with other CNS depressants, antidepressants, antihistamines, narcotics, or sedative/hypnotics. ▪ Additive anticholinergic effects may occur if hydroxyzine is used with other drugs that have anticholinergic properties.

Patients who present with irrational behavior may do so because of disease or injury process, not because of mental illness. For example, head injury, drug abuse, or a severe diabetic episode can lead to behavior suggestive of a psychotic disorder. If possible, the patient who presents with psychotic behavior should be assessed for other medical or physical causes. For example, giving an antipsychotic drug to an individual suffering from an overdose of crack cocaine would not help and could be harmful. If the patient's problem is in fact of psychiatric origin, treat the patient appropriately.

It is more appropriate to give antipsychotic drugs in the hospital setting, which is a more controlled environment. However, there may be occasions when prehospital antipsychotic drug therapy is ordered before transport to an emergency facility is complete. As with any emergency situation, follow local protocols.

STUDY QUESTIONS

1. Chlorpromazine and haloperidol are classified as antipsychotics, and their use is contraindicated for patients
   a. In mild alcohol withdrawal.
   b. With CNS depression.
   c. With a history of acute psychotic episodes.
   d. With a history of seizure disorders.

2. The recommended adult dose for chlorpromazine is
   a. 15 mg.
   b. 20 mg.
   c. 25 mg.
   d. 30 mg.

3. What dose of haloperidol would you expect medical control to order for an 11-year-old patient suffering from chronic psychosis?
   a. 0.55 mg/kg.
   b. 2–5 mg.
   c. 25 mg.
   d. None.

4. You have a pediatric patient who weighs 46 lb. Medical control instructs you to administer hydroxyzine to this patient for the treatment of anxiety. What dose of hydroxyzine would you give?
   a. 21 mg.
   b. 30 mg.
   c. 46 mg.
   d. 101 mg.

CASE STUDIES

1. At 5:30 AM you are called to the home of a man "not breathing." On arrival you determine that the individual has been down too long, and resuscitative efforts should not be initiated. When you tell the wife, she becomes hysterical. You attempt to calm her down, but nothing you do seems to help. After your calming efforts fail, you call medical control and explain the situation, and add that you are afraid to leave her. The physician agrees and orders sedation and transport. Which drug(s) should the physician order for sedation?

a. Chlorpromazine.
b. Haloperidol.
c. Diazepam.
d. Hydroxyzine.

2. You are called to the home of an individual who has previously experienced psychotic episodes and seizures. On arrival, the patient is displaying bizarre and aggressive behavior. The more you attempt to calm him down, the more aggressive he seems to become. Medical control is familiar with this patient, and instructs you to give him 25 mg of chlorpromazine to treat his psychosis. In this situation, what other drug should you have readily available?
a. Haloperidol.
b. Diazepam.
c. Hydroxyzine.
d. $D_{50}W$.

EXTENDED CASE STUDY: Psychotic Emergency

You respond to a local warehouse for a "man acting bizarre." While en route to the scene, you request that the police also respond.

On your arrival, the warehouse foreman tells you that the patient is an excellent employee and has never before caused any problems. However, today he has been very loud, has broken several pieces of equipment, and has been rude to several of his fellow workers. He is now sitting quietly at a table in the corner. His wife is in the foreman's office, confused and scared.

Before making any attempt to approach the patient, try to obtain information about the patient from his wife. Family members can frequently provide some clues as to the nature of the patient's problem. The police can stand by (ideally out of sight) while you speak with the patient's wife.

The patient's wife says that her husband has been under a lot of stress at work lately, because of increased project deadlines. He is 40, in good health, takes no medications, and has no history of psychiatric disorders.

It is very difficult for a prehospital emergency care professional to eliminate probable causes of behavior emergencies in the prehospital setting. It is not appropriate to draw any definite conclusions based solely on information gathered from history, which is often only suggestive at best.

Approach the patient with a suspected mental disorder in a slow, calm, deliberate manner. Calmly explain why you were called, and assure him or her that you are there to help in any way that you can.

It can be frustrating to try to communicate with this type of patient, who may not be dealing in reality. A commonsense approach to the patient, combining reinforcement of factual information and reassurance, is recommended.

So far, your patient has exhibited no aggressive behavior. He allowed his vital signs to be taken; they are:

- *Level of consciousness:* Alert, disoriented.
- *Respirations:* 16 breaths/min.
- *Pulse:* 82 beats/min, regular.
- *Blood pressure:* 156/96.

There are no other obvious signs of trauma or medical problems.

While you are helping the patient to the ambulance, he suddenly goes into a grand mal seizure. Your immediate course of action should be to protect the patient from injuring himself and to protect the airway during the seizure. The seizure is clonic and subsides after approximately 2 min. The patient remains unconscious. At this point, place the patient in the ambulance and administer humidified oxygen.

While en route to the hospital, the patient goes into another seizure, which also lasts approximately 2 min. Medical control orders an IV of D_5W at a keep-open rate and 5 mg of diazepam by slow IV bolus. If necessary, another 5 mg can be given.

Patients with mental disorders are rarely sedated in the prehospital setting. In this case, the diazepam is primarily to help control seizure activity. Diazepam depresses the CNS, causing seizure activity to subside.

During transport, you monitor the patient closely, alert for any changes. The patient is still unconscious. His reflexes are normal, his vital signs are stable, and his pupils are equal and reactive.

Patients with mental disorders are usually difficult to manage. The role of the prehospital emergency care professional is primarily supportive. Occasionally these patients exhibit aggressive behavior and may perceive you as a threat to their safety or an ally of their enemies. A calm, nonthreatening approach can work toward patient confidence, regardless of whether the patient is behaving aggressively or passively. Expressing a desire to help frequently produces positive results.

Patients who experience severe psychotic episodes in the prehospital setting may require antipsychotic drugs such as chlorpromazine or haloperidol. These drugs block dopamine receptors in the brain associated with behavior and mood. The adult dose of chlorpromazine is 25 mg IM, and the adult dose of haloperidol is 2–5 mg, also IM. Although it is rare for these drugs to be administered in the prehospital setting, it is important for you to be familiar with them, because you may administer them while working in the hospital setting.

In most cases when a mental disorder is suspected, quiet transport to the emergency department is called for. The siren can be disturbing for the patient, and it should not be used unless a life-threatening emergency exists.

Appendix A

Drugs (Generic and Trade Names) and Their Therapeutic Classifications*

Drug Name	Therapeutic Classification(s)
A-Methapred (methylprednisolone)	Anti-inflammatory, immunosuppressant
Abeneton (biperiden)	Antiparkinsonian
acebutolol	Antihypertensive, antiarrhythmic
Acephen (acetaminophen)	Non-narcotic analgesic, antipyretic
acetaminophen	Non-narcotic analgesic, antipyretic
acetazolamide	Anticonvulsant, diuretic
acetohexamide	Antidiabetic
acetophenazine	Antipsychotic
Activase (alteplase)	Antithrombolytic enzyme
Adalat (nifedipine)	Antianginal
Adapin (doxepin)	Antidepressant
Adrenalin Chloride (epinephrine hydrochloride)	Bronchodilator, vasopressor, cardiac stimulant, local anesthetic adjunct, topical antihemorrhagic, antiglaucoma agent
Aerolate (theophylline)	Bronchodilator
Akineton (biperiden)	Antiparkinsonian
Ak-Zol (acetazolamide)	Anticonvulsant, diuretic
Alalat (nifedipine)	Antianginal
Alazsine Tabs (hydralazine)	Antihypertensive
albuterol	Bronchodilator
Aldactone (spironolactone)	Antihypertensive, diuretic
Alphancaine (lidocaine)	Ventricular antiarrhythmic, local anesthetic
alprazolam	Antianxiety agent—controlled substance, Schedule IV
alteplase	Thrombolytic enzyme
Alupent (metaproterenol)	Bronchodilator
Alzapam (lorazepam)	Antianxiety agent, sedative/hypotic—controlled substance, Schedule IV
A-methapred (methylprednisolone)	Anti-inflammatory
Amcill (ampicillin)	Antibiotic
Aminophyllin (aminophylline)	Bronchodilator

* Drug names beginning with a capital letter are trade; drug names beginning with a lowercase letter are generic.

236

Drug Name	Therapeutic Classification(s)
aminophylline	Bronchodilator
amiodarone	Ventricular and supraventricular antiarrhythmic
amitriptyline	Antidepressant
amobarbital	Sedative/hypnotic, anticonvulsant—controlled substance, Schedule II
Amodopa Tabs (methyldopa)	Antihypertensive
Amoline (aminophylline)	Bronchodilator
amoxapine	Antidepressant
amoxicillin	Antibiotic
Amoxil (amoxicillin)	Antibiotic
amphotericin B	Antifungal
ampicillin	Antibiotic
amrinone	Inotropic, vasodilator
amyl nitrite	Cyanide poisoning adjunct
Amytal (amobarbital)	Sedative/hypnotic, anticonvulsant—controlled substance, Schedule II
Anacin-3 (acetaminophen)	Non-narcotic analgesic, antipyretic
Anestucon (lidocaine)	Ventricular antiarrhythmic, local anesthetic
Ang-O-Span (nitroglycerin [oral])	Antianginal, vasodilator
Anspor (cephradine)	Antibiotic
Antilirium (physostigmine)	Antimuscarinic
Apo-Amitriptyline (amitriptyline)	Antidepressant
Apresoline (hydralazine)	Antihypertensive
Aprozide (hydrochlorothiazide)	Diuretic, antihypertensive
Aquachloral (chloral hydrate)	Sedative/hypnotic—controlled substance, Schedule IV
Aquatensen (methyclothiazide)	Diuretic, antihypertensive
Arm-a-Med (isoetharine)	Bronchodilator
Asendin (amoxapine)	Antidepressant
Asthma Nefrin (epinephrine hydrochloride)	Bronchodilator, vasopressor, cardiac stimulant, local anesthetic adjunct, topical antihemorrhagic, antiglaucoma agent
AsthmaHaler (epinephrine bitartrate)	Bronchodilator, vasopressor, cardiac stimulant, local anesthetic adjunct, topical antihemorrhagic, antiglaucoma agent
Astromorph (morphine)	Analgesic—controlled substance, Schedule II
Atarax (hydroxyzine)	Antianxiety agent, sedative
atenolol	Antihypertensive, antianginal
atropine	Antiarrhythmic
Atrovent (ipratropium)	Bronchodilator
Auto-Injector (lidocaine)	Ventricular antiarrhythmic, local anesthetic
Aventyl (nortriptyline)	Antidepressant

* Drug names beginning with a capital letter are trade; drug names beginning with a lowercase letter are generic.

Drug Name	Therapeutic Classification(s)
Bacampicillin	Antibiotic
Barbased (bitabarbital)	Sedative/hypnotic—controlled substance, Schedule III
Barbita (phenobarbital)	Anticonvulsant, sedative/hypnotic—controlled substance, Schedule IV
beclomethasone	Anti-inflammatory, antiasthmatic
Beclovent (beclomethasone)	Anti-inflammatory, antiasthmatic
Beconase (beclomethasone)	Anti-inflammatory,antiasthmatic
Beef Regular Iletin II (insulin [regular])	Antidiabetic agent
Beldin (diphenhydramine)	Antihistamine, antiemetic and antivertigo agent, antitussive, sedative/hypnotic, topical anesthetic
Benadryl (diphenhydramine)	Antihistamine, antiemetic and antivertigo agent, antitussive, sedative/hypnotic, topical anesthetic
Benadryl Children's Allergy (diphenhydramine)	Antihistamine, antiemetic and antivertigo agent, antitussive, sedative/hypnotic, topical anesthetic
Benadryl Complete Allergy (diphenhydramine)	Antihistamine, antiemetic and antivertigo agent, antitussive, sedative/hypnotic, topical anesthetic
Bendylate (diphenhydramine)	Antihistamine, antiemetic and antivertigo agent, antitussive, sedative/hypnotic, topical anesthetic
Benylin (diphenhydramine)	Antihistamine, antiemetic and antivertigo agent, antitussive, sedative/hypnotic, topical anesthetic
Benylin DM Cough (dextromethorphan)	Non-narcotic antitussive
benzphetamine	Anorexigenic agent
Beta-2 (isoetharine)	Bronchodilator
biperiden	Antiparkinsonian
Bisorine (isoetharine)	Bronchodilator
Bitolterol	Bronchodilator
Blocadren (timolol)	Antihypertensive, antiglaucoma agent
Brethine (terbutaline)	Bronchodilator
bretylium tosylate	Antiarrhythmic
Bretylol (bretylium)	Antiarrhythmic
Bricanyl (terbutaline)	Bronchodilator
Bromo-Seltzer (acetaminophen)	Non-narcotic analgesic, antipyretic
bromocriptine	Antiparkinsonian agent
Bronitin Mist (epinephrine bitartrate)	Bronchodilator, vasopressor, cardiac stimulant, local anesthetic adjunct, topical antihemorrhagic, antiglaucoma agent

* Drug names beginning with a capital letter are trade; drug names beginning with a lowercase letter are generic.

Drug Name	Therapeutic Classification(s)
Bronkaid Mist (epinephrine)	Bronchodilator, vasopressor, cardia stimulant, local anesthetic adjunct, topical antihemorrhagic, antiglaucoma agent
Bronkaid Mist Suspension (epinephrine bitartrate)	Bronchodilator, vasopressor, cardiac stimulant, local anesthetic adjunct, topical antihemorrhagic, antiglaucoma agent
Bronkodyl (theophylline)	Bronchodilator
Bronkosol (isoetharine)	Bronchodilator
bumetanide	Antihypertensive, diuretic
Bumex	Antihypertensive, diuretic
butabarbital	Sedative/hypnotic—controlled substance, Schedule III
Butalan (butabarbital)	Sedative/hypnotic—controlled substance, Schedule III
Butatran (butabarbital)	Sedative/hypnotic—controlled substance, Schedule III
Buticaps (butabarbital)	Sedative/hypnotic—controlled substance, Schedule III
Butisol (butabarbital)	Sedative/hypnotic—controlled substance, Schedule III
butorphanol	Narcotic agonist-antagonist, opioid partial agonist
Calan (verapamil)	Antianginal, antiarrhythmic, antihypertensive
Capoten (captopril)	Antihypertensive
calcium chloride	Electrolyte modifier
calcium gluceptate	Electrolyte modifier
calcium gluconate	Electrolyte modifier
captopril	Antihypertensive
carbamazepine	Anticonvulsant, analgesic
carbenicillin	Antibiotic
Cardizem (diltiazem)	Antianginal
Catapres (clonidine)	Antihypertensive
Catapres-TTS (clonidine)	Antihypertensive
Ceclor (cefaclor)	Antibiotic
Cedilanid-D Injections (deslanoside)	Antiarrhythmic, inotropic
cefaclor	Antibiotic
Celontin Half Strength Kapseals (methsuximide)	Anticonvulsant
Celontin Kapseals (methsuximide)	Anticonvulsant
Centrax (prazepam)	Antianxiety agent-—controlled substance, Schedule IV
cephradine	Antibiotic

* Drug names beginning with a capital letter are trade; drug names beginning with a lowercase letter are generic.

Drug Name	Therapeutic Classification(s)
chloral hydrate	Sedative/hypnotic—controlled substance, Schedule IV
Chlorpazine (prochlorpazine)	Antipsychotic, antiemetic, antianxiety agent
chlordiazepoxide	Antianxiety agent, anticonvulsant, sedative/hypnotic—controlled substance, Schedule IV
chlorothiazide	Diuretic, antihypertensive
chlorpromazine	Antipsychotic, antiemetic
chlorpropamide	Antidiabetic, antidiuretic agent
chlorprothixene	Antipsychotic
chlorthalidone	Diuretic, antihypertensive
Chlorzide (hydrochlorothiazide)	Diuretic, antihypertensive
Chlorzine (chlorpromazine)	Antipsychotic, antiemetic
Choledyl (oxtriphylline)	Bronchodilator
Cin-Quin (quinidine)	Ventricular and supraventricular antiarrhythmic, atrial antiarrhythmic
clemastine	Antihistamine
clonazepam	Anticonvulsant—controlled substance, Schedule IV
clonidine	Antihypertensive
clorazepate	Antianxiety agent, anticonvulsant, sedative/hypnotic—controlled substance, Schedule IV
codeine	Analgesic, antitussive—controlled substance, Schedule II
Compazine (prochlorperazine)	Antipsychotic, antiemetic, antianxiety agent
Compazine Spansule (prochlorperazine)	Antipsychotic, antiemetic, antianxiety agent
Compoz (diphenhydramine)	Antihistamine, antiemetic and antivertigo agent, antitussive, sedative/hypnotic, topical anesthetic
Congesprin (dextromethorphan)	Non-narcotic antitussive
Constant-T (theophylline)	Bronchodilator
Cordarone (amiodarone)	Ventricular and supraventricular antiarrhythmic
Corgard (nadolol)	Antihypertensive, antianginal
Cortef (hydrocortisone)	Anti-inflammatory
Cortisol (hydrocortisone)	Anti-inflammatory
Coumadin (warfarin)	Anticoagulant
Cremacoat 1 (dextromethorphan)	Non-narcotic antitussive
Crystodigin (digitoxin)	Antiarrhythmic agent, inotropic agent
Dalcaine (lidocaine)	Ventricular antiarrhythmic, local anesthetic

* Drug names beginning with a capital letter are trade; drug names beginning with a lowercase letter are generic.

Drug Name	Therapeutic Classification(s)
Dalmane (flurazepam)	Sedative/hypnotic—controlled substance, Schedule IV
Darvon (propoxyphene)	Analgesic—controlled substance, Schedule IV
Datril (acetaminophen)	Non-narcotic analgesic, antipyretic
Datril-500 (acetaminophen)	Non-narcotic analgesic, antipyretic
Decadron (dexamethasone)	Anti-inflammatory
Delsym (dextromethorphan)	Non-narcotic antitussive
Demerol (meperidine)	Analgesic—controlled substance, Schedule II
Depakene (valproic acid)	Anticonvulsant
desipramine	Antidepressant, antianxiety agent
deslanoside	Antiarrhythmic, inotropic
dexamethasone	Anti-inflammatory
dextromethorphan	Non-narcotic antitussive
dextrose 50% in water	Hyperglycemic
Dey-Dose (isoetharine)	Bronchodilator
Dey-Lute (isoetharine)	Bronchodilator
DiaBeta (glyburide)	Antidiabetic
Diabinese (chlorpropamide)	Antidiabetic, antidiuretic agent
Diachlor (chlorothiazide)	Diuretic, antihypertensive
Diahist (diphenhydramine)	Antihistamine, antiemetic and antivertigo agent, antitussive, sedative/hypnotic, topical anesthetic
Diamox (acetazolamide)	Anticonvulsant, diuretic
Diamox Sequels (acetazolamide)	Anticonvulsant, diuretic
Diaqua (hydrochlorothiazide)	Diuretic, antihypertensive
diazepam	Antianxiety agent, skeletal muscle relaxant, amnesic agent, anticonvulsant, sedative/hypnotic
diazoxide	Antihypertensive
Didrex (benzphetamine)	Anorexigenic agent
digitoxin	Antiarrhythmic, inotropic
digoxin	Antiarrhythmic, inotropic
Dilantin (phenytoin)	Anticonvulsant, antiarrhythmic
Dilaudid (hydromorphone)	Analgesic, antitussive
Dilocaine (lidocaine)	Ventricular antiarrhythmic, local anesthetic
diltiazem	Antianginal
Diphen (diphenhydramine)	Antihistamine, antiemetic and antivertigo agent, antitussive, sedative/hypnotic,
Diphen (diphenhydramine)	topical anesthetic
Diphenadril (diphenhydramine)	Antihistamine, antiemetic and antivertigo agent, antitussive, sedative/hypnotic, topical anesthetic

* Drug names beginning with a capital letter are trade; drug names beginning with a lowercase letter are generic.

Drug Name	Therapeutic Classification(s)
diphenhydramine	Antihistamine, antiemetic and antivertigo agent, antitussive, sedative/hypnotic, topical anesthetic
dipyridamole	Coronary vasodilator, platelet aggregation inhibitor
disopyramide	Ventricular/supraventricular antiarrhythmia, atrial antitachyarrhythmic
Dispos-a-Med (isoetharine)	Bronchodilator
Diuril (chlorothiazide)	Diuretic, antihypertensive
DM Cough (dextromethorphan)	Non-narcotic antitussive
dobutamine	Inotropic
Dobutrex (dobutamine)	Intropic
Dolene (propoxyphene)	Analgesic—controlled substance, Schedule IV
Dolophine (methadone)	Analgesic, narcotic detoxification adjunct—controlled substance, Schedule II
dopamine	Inotropic, vasopressor
Dopastat (dopamine)	Inotropic, vasopressor
Doriden (glutethimide)	Sedative/hypnotic—controlled substance, Schedule III
Doriglute (glutethimide)	Sedative/hypnotic—controlled substance, Schedule III
Doxaphene (propoxyphene)	Analgesic—controlled substance, Schedule IV
doxepin	Antidepressant
Duramorph (morphine)	Analgesic—controlled substance, Schedule II
Durapam (flurazepam)	Sedative/hypnotic—controlled substance, Schedule IV
Dymelor (acetohexamide)	Antidiabetic
Edecrin (ethacrynic acid)	Diuretic
edrophonium	Antiarrhythmic, cholinergic agonist
Elavil (amitriptyline)	Antidepressant
Elixophyllin (theophylline)	Bronchodilator
Emitrip (amitriptyline)	Antidepressant
Endep (amitriptyline)	Antidepressant
Enduron (methyclothiazide)	Diuretic, antihypertensive
Enovil (amitriptyline)	Antidepressant
Epifrin (epinephrine hydrochloride)	Bronchodilator, vasopressor, cardiac stimulant, local anesthetic adjunct, topical antihemorrhagic, antiglaucoma agent
epinephrine	Bronchodilator, vasopressor, cardiac stimulant, local anesthetic adjunct, topical antihemorrhagic, antiglaucoma agent

* Drug names beginning with a capital letter are trade; drug names beginning with a lowercase letter are generic.

Drug Name	Therapeutic Classification(s)
epinephrine bitartrate	Bronchodilator, vasopressor, cardiac stimulant, local anesthetic adjunct, topical antihemorrhagic, antiglaucoma agent
epinephrine hydrochloride	Bronchodilator, vasopressor, cardiac stimulant, local anesthetic adjunct, topical antihemorrhagic, antiglaucoma agent
EpiPen (epinephrine)	Bronchodilator, vasopressor, cardiac stimulant, local anesthetic adjunct, topical antihemorrhagic, antiglaucoma agent
EpiPen Jr. (epinephrine)	Bronchodilator, vasopressor, cardiac stimulant, local anesthetic adjunct, topical antihemorrhagic, antiglaucoma agent
Epitol (carbamazepine)	Anticonvulsant, analgesic
Epitrate (epinephrine bitartrate)	Bronchodilator, vasopressor, cardiac stimulant, local anesthetic adjunct, topical antihemorrhagic, antiglaucoma agent
Equanil (meprobamate)	Antianxiety agent—controlled substance, Schedule IV
Esidrix (hydrochlorothiazide)	Diuretic, antihypertensive
Eskalith (lithium)	Antimanic, antipsychotic
Eskalith CR (lithium)	Antimanic, antipsychotic
ethacrynic acid	Diuretic
ethchlorvynol	Sedative/hypnotic—controlled substance, Schedule IV
ethosuximide	Anticonvulsant
Eutonil (pargyline)	Antihypertensive
Extentabs (quinidine)	Ventricular and supraventricular antiarrhythmic, atrial antiarrhythmic
Fenylhist (diphenhydramine)	Antihistamine, antiemetic and antivertigo agent, antitussive, sedative/hypnotic, topical anesthetic
flecainide	Ventricular antiarrhythmic
flurazepam	Sedative/hypnotic—controlled substance, Schedule IV
Fortrol (pentazocine)	Analgesic—controlled substance, Schedule IV
Fungizone (amphotericin B)	Antifungal
furosemide	Diuretic, antihypertensive
Fynex (diphenhydramine)	Antihistamine, antiemetic and antivertigo agent, antitussive, sedative/hypnotic, topical anesthetic
Geopen (carbenicillin)	Antibiotic
Glaucon (epinephrine hydrochloride)	Bronchodilator, vasopressor, cardiac stimulant, local anesthetic adjunct, topical antihemorrhagic, antiglaucoma agent

* Drug names beginning with a capital letter are trade; drug names beginning with a lowercase letter are generic.

Drug Name	Therapeutic Classification(s)
glipizide	Antidiabetic agent
Glucamide (chlorpropamide)	Antidiabetic, antidiuretic agent
Glucotrol (glipizide)	Antidiabetic agent
glutethimide	Sedative/hypnotic—controlled substance, Schedule III
glyburide	Antidiabetic
guanabenz	Antihypertensive
guanethidine	Antihypertensive
halazepam	Antianxiety agent—controlled substance, Schedule IV
Halcion (triazolam)	Sedative/hypnotic—controlled substance, Schedule III
Haldol (haloperidol)	Antipsychotic
haloperidol	Antipsychotic
Hexadrol (dexamethasone)	Anti-inflammatory
Hold (dextromethorphan)	Non-narcotic antitussive
Humulin R (insulin [regular])	Antidiabetic agent
hydralazine	Antihypertensive
Hydramine (diphenhydramine)	Antihistamine, antiemetic and antivertigo agent, antitussive, sedative/hypnotic, topical anesthetic
Hydril (diphenhydramine)	Antihistamine, antiemetic and antivertigo agent, antitussive, sedative/hypnotic, topical anesthetic
Hydro DIURIL (hydrochlorothiazide)	Diuretic, antihypertensive
Hydro-Z-50 (hydrochlorothiazide)	Diuretic, antihypertensive
hydrochlorothiazide	Diuretic, antihypertensive
hydrocortisone	Anti-inflammatory
Hydrocortone (hydrocortisone)	Anti-inflammatory
Hydromal (hydrochlorothiazide)	Diuretic, antihypertensive
hydromorphone	Analgesic, antitussive
hydroxyzine	Antianxiety agent, sedative
Hygroton (chlorthalidone)	Diuretic, antihypertensive
Hyperstat (diazoxide)	Antihypertensive
Hylidone (chlorthalidone)	Diuretic, antihypertensive
Inderal (propranolol)	Antihypertensive, antianginal, antiarrhythmic
Inderal LA (propranolol)	Antihypertensive, antianginal, antiarrhythmic
Inocor (amrinone)	Inotropic, vasodilator
insulin (regular)	Antidiabetic agent
Intropin (dopamine)	Inotropic, vasopressor
ipratropium	Bronchodilator
Ismelin (guanethidine)	Antihypertensive

* Drug names beginning with a capital letter are trade; drug names beginning with a lowercase letter are generic.

Drug Name	Therapeutic Classification(s)
Isomotic (isosorbide)	Antiglaucoma agent
isocarboxazid	Antidepressant
isoetharine	Bronchodilator
isoproterenol	Antiarrhythmic, bronchodilator, cardiac stimulant
Isoptin (verapamil)	Antianginal, antihypertensive, antiarrhythmic
isosorbide	Antiglaucoma agent
Klavikordal (nitroglycerin [oral])	Antianginal, vasodilator
Klonopin (clonazepam)	Anticonvulsant—controlled substance, Schedule IV
L-caine (lidocaine)	Ventricular antiarrhythmic, local anesthetic
labetalol	Antihypertensive
Lanoxicaps (digoxin)	Antiarrhythmic agent, inotropic agent
Lanoxin (digoxin)	Antiarrhythmic, inotropic
Lasix (furosemide)	Diuretic, antihypertensive
Levoprome (methotrimeprazine)	Sedative, analgesic agent, antipruritic
Librium (chlordiazepoxide)	Antianxiety agent, anticonvulsant, sedative/hypnotic—controlled substance, Schedule IV
lidocaine	Ventriculr antiarrhythmic, local anesthetic
Lidoject (lidocaine)	Ventricular antiarrhythmic, local anesthetic
LidoPen (lidocaine)	Ventricular antiarrhythmic, local anesthetic
Lipoxide (chlordiazepoxide)	Antianxiety agent, anticonvulsant, sedative/hypnotic—controlled substance, Schedule IV
Lithane (lithium)	Antimanic, antipsychotic
lithium	Antimanic, antipsychotic
Lithobid (lithium)	Antimanic, antipsychotic
Lithonate (lithium)	Antimanic, antipsychotic
Lithotabs (lithium)	Antimanic, antipsychotic
Loniten (minoxidil)	Antihypertensive
Loraz (lorazepam)	Antianxiety agent, sedative/hypnotic—controlled substance, Schedule IV
lorazepam	Antianxiety agent, sedative/hypnotic—controlled substance, Schedule IV
Lopressor (metoprolol)	Antihypertensive
Ludiomil (maprotiline)	Antidepressant
Luminal (phenobarbital)	Anticonvulsant, sedative/hypnotic—controlled substance, Schedule IV
mannitol	Diuretic
maprotiline	Antidepressant
Marplan (isocarboxazid)	Antidepressant

* Drug names beginning with a capital letter are trade; drug names beginning with a lowercase letter are generic.

Drug Name	Therapeutic Classification(s)
Mazepine (carbamazepine)	Anticonvulsant, analgesic
Mebaral (mephobarbital)	Anticonvulsant—controlled substance, Schedule IV
Medihaler-Epi (epinephrine bitartrate) .	Bronchodilator, vasopressor, cardiac stimulant, local anesthetic adjunct, topical antihemorrhagic, antiglaucoma agent
Mediquell (dextromethorphan)	Non-narcotic antitussive
Medrol (methylprednisolone)	Anti-inflammatory, immunosuppressant
Mellaril-S (thioridazine)	Antipsychotic
Mentaban (mephobarbital)	Anticonvulsant—controlled substance, Schedule IV
meperidine	Analgesic—controlled substance, Schedule II
mephenytoin	Anticonvulsant
mephobarbital	Anticonvulsant—controlled substance, Schedule IV
meprobamate	Antianxiety agent—controlled substance, Schedule IV
Meprospan (meprobamate)	Antianxiety agent—controlled substance, Schedule IV
Mesantoin (mephenytoin)	Anticonvulsant
mesoridazine	Antipsychotic
Metaprel (metaproterenol)	Bronchodilator
metaprolol	Antihypertensive
metaproterenol	Bronchodilator
methadone	Analgesic, narcotic detoxification adjunct—controlled substance, Schedule II
Methadose (methadone)	Analgesic, narcotic detoxification adjunct—controlled substance, Schedule II
Methidate (methylpenidate)	CNS stimulant—controlled substance, Schedule II
methotrimeprazine	Sedative, analgesic agent, antipruritic
methyclothiazide	Diuretic, antihypertensive
methyldopa	Antihypertensive
methylphenidate	CNS stimulant—controlled substance, Schedule II
methylprednisolone	Anti-inflammatory
methyprylon	Sedative/hypnotic—controlled substance, Schedule III
metoprolol	Antihypertensive
mexiletine	Ventricular antiarrhythmic
Mexitil (mexiletine)	Ventricular antiarrhythmic

* Drug names beginning with a capital letter are trade; drug names beginning with a lowercase letter are generic.

Drug Name	Therapeutic Classification(s)
Micronase (glyburide)	Antidiabetic
MicroNefrin (epinephrine hydrochloride)	Bronchodilator, vasopressor, cardiac stimulant, local anesthetic adjunct, topical antihemorrhagic, antiglaucoma agent
Milontin (phensuximide)	Anticonvulsant
Miltown (meprobamate)	Antianxiety agent—controlled substance, Schedule IV
Minipress (prazosin)	Antihypertensive
minoxidil	Antihypertensive
morphine	Analgesic—controlled substance, Schedule II
MS Contin (morphine)	Analgesic—controlled substance, Schedule II
Murcil (chlordiazepoxide)	Antianxiety agent, anticonvulsant, sedative/hypnotic—controlled substance, Schedule IV
Myidone (primidone)	Anticonvulsant
Mysoline (primidone)	Anticonvulsant
N-G-C (nitroglycerin [oral])	Antianginal, vasodilator
nadolol	Antihypertensive, antianginal
nalbuphine	Analgesic
Nalicaine (lidocaine)	Ventricular antiarrhythmic, local anesthetic
naloxone	Narcotic antagonist
Napamide (disopyramide)	Ventricular/supraventricular antiarrhythmia, atrial antitachyarrhythmic
Narcan (naloxone)	Narcotic antagonist
nardil (phenelzine)	Antidepressant
Navane (thiothixene)	Antipsychotic
Nembutal (pentobarbital)	Anticonvulsant, sedative/hypnotic—controlled substance, Schedule II; suppositories under Schedule III
Nervine (diphenhydramine)	Antihistamine, antiemetic and antivertigo agent, antitussive, sedative/hypnotic, topical anesthetic
Nervocaine (lidocaine)	Ventricular antiarrhythmic, local anesthetic
Neuramate (meprobamate)	Antianxiety agent—contorlled substance, Schedule IV
Neurate (meprobamate)	Antianxiety agent—controlled substance, Schedule IV
nifedipine	Antianginal
Nighttime Sleep-Aid (diphenhydramine)	Antihistamine, antiemetic and antivertigo agent, antitussive, sedative/hypnotic, topical anesthetic
Niong (nitroglycerin [oral])	Antianginal, vasodilator

* Drug names beginning with a capital letter are trade; drug names beginning with a lowercase letter are generic.

Drug Name	Therapeutic Classification(s)
Nitro-bid (nitroglycerin [oral])	Antianginal, vasodilator
Nitrobid (nitroglycerin [topical])	Antianginal, vasodilator
Nitrocap (nitroglycerin [oral])	Antianginal, vasodilator
Nitrocap T.D. (nitroglycerin [oral])	Antianginal, vasodialtor
nitroglycerin (oral)	Antianginal, vasodilator
nitroglycerin (sublingual)	Antianginal, vasodilator
nitroglycerin (topical)	Antianginal, vasodilator
Nitroglyn (nitroglycerin [oral])	Antianginal, vasodilator
Nitrol (nitroglycerin [topical])	Antianginal, vasodilator
Nitrolin (nitroglycerin [oral])	Antianginal, vasodilator
Nitronet (nitroglycerin [oral])	Antianginal, vasodilator
Nitrong (nitroglycerin [oral])	Antianginal, vasodilator
Nitrong (nitroglycerin [topical])	Antianginal, vasodilator
Nitropress (nitroprusside)	Antihypertensive
Nitroprusside	Antihypertensive
Nitrospan (nitroglycerin [oral])	Antianginal, vasodilator
Nitrostat (nitroglycerin [sublingual])	Antianginal, vasodilator
Nitrostat (nitroglycerin [topical])	Antianginal, vasodilator
Nitrostat SR (nitroglycerin [oral])	Antianginal, vasodilator
Noctec (chloral hydrate)	Sedative/hypnotic—controlled substance, Schedule IV
Noludar (methyprylon)	Sedative/hypnotic—controlled substance, Schedule III
Nordryl (diphenhydramine)	Antihistamine, antiemetic and antivertigo agent, antitussive, sedative/hypnotic, topical anesthetic
Normodyne (labetalol)	Antihypertensive
Norpace (disopyramide)	Ventricular/supraventricular antiarrhythmic, atrial antitachyarrhythmic
Norpace CR (disopyramide)	Ventricular/supraventricular antiarrhythmic, atrial antitachyarrhythmic
Norpramin (desipramine)	Antidepressant, antianxiety agent
nortriptyline	Antidepressant
Novochlorhydrate (chloral hydrate)	Sedative/hypnotic—controlled substance, Schedule IV
Novolin (insulin [regular])	Antidiabetic agent
Nubain (nalbuphine)	Analgesic
Numorphan (oxymorphone)	Analgesic—controlled substance, Schedule II

---

* Drug names beginning with a capital letter are trade; drug names beginning with a lowercase letter are generic.

Drug Name	Therapeutic Classification(s)
Nytol with DPH (diphenhydramine)	Antihistamine, antiemetic and antivertigo agent, antitussive, sedative/hypnotic, topical anesthetic
Omnipen (ampicillin)	Antibiotic
Oramide (tolbutamide)	Antidiabetic agent
Oretic (hydrochlorothiazide)	Diuretic, antihypertensive
Orinase (tolbutamide)	Antidiabetic agent
Ormayine (chlorpromazine)	Antipsychotic, antiemetic
Osmitrol (mannitol)	Diuretic
oxazepam	Antianxiety, sedative/hypnotic—controlled substance, Schedule IV
oxtriphylline	Bronchodilator
oxymorphone	Analgesic—controlled substance, Schedule II
oxytocin	Oxytocic
Pamelor (nortriptyline)	Antidepressant
Panwarfin (warfarin)	Anticoagulant
Parlodel (bromocriptine)	Antiparkinsonian agent
Parnate (tranylcypromine)	Antidepressant
Paxipam (halazepam)	Antianxiety agent—controlled substance, Schedule IV
Pedia Care (dextromethorphan)	Non-narcotic antitussive
pentazocine	Analgesic—controlled substance, Schedule IV
pentobarbital	Anticonvulsant, sedative/hypnotic—controlled substance, Schedule II; suppositories under Schedule III
perphenazine	Antipsychotic, antiemetic
Persantine (dipyridamole)	Coronary vasodilator, platelet aggregation inhibitor
Pertofrane (desipramine)	Antidepressant, antianxiety agent
Pertussin 8 Hour Cough Formula (dextromethorphan)	Non-narcotic antitussive
phenelzine	Antidepressant
phenobarbital	Anticonvulsant, sedative/hypnotic—controlled substance, Schedule IV
phensuximide	Anticonvulsant
phenytoin	Anticonvulsant, antiarrhythmic
Phyllocontin (aminophylline)	Bronchodilator
physostigmine	Antimuscarinic
pindolol	Antihypertensive
Pitocin (oxytocin)	Oxytocic

* Drug names beginning with a capital letter are trade; drug names beginning with a lowercase letter are generic.

250   *Pharmacology for Prehospital Emergency Care*

Drug Name	Therapeutic Classification(s)
Placidyl (ethchlorvynol)	Sedative/hypnotic—controlled substance, Schedule IV
Polycillin (ampicillin)	Antibiotic
Polymox (amoxicillin)	Antibiotic
Pork Regular Iletin II (insulin [regular])	Antidiabetic agent
pralidoxime	Anticholinesterase inhibitor
prazepam	Antianxiety agent—controlled substance, Schedule IV
prazosin	Antihypertensive
Primatene Mist Solution (epinephrine)	Bronchodilator, vasopressor, cardiac stimulant, local anesthetic adjunct, topical antihemorrhagic, antiglaucoma agent
Primatene Mist Suspension (epinephrine bitartrate)	Bronchodilator, vasopressor, cardiac stimulant, local anesthetic adjunct, topical antihemorrhagic, antiglaucoma agent
primidone	Anticonvulsant
Principen (ampicillin)	Antibiotic
procainamide	Ventricular and supraventricular antiarrhythmic, atrial antitachyarrhythmic
Procan SR (procainamide)	Ventricular and supraventricular antiarrhythmic, atrial antitachyarrhythmic
Procardia (nifedipine)	Antianginal
prochlorperazine	Antipsychotic, antiemetic, antianxiety agent
Profene (propoxyphene)	Analgesic—controlled substance, Schedule IV
Proglycem (diazoxide)	Antihypertensive
Promapar (chlorpromazine)	Antipsychotic, antiemetic
Promay (chlorpromazine)	Antipsychotic, antiemetic
promazine	Antipsychotic, antiemetic, analgesic—controlled substance, Schedule IV
Promine (procainamide)	Ventricular and supraventricular antiarrhythmic, atrial antitachyarrhythmic
Pronestyl (procainamide)	Ventricular and supraventricular antiarrhythmic, atrial antitachyarrhythmic
Pronestyl-SR (procainamide)	Ventricular and supraventricular antiarrhythmic, atrial antitachyarrhythmic
propoxyphene	Analgesic—controlled substance, Schedule IV
propranolol	Antihypertensive, antianginal, antiarrhythmic
Protopam (pralidoxime)	Anticholinasterase inhibitor
protriptyline	Antidepressant
Proventil (albuterol)	Bronchodilator
Proventil Syrup (albuterol)	Bronchodilator
Prozine (promazine)	Antipsychotic, antiemetic, analgesic—controlled substance, Schedule IV

* Drug names beginning with a capital letter are trade; drug names beginning with a lowercase letter are generic.

Drug Name	Therapeutic Classification(s)
Purodigin (digitoxin)	Antiarrhythmic agent, inotropic agent
Pyopen (carbenicillin)	Antibiotic
Pyridamole (dipyridamole)	Coronary vasodilator, platelet aggregation inhibitor
Quinidex (quinidine)	Ventricular and supraventricular antiarrhythmic, atrial antiarrhythmic
quinidine	Ventricular and supraventricular antiarrhythmic, atrial antiarrhythmic
Quinora (quinidine)	Ventricular and supraventricular antiarrhythmic, atrial antiarrhythmic
Razepam (temazepam)	Sedative/hypnotic—controlled substance, Schedule IV
Regular Iletin I (insulin [regular])	Antidiabetic agent
Regular Iletin II (insulin [regular])	Antidiabetic agent
Regular Pork Insulin (insulin [regular])	Antidiabetic agent
Reposans-10 (chlordiazepoxide)	Antianxiety agent, anticonvulsant, sedative/hypnotic—controlled substance, Schedule IV
reserpine	Antihypertensive, antipsychotic
Restoril (temazepam)	Sedative/hypnotic—controlled substance, Schedule IV
Rhythmin (procainamide)	Ventricular and supraventricular antiarrhythmic, atrial antitachyarrhythmic
Ritalin (methylphenidate)	CNS stimulant—controlled substance, Schedule II
Ritalin SR (methylphenidate)	CNS stimulant—controlled substance, Schedule II
Rivotril (clonazepam)	Anticonvulsant—controlled substance, Schedule IV
RMS Uniserts (morphine)	Analgesic—controlled substance, Schedule II
Ro-Chlorozide (chlorothiazide)	Diuretic, antihypertensive
Ro-Hydrazide (hydrochlorothiazide)	Diuretic, antihypertensive
Roampicillin (ampicillin)	Antibiotic
Robalyn (diphenhydramine)	Antihistamine, antiemetic and antivertigo agent, antitussive, sedative/hypnotic, topical anesthetic
Ronase (tolazamide)	Antidiabetic agent
Roxanol (morphine)	Analgesic—controlled substance, Schedule II
S-2 Inhalant (epinephrine hydrochloride)	Bronchodilator, vasopressor, cardiac stimulant, local anesthetic adjunct, topical antihemorrhagic, antiglaucoma agent
Sandril (reserpine)	Antihypertensive, antipsychotic
Sarisol No. 2 (butabarbital)	Sedative/hypnotic—controlled substance, Schedule III

* Drug names beginning with a capital letter are trade; drug names beginning with a lowercase letter are generic.

Drug Name	Therapeutic Classification(s)
Seconal (secobarbital)	Sedative/hypnotic, anticonvulsant—controlled substance, Schedule II; suppositories are under Schedule III
secobarbital	Sedative/hypnotic, anticonvulsant—controlled substance, Schedule II; suppositories are under Schedule III
Sectral (acebutolol)	Antihypertensive, antiarrhythmic
Sedabamate (meprobamate)	Antianxiety agent—controlled substance, Schedule IV
Serax (oxazepam)	Antianxiety, sedative/hypnotic—controlled substance, Schedule IV
Sereen (chlordiazepoxide)	Antianxiety agent, anticonvulsant, sedative/hypnotic—controlled substance, Schedule IV
Serentil (mesoridazine)	Antipsychotic
Serpanray (reserpine)	Antihypertensive, antipsychotic
Serpasil (reserpine)	Antihypertensive, antipsychotic
Serpate (reserpine)	Antihypertensive, antipsychotic
Serpolan (reserpine)	Antihypertensive, antipsychotic
Sertan (primidone)	Anticonvulsant
Sinequan (doxepin)	Antidepressant
Sintocine (oxytocin)	Oxytocic
SK-Amitriptyline (amitriptyline)	Antidepressant
SK-Bamate (meprobamate)	Antianxiety agent—controlled substance, Schedule IV
SK-Chlorozide (chlorothiazide)	Diuretic, antihypertensive
SK-Hydrochlorothiazide (hydrochlorothiazide)	Diuretic, antihypertensive
SK-Lasix (furosemide)	Diuretic, antihypertensive
SK-Lygen (chlordiazepoxide)	Antianxiety agent, anticonvulsant, sedative/hypnotic—controlled substance, Schedule IV
SK-Quinidine Sulfate (quinidine)	Ventricular and supraventricular antiarrhythmic, atrial antiarrhythmic
SK-Tolbutamide (tolbutamide)	Antidiabetic agent
Sleep-Eye 3 (diphenhydramine)	Antihistamine, antiemetic and antivertigo agent, antitussive, sedative/hypnotic, topical anesthetic
Slo-bid (theophylline)	Bronchodilator
Slo-Phyllin (theophylline)	Bronchodilator
Sofarin (warfarin)	Anticoagulant
Solfoton (phenobarbital)	Anticonvulsant, sedative/hypnotic—controlled substance, Schedule IV

* Drug names beginning with a capital letter are trade; drug names beginning with a lowercase letter are generic.

Drug Name	Therapeutic Classification(s)
Solu-Medrol	Anti-inflammatory, immunosuppressant
Sominex Formula 2 (diphenhydramine)	Antihistamine, antiemetic and antivertigo agent, antitussive, sedative/hypnotic, topical anesthetic
Somophyllin-T (theophylline)	Bronchodilator
Somophyllin (aminophylline)	Bronchodilator
Sonayine (chlorpromazine)	Antipsychotic, antiemetic
Sparine (promazine)	Antipsychotic, antiemetic, analgesic—controlled substance, Schedule IV
Spectrobid (bacampicillin)	Antibiotic
spironolactone	Antihypertensive, diuretic
St. Joseph for Children (dextromethorphan)	Non-narcotic antitussive
Stadol (butorphanol)	Narcotic agonist-antagonist, opioid partial agonist
Stelazine (trifluoperazine)	Antipsychotic, antiemetic
streptokinase	Thrombolytic
Sucrets Cough Control (dextromethorphan)	Non-narcotic antitussive
Super Totacillian (ampicillin)	Antibiotic
Suprazine (trifluoperazine)	Antipsychotic, antiemetic
Sus-Phrine (epinephrine)	Bronchodilator, vasopressor, cardiac stimulant, local anesthetic adjunct, topical antihemorrhagic, antiglaucoma agent
Sustaire (theophylline)	Bronchodilator
Talwin-NX (pentazocine)	Analagesic—controlled substance, Schedule IV
Tambocor (flecainide)	Ventricular antiarrhythmic
Taractan (chlorprothixene)	Antipsychotic
Tavist (clemastine)	Antihistamine
Tavist-1 (clemastine)	Antihistamine
Tegretol (carbamazepine)	Anticonvulsant, analgesic
temazepam	Sedative/hypnotic—controlled substance, Schedule IV
Tempay (temazepam)	Sedative/hypnotic—controlled substance, Schedule IV
Tempra (acetaminophen)	Non-narcotic analgesic, antipyretic
Tenormin (atenolol)	Antihypertensive, antianginal
Tensilon (edrophonium)	Antiarrhythmic, cholinergic agonist
terbutaline	Bronchodilator
Thalitone (chlorthalidone)	Diuretic, antihypertensive
Theo-24 (theophylline)	Bronchodilator

* Drug names beginning with a capital letter are trade; drug names beginning with a lowercase letter are generic.

Drug Name	Therapeutic Classification(s)
Theo-Dur (theophylline)	Bronchodilator
Theobid (theophylline)	Bronchodilator
Theoclear (theophylline)	Bronchodilator
Theophyl (theophylline)	Bronchodilator
theophylline	Bronchodilator
Theospan-SR (theophylline)	Bronchodilator
Theovent (theophylline)	Bronchodilator
thioridazine	Antipsychotic
thiothixene	Antipsychotic
Thor-Prom (chlorpromazine)	Antipsychotic, antiemetic
Thorayine (chlorpromazine)	Antipsychotic, antiemetic
timolol	Antihypertensive, antiglaucoma agent
Timoptic (timolol)	Antihypertensive, antiglaucoma agent
Tindal (acetophenazine)	Antipsychotic
tocainide	Ventricular antiarrhythmic
tolazamide	Antidiabetic agent
tolbutamide	Antidiabetic agent
Tolinase (tolazamide)	Antidiabetic agent
Tonocard (tocainide)	Ventricular antiarrhythmic
Tornalate (bitolterol)	Bronchodilator
Trandate (labetalol)	Antihypertensive
Tranmep (meprobamate)	Antianxiety agent—controlled substance, Schedule IV
Tranxene-SD (clorazepate)	Antianxiety agent, anticonvulsant, sedative/hypnotic—controlled substance, Schedule IV
Tranxene-SD Half Strength (clorazepate)	Antianxiety agent, anticonvulsant, sedative/hypnotic—controlled substance, Schedule IV
tranylcypromine	Antidepressant
triazolam	Sedative/hypnotic—controlled substance, Schedule III
Tridione (trimethadione)	Anticonvulsant
trifluoperazine	Antipsychotic, antiemetic
Trilafon (perphenazine)	Antipsychotic, antiemetic
trimethadione	Anticonvulsant
Trimox (amoxicillin)	Antibiotic
Triptil (protriptyline)	Antidepressant
Truphylline (aminophylline)	Bronchodilator
Tusstat (diphenhydramine)	Antihistamine, antiemetic and antivertigo agent, antitussive, sedative/hypnotic, topical anesthetic

* Drug names beginning with a capital letter are trade; drug names beginning with a lowercase letter are generic.

Drug Name	Therapeutic Classification(s)
Twilite (diphenhydramine)	Antihistamine, antiemetic and antivertigo agent
Tylenol (acetaminophen)	Nonarcotic analgesic, antipyretic
Uniphyl (theophylline)	Bronchodilator
Utimox (amoxicillin)	Antibiotic
Valadol (acetaminophen)	Nonarcotic analgesic, antipyretic
Valdrene (diphenhydramine)	Antihistamine, antiemetic and antivertigo agent, antitussive, sedative/hypnotic, topical anesthetic
Valium (diazepam)	Antianxiety agent, skeletal muscle relaxant, amnesic, anticonvulsant, sedative/hypnotic
Valorin (acetaminophen)	Nonarcotic analgesic, antipyretic
valproic acid	Anticonvulsant
Valrelease (diazepam)	Antianxiety agent, skeletal muscle relaxant, amnesic agent, anticonvulsant, sedative/hypnotic
Vancerase (beclomethasone)	Anti-inflammatory, antiasthmatic
Vanceril (beclomethasone)	Anti-inflammatory, antiasthmatic
Vaponefrin (epinephrine hydrochloride)	Bronchodilator, vasopressor, cardiac stimulant, local anesthetic adjunct, topical antihemorrhagic, antiglaucoma agent
Velosef (cephradine)	Antibiotic
Velosulin (insulin [regular])	Antidiabetic agent
Velosulin Human (insulin [regular])	Antidiabetic agent
Ventolin (albuterol)	Bronchodilator
Ventolin Syrup (albuterol)	Bronchodilator
verapamil	Antianginal, antihypertensive, antiarrhythmic
Viscous (lidocaine)	Ventricular antiarrhythmic, local anesthetic
Visken (pindolol)	Antihypertensive
Vistaril (hydroxyzine)	Antianxiety agent, sedative
Vivactil (protriptyline)	Antidepressant
warfarin	Anticoagulant
Wymox (amoxicillin)	Antibiotic
Wytensin (guanabenz)	Antihypertensive
Xanax (alprozolam)	Antianxiety agent—controlled substance, Schedule IV
Xylocaine (lidocaine)	Ventricular antiarrhythmic, local anesthetic
Zarontin (ethosuximide)	Anticonvulsant
Zepine (reserpine)	Antihypertensive, antipyschotic

---

* Drug names beginning with a capital letter are trade; drug names beginning with a lowercase letter are generic.

Appendix B

Intubation

During an emergency it may not be possible to start an IV, or the IV may be delayed. This situation can cause a delay in the administration of life-saving drugs. An alternative route for giving drugs is down the ET. Five drugs can be given down the ET: naloxone, atropine, diazepam, epinephrine, and lidocaine. Endotracheal intubation is not a difficult procedure. If skill levels are not maintained, however, success rates will be compromised.

METHOD FOR ENDOTRACHEAL INTUBATION

The actual intubation procedure should take less than 30 sec.

- Place the patient in the "sniffing" position. This is accomplished by extending the head and flexing the neck. When proper head position is achieved, three axes—the mouth, the pharynx, and the trachea—will be aligned, permitting direct visualization of the larynx.
- Establish ventilations using high-flow 100% oxygen.
- Prepare and check equipment.
- Hyperventilate the patient for approximately 2 to 3 min.
- While holding the laryngoscope in the left hand, carefully insert the blade. There are two acceptable methods of inserting the laryngoscope blade:
  1. The laryngoscope blade is inserted in the right side of the mouth, displacing the tongue to the left. The blade is then moved toward the midline, advancing to the base of the tongue.
  2. The laryngoscope blade is inserted over the tongue in the midline and then moved to the right side of the mouth, displacing the tongue to the left. The blade is then advanced to the base of the tongue. This method is less likely to damage mucous membranes.

Follow local protocols as to which method to use when inserting the laryngoscope blade.

- Once the laryngoscope blade is in proper placement, visualization of the vocal cords will be possible. Figure B–1 illustrates proper placement of the curved laryngoscope blade, Figure B–2 illustrates proper placement of the straight laryngoscope blade, and Figure B–3 illustrates direct exposure of the larynx.
- Insert the ET and remove the laryngoscope blade. The ET should be inserted approximately 3 cm past the tube cuff. Inflate the cuff until resistance is met.
- Check tube placement. This is done by auscultation over both lungs and the gastric area.
- Insert an oropharyngeal airway and tape the ET in place.

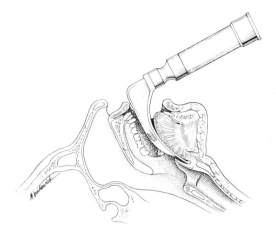

Figure B–1. Direct laryngoscopy using a curved blade. (From Finucane, BT and Santora, AH: Principles of Airway Management. F. A. Davis, Philadelphia, 1986, p 131, with permission.)

There are three methods in estimating the size of an ET for pediatric patients.

1. $\dfrac{Age\ (y)}{4} + 4$

2. $\dfrac{16 + Age\ (y)}{4}$

3. Estimate by using the tip of the patient's little finger.

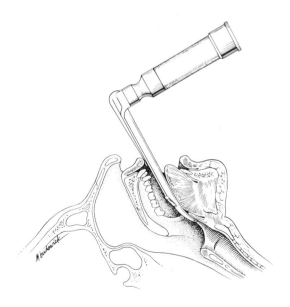

Figure B–2. Direct laryngoscopy using a straight blade. (From Finucane, BT and Santora, AH: Principles of Airway Management. F. A. Davis, Philadelphia, 1986, p 137, with permission.)

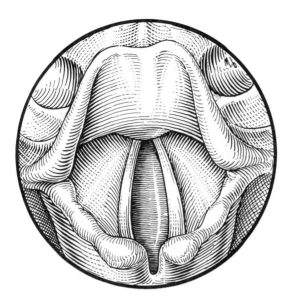

Figure B–3. Direct exposure of the larynx. (From Finucane, BT and Santora, AH: Principles of Airway Management. F. A. Davis, Philadelphia, 1986, p 132, with permission.)

PARALYSIS FOR ENDOTRACHEAL INTUBATION

Situations may arise where an IV has been established, but endotracheal intubation is not immediately possible. For example, a patient may resist ventilation because of pain. A semiconscious or combative patient may also resist ventilation. In situations such as these, it may be appropriate to administer a neuromuscular blocking drug to temporarily paralyze the patient so an ET can be inserted. As with all drug therapy, this treatment must be at the order of medical control and local protocols. The prehospital drug of choice to accomplish paralysis for intubation is succinylcholine.

SUCCINYLCHOLINE
Anectine, Quelicin, Sucostrin

CLASSIFICATIONS
Pharmacologic: Depolarizing
  neuromuscular blocking drug
Therapeutic: Skeletal muscle
  relaxant

MECHANISM OF ACTION: Succinylcholine is a rapid-acting neuromuscular blocking drug. It binds to acetylcholine receptors at nerve terminal endings on skeletal muscles. Succinylcholine makes muscles unable to be stimulated by any stimulating nerve impulses.

THERAPEUTIC BENEFIT: Succinylcholine causes skeletal muscle relaxation to aid in endotracheal intubation.

INDICATIONS FOR PREHOSPITAL USE: Succinylcholine is used for rapid skeletal muscle relaxation to assist in endotracheal intubation.

CONTRAINDICATIONS: ▪ Do not administer succinylcholine to patients with: ▪ Hypersensitivity to the drug. ▪ Narrow-angle glaucoma or penetrating eye injuries (succinylcholine raises intraocular pressure).

PRECAUTIONS: Succinylcholine should be used with caution in patients who have sustained extensive or severe burns.

ROUTE AND DOSAGE

Adult: 1-2 mg/kg by IV bolus. Repeated once, if needed.

Pediatric: 1-2 mg/kg by IV bolus.
Usually muscle paralysis will last approximately 5-16 min. Diazepam should be available if sedation is necessary.

ADVERSE REACTIONS AND SIDE EFFECTS

- Respiratory: Respiratory depression, apnea, wheezing.
- Cardiovascular: Arrhythmias, sinus arrest, hypertension or hypotension.
- Eyes: Increased intraocular pressure.

PARAMEDIC IMPLICATIONS: ▪ Succinylcholine changes a patient with a poor airway into a patient with no airway. Therefore, make sure that intubation is possible before administering succinylcholine. ▪ Succinylcholine causes paralysis without affecting the patient's level of consciousness. Therefore, sedation may be necessary. ▪ As with any intubated patient, assisted ventilation with 100% oxygen is necessary before succinylcholine is given.

DRUG INTERACTIONS: Using succinylcholine simultaneously with glycosides may cause arrhythmias.

PREMEDICATION PROCEDURES DURING ENDOTRACHEAL INTUBATION: There may be situations when Medical Control may order you to premedicate your patient before insertion of the endotracheal tube. During your sequence of steps while preparing your patient for intubation:

- Allow the patient to breathe 100% humidified oxygen by mask or assist ventilations as appropriate.
- Ensure that the patient has a functioning IV line in place.
- Ensure that the patient is connected to a cardiac monitor.
- Premedicate as follows:
  - *Diazepam:* 3-5 mg by slow IV bolus. This is given for sedation of conscious patients.
  - *Atropine:* 0.01-0.02 mg/kg by IV bolus. This is for control of possible bradycardia which may develop due to vagal stimulation during intubation in **pediatric** patients.
  - *Lidocaine:* 1 mg/kg by IV bolus. This is given for intracranial pressure control in head-injured patients with central nervous system (CNS) injury.
  - *Succinylcholine:* 1-2 mg/kg by IV bolus.
- Proceed with intubation.

Appendix C

Pediatric Normal Values, Dosages, and Infusion Rates

Age	Average Weight*	Respiratory Rate	Pulse Rate	Blood Pressure†
Birth–6 wk	4–5 kg (9–11 lb)	30–50 breaths/min	120–160 beats/min	74–100 mm Hg 50–68 mm Hg
7 wk–1 y	4–11 kg (9–24 lb)	20–30 breaths/min	80–140 beats/min	84–106 mm Hg 45–70 mm Hg
1–2 y	11–14 kg (24–31 lb)	20–30 breaths/min	80–130 beats/min	98–106 mm Hg 58–70 mm Hg
2–6 y	14–25 kg (31–55 lb)	20–30 breaths/min	80–120 beats/min	98–112 mm Hg 64–70 mm Hg
6–13 y	25–63 kg (55–139 lb)	12–20 breaths/min	60–100 beats/min	104–124 mm Hg 64–80 mm Hg
13–16 y	62–80 kg (136–176 lb)	12–20 breaths/min	60–100 beats/min	118–132 mm Hg 70–82 mm Hg

* Weight estimation : 8 + (12 × age [y]) = weight in kg.
† Systolic blood pressure estimation: 80 + (2 × age [y]) = approx systolic B/P.

PEDIATRIC DRUG DOSAGES

	BODY WEIGHT (kg/lb)†				
Drug	1 kg/2 lb	2 kg/4 lb	3 kg/7 lb	4 kg/9 lb	5 kg/11 lb
Aminophylline	6 mg	12 mg	18 mg	24 mg	30 mg
Atropine	0.02 mg	0.04 mg	0.06 mg	0.08 mg	0.10 mg
Bretylium	5 mg	10 mg	15 mg	20 mg	25 mg
Calcium chloride	20 mg	40 mg	60 mg	80 mg	100 mg
Dextrose 50% in water	0.5–1 mg	1–2 mg	1.5–3 mg	2–4 mg	2.5–5 mg
Diazoxide	1–3 mg	2–6 mg	3–9 mg	4–12 mg	5–15 mg
Diphenhydramine	2–5 mg	4–10 mg	6–15 mg	8–20 mg	10–25 mg
Dopamine	2–20 µg/min	4–40 µg/min	6–60 µg/min	8–80 µg/min	10–100 µg/min
Epinephrine (1:10,000)	0.01 mg	0.02 mg	0.03 mg	0.04 mg	0.05 mg

* Doses are the usual initial single dose.
† Pounds have been rounded to the nearest pound.

260

PEDIATRIC DRUG DOSAGES (Continued)

Drug	1 kg/2 lb	2 kg/4 lb	3 kg/7 lb	4 kg/9 lb	5 kg/11 lb
			BODY WEIGHT (kg/lb)†		
Furosemide	1 mg	2 mg	3 mg	4 mg	5 mg
Isoproterenol	0.1–0.2 μg/min	0.2–0.4 μg/min	0.3–0.6 μg/min	0.4–0.8 μg/min	0.5–1 μg/min
Lidocaine	1 mg	2 mg	3 mg	4 mg	5 mg
Naloxone	0.01 mg	0.02 mg	0.03 mg	0.04 mg	0.05 mg
Propranolol	0.01 mg	0.02 mg	0.03 mg	0.04 mg	0.05 mg
Sodium bicarbonate	1 mEq	2 mEq	3 mEq	4 mEq	5 mEq
Verapamil	0.1–0.3 mg	0.2–0.6 mg	0.3–0.9 mg	0.4–1.2 mg	0.5–1.5 mg

	6 kg/13 lb	7 kg/15 lb	8 kg/18 lb	9 kg/20 lb	10 kg/22 lb
Aminophylline	36 mg	42 mg	48 mg	54 mg	60 mg
Atropine	0.12 mg	0.14 mg	0.16 mg	0.18 mg	0.2 mg
Bretylium	30 mg	35 mg	40 mg	45 mg	50 mg
Calcium chloride	120 mg	140 mg	160 mg	180 mg	200 mg
Dextrose 50% in water	3–6 mg	3.5–7 mg	4–8 mg	4.6–9 mg	5–10 mg
Diazoxide	6–18 mg	7–21 mg	8–24 mg	9–27 mg	10–30 mg
Diphenhydramine	12–30 mg	14–35 mg	16–40 mg	18–45 mg	20–50 mg
Dopamine	12–120 μg/min	14–140 μg/min	16–160 μg/min	18–180 μg/min	20–200 μg/min
Epinephrine (1:10,000)	0.06 mg	0.07 mg	0.08 mg	0.09 mg	0.1 mg
Furosemide	6 mg	7 mg	8 mg	9 mg	10 mg
Isoproterenol	0.6–1.2 μg/min	0.7–1.4 μg/min	0.8–1.6 μg/min	0.9–1.8 μg/min	1.0–2 μg/min
Lidocaine	6 mg	7 mg	8 mg	9 mg	10 mg
Naloxone	0.06 mg	0.07 mg	0.08 mg	0.09 mg	0.1 mg
Propranolol	0.06 mg	0.07 mg	0.08 mg	0.09 mg	0.1 mg
Sodium bicarbonate	6 mEq	7 mEq	8 mEq	9 mEq	10 mEq
Verapamil	0.6–1.8 g	0.7–2.1 mg	0.8–2.4 mg	0.9–2.7 mg	1–3 mg

	12.5 kg/28 lb	15 kg/33 lb	17.5 kg/39 lb	20 kg/44 lb	20.5 kg/50 lb
Aminophylline	75 mg	90 mg	105 mg	120 mg	135 mg
Atropine	0.25 mg	0.30 mg	0.35 mg	0.4 mg	0.45 mg
Bretylium	62.5 mg	75 mg	87.5 mg	100 mg	112.5 mg
Calcium chloride	250 mg	300 mg	350 mg	400 mg	410 mg
Dextrose 50% in water	6.25–12.5 g	7.5–15 g	8.75–17.5 g	10–20 g	11.25–22.5 g
Diazoxide	12.5–37.5 mg	15–45 mg	17.5–52.5 mg	20–60 mg	22.5–67.5 mg
Diphenhydramine	25–62.5 mg	30–75 mg	35–87.5 mg	40–100 mg	45–112.5 mg
Dopamine	25–250 μg/min	30–300 μg/min	35–350 μg/min	40–400 μg/min	41–410 μg/min
Epinephrine (1:10,000)	0.125 mg	0.15 mg	0.175 mg	0.2 mg	0.225 mg
Furosemide	12.5 mg	15 mg	17.5 mg	20 mg	22.5 mg
Isoproterenol	1.25–2.5 μg/min	1.5–3 μg/min	1.75–3.5 μg/min	2–4 μg/min	2.25–4.5 μg/min

* Doses are the usual initial single dose.
† Pounds have been rounded to the nearest pound.

PEDIATRIC DRUG DOSAGES (*Continued*)

Drug	BODY WEIGHT (kg/lb)†				
	12.5 kg/28 lb	15 kg/33 lb	17.5 kg/39 lb	20 kg/44 lb	20.5 kg/50 lb
Lidocaine	12.5 mg	15 mg	17.5 mg	20 mg	22.5 mg
Naloxone	0.125 mg	0.15 mg	0.175 mg	0.2 mg	0.225 mg
Propranolol	0.125 mg	0.15 mg	0.175 mg	0.2 mg	0.225 mg
Sodium bicarbonate	12.5 mEq	15 mEq	17.5 mEq	20 mEq	22.5 mEq
Verapamil	1.25–3.75 mg	1.5–4.5 mg	1.75–5 mg	2–5 mg	2–5 mg
	25 kg/55 lb	**30 kg/66 lb**	**35 kg/77 lb**	**40 kg/88 lb**	**45 kg/99 lb**
Aminophylline	150 mg	180 mg	210 mg	240 mg	270 mg
Atropine	0.5 mg	0.5 mg	0.5 mg	0.5 mg	0.5 mg
Bretylium	125 mg	150 mg	175 mg	200 mg	225 mg
Calcium chloride	500 mg	600 mg	700 mg	800 mg	900 mg
Dextrose 50% in water	12.5–25 g	15–30 g	17.5–35 g	20–40 g	22.5–45 g
Diazoxide	25–75 mg	30–90 mg	35–105 mg	40–120 mg	45–135 mg
Diphenhydramine	50–125 mg	60–150 mg	70–176 mg	80–200 mg	90–225 mg
Dopamine	50–500 μg/min	60–600 μg/min	70–700 μg/min	80–800 μg/min	90–900 μg/min
Epinephrine (1:10,000)	0.25 mg	0.3 mg	0.35 mg	0.4 mg	0.45 mg
Furosemide	25 mg	30 mg	35 mg	40 mg	45 mg
Isoproterenol	2.5–5 μg/min	3–6 μg/min	3.5–7 μg/min	4–8 μg/min	4.5–9 μg/min
Lidocaine	25 mg	30 mg	35 mg	40 mg	45 mg
Naloxone	0.25 mg	0.3 mg	0.35 mg	0.4 mg	0.45 mg
Propranolol	0.25 mg	0.3 mg	0.35 mg	0.4 mg	0.45 mg
Sodium bicarbonate	25 mEq	30 mEq	35 mEq	40 mEq	45 mEq
Verapamil	2.5–7.5 mg	3–9 mg	3.5–10.5 mg	4–12 mg	4.5–13.5 mg
	50 kg/110 lb	**55 kg/121 lb**	**60 kg/132 lb**	**65 kg/143 lb**	**70 kg/154 lb**
Aminophylline	300 mg	330 mg	360 mg	390 mg	420 mg
Atropine	0.5 mg	0.5 mg	0.5 mg	0.5 mg	0.5 mg
Bretylium	250 mg	275 mg	300 mg	325 mg	350 mg
Calcium chloride	1 g	1.1 g	1.2 g	1.3 g	1.4 g
Dextroxe 50% in water	25–50 g	27.5–55 g	30–60 g	32.5–65 g	35–70 g
Diazoxide	50–150 mg	55–150 mg	60–150 mg	65–150 mg	70–150 mg
Diphenhydramine	100–250 mg	110–275 mg	120–300 mg	130–325 mg	140–350 mg
Dopamine	100–1000 μg/min	110–1100 μg/min	120–1200 μg/min	130–1300 μg/min	140–1400 μg/min
Epinephrine (1:10,000)	0.5 mg	0.55 mg	0.6 mg	0.65 mg	0.7 mg
Furosemide	50 mg	55 mg	60 mg	65 mg	70 mg
Isoproterenol	5–10 μg/min	5.5–11 μg/min	6–12 μg/min	6.5–13 μg/min	7–14 μg/min

* Doses are the usual initial single dose.
† Pounds have been rounded to the nearest pound.

PEDIATRIC DRUG DOSAGES (*Continued*)

	BODY WEIGHT (kg/lb)†				
Drug	50 kg/110 lb	55 kg/121 lb	60 kg/132 lb	65 kg/143 lb	70 kg/154 lb
Lidocaine	50 mg	55 mg	60 mg	65 mg	70 mg
Naloxone	0.5 mg	0.55 mg	0.6 mg	0.65 mg	0.7 mg
Propranolol	0.5 mg	0.55 mg	0.6 mg	0.65 mg	0.7 mg
Sodium bicarbonate	50 mEq	55 mEq	60 mEq	65 mEq	70 mEq
Verapamil	2–5 mg	2–5 mg	2–5 mg	2–5 mg	2–5 mg

* Doses are the usual initial single dose.
† Pounds have been rounded to the nearest pound.

CALCULATING DRUG CONCENTRATIONS AND INFUSION RATES FOR COMMON PEDIATRIC MEDICATIONS

Drug	Commonly Found Drug Concentration	Desired Rate of Administration	Amount of Drug Solution to Add to 100 mL of D_5W
Isoproterenol	0.2 mg/mL	0.1 μg/kg/min	3 mL
Epinephrine	1:1000 (1 mg/mL)	0.1 μg/kg/min	0.6 mL
Dopamine	40 mg/mL	10 μg/kg/min	1.5 mL
Dobutamine	25 mg/mL	10 μg/kg/min	2.4 mL
Lidocaine	1% (10 mg/mL)	20 μg/kg/min	12 mL

Listed above are five prehospital pediatric drugs. The chart shows, for each drug, the drug's concentration in its most common preparation and the rate of administration that medical control usually orders for the drug. The last column shows the amount of drug preparation to add to 100 mL of D_5W. By infusing the resulting solution at the rate of administration indicated on the body weight chart below, you will achieve the desired rate of drug administration.

WEIGHT			WEIGHT		
kg	lb	Infusion Rate (mL/h)	kg	lb	Infusion Rate (mL/h)
3	6.6	3	30	66	30
7	15.4	7	35	77	35
10	22	10	40	88	40
12.5	27.5	12.5	45	99	45
15	33	15	55	110	50
17.5	38.5	17.5	55	121	55
20	44	20	60	132	60
22.5	49.5	22.5	65	143	65
25	55	25	70	154	70

DRUGS USED IN PEDIATRIC ADVANCED LIFE SUPPORT*

Drug	Dose	Remarks
Adenosine	0.1 to 0.2 mg/kg Maximum single dose: 12 mg	Rapid IV bolus
Atropine sulfate	0.02 mg/kg per dose	Minimum dose: 0.1 mg Maximum single dose: 0.5 mg in child, 1.0 mg in adolescent
Bretylium	5 mg/kg; may be increased to 10 mg/kg	Rapid IV
Calcium chloride 10%	20 mg/kg per dose	Give slowly
Dopamine hydrochloride	2–20 µg/kg/min	α-Adrenergic action dominates at ≥ 15–20 µg/kg/min
Dobutamine hydrochloride	2–20 µg/kg/min	Titrate to desired effect
Epinephrine For bradycardia	IV/IO; 0.01 mg/kg (1:10,000) ET: 0.1 mg/kg (1:1000)	Be aware of effective dose of preservatives administered (if preservatives are present in epinephrine preparation) when high doses are used
For asystolic or pulseless arrest	First dose: IV/IO: 0.01 mg/kg (1:10,000) ET: 0.1 mg/kg (1:1000) Doses as high as 0.2 mg/kg may be effective Subsequent doses: IV/IO/ET: 0.1 mg/kg (1:1000) Doses as high as 0.2 mg/kg may be effective	Be aware of effective dose of preservative administered (if preservatives present in epinephrine preparation) when high doses are used
Epinephrine infusion	Initial at 0.1 µg/kg/min Higher infusion dose used if asystole present	Titrate to desired effect (0.1–1.0 µg/kg/min)
Lidocaine	1 mg/kg per dose	
Lidocaine infusion	20–50 µg/kg/min	
Sodium bicarbonate	1 mEq/kg per dose or 0.3 × kg × base deficit	Infuse slowly and only if ventilation is adequate

*IV indicates intravenous route; IO, intraosseous route; and ET, endotracheal route.

Answers to Study Questions and Case Study Questions

CHAPTER 1

1. **(1) Plants.** Leaves, roots, seeds, and other plant parts are processed for use as drugs. Atropine, a drug used to treat symptomatic bradycardia, is obtained from the plant called deadly nightshade (scientific name *Atropa belladonna*). **(2) Animal.** Some of the most powerful drugs are extracted from animal tissue. These drugs are often used to replace insufficient human glandular secretions. Oxytocin is a pituitary hormone used in prehospital emergency care to control postpartum hemorrhage. **(3) Inorganic.** Elements such as sulfur, iodine, and mineral salts are commonly used to manufacture drugs. Magnesium sulfate, used to treat eclampsia, is a naturally occurring mineral element obtained from well and sea water. **(4) Synthetic.** Synthetic drugs are man-made by chemical processes. Most drugs currently used are produced synthetically.

2. **(1).** *Explanation:* During the first 10 years of the 20th century, the use of chemicals in medicine increased rapidly, bringing with it an increased use of dangerous ingredients and complex formulas. Drug companies used poor quality control and made unproved claims for their products. This situation made it necessary to develop national standards and government regulations to guarantee that drugs sold to the public were accurately identified and of uniform strength and purity.

3. **(1) Chemical name.** A drug's chemical name is an exact description of the drug's structure and composition. **(2) Generic name.** A drug's generic name is the name given by the company that first formulated it. **(3) Trade name.** A trade name is the name registered by the company that manufactures the drug. A trade name is designated in print by its initial capital letter and a raised registered symbol ® following the name. **(4) Official name.** A drug's official name is published in the *United States Pharmacopeia* and *National Formulary* when the drug has met specific standard for quality, strength, purity, packaging, and labeling. Drugs meeting these standards are designated by the letters "USP" following their name. Table 1–2 gives examples of all four drug names.

CHAPTER 2

1. **(1) Circulatory status.** Poor circulation results in slow drug absorption, and, therefore, inadequate therapeutic response. **(2) Solubility.** The more soluble a drug is, the faster it enters the bloodstream. **(3) Body pH.** Acidosis can delay drug absorption. Poor ventilation and/or chest compressions produces an acidotic state. **(4)**

Drug concentration. In general, the higher the percentage of drug in the preparation administered, the faster the rate of absorption.

2. **c.** *Explanation: Affinity* means "attraction." To say that a drug has an affinity for a receptor means that it tends to combine with that receptor. Efficacy means the power to produce a desired effect. Tolerance is the progressive decrease in the effectiveness or response to a drug. Cumulative drug effects are the effects of small but repeated doses of drugs.

3. **(1) Administration phase.** The administration phase is the actual administration of a drug. **(2) Pharmaceutical phase.** During the pharmaceutical phase, the drug dissolves so it can be made available for absorption. Drugs given by the intravenous, endotracheal, and intraosseous routes bypass the pharmaceutical phase. **(3) Pharmacokinetic phase.** Once dissolved, drugs begin the pharmacokinetic phase. During this phase, free drugs are capable of reaching their receptors. **(4) Pharmacodynamic phase.** Once drugs reach their receptors, the pharmacodynamic phase of drug activity occurs. It is only when the drug binds to its receptor that the pharmacologic effect occurs.

4. A drug concentration below the minimum therapeutic concentration will not produce an effective response; conversely, drug concentrations that are too high may produce toxic effects or may even be fatal. Most drug dosages are calculated by body weight or administered at a predetermined standard dosage. Dosage guidelines are established to achieve minimum therapeutic concentrations. Therefore, the goal for drug therapy is to give the minimum concentration of a drug to obtain the effective desired therapeutic response.

CHAPTER 3

1. **a.** *Explanation:* The major nerves of the parasympathetic nervous system are the two vagus nerves. Vagus nerve stimulation causes
   - Salivation.
   - Bradycardia.
   - Decreased strength of cardiac contractions.
   - Hypotension.
   - Increased blood flow to the stomach and intestines.
   - An increase in glandular secretions of digestive juices.

   Stimulation of sympathetic nervous system causes
   - Dry mouth.
   - Tachycardia.
   - Increased strength of cardiac contractions.
   - Hypertension.
   - Dilation of pupils.
   - Vasoconstriction of the skin, kidneys, and digestive organs.

   The sympathetic nervous system has specific effects on the heart, which include
   - Increased firing rate of the sinoatrial node.
   - Increased atrial muscle contractility and conduction velocity.
   - Increased conduction rate of the atrioventricular node.

- Increased contractility and automaticity in the left ventricle.
- Increased stroke volume.

2. **c.** *Explanation:* Alpha$_1$ receptors are postsynaptic and located on the vascular smooth muscle. When stimulated, alpha$_1$ receptors cause vasoconstriction, mainly peripheral and coronary vasoconstriction.

   Alpha$_2$ receptors are presynaptic and, when stimulated, inhibit the release of additional norepinephrine. Beta$_1$ receptor sites are located mainly in the heart. Beta$_1$ stimulation causes increased heart rate, increased contractility, and an increase in atrioventricular conduction. Beta$_2$ receptors are located mainly in bronchial and vascular smooth muscle. Beta$_2$ stimulation causes vasodilation, bronchodilation, and uterine contraction.

3. **b.** *Explanation:* A neurotransmitter is a body-produced chemical located on a presynaptic neuron. An electrical signal travels along the neuron and causes the release of a neurotransmitter from the presynaptic neuron. The neurotransmitter moves across the synaptic space and combines with receptors on the postsynaptic neuron. These actions cause an electrical change in membrane ion permeability, which then starts an action impulse potential in the postsynaptic neuron of the effector organ. Acetylcholine (ACh), norepinephrine, and epinephrine are the primary neurotransmitters of the autonomic nervous system.

4. **a.** *Explanation:* Adrenergic is synonymous with sympathetic, and cholinergic is synonymous with parasympathetic. Neurons and effector organs that are activated by epinephrine are called adrenergic. Neurons and effector organs that are activated by acetylcholine are called cholinergic. Adrenergic drugs imitate the action of epinephrine, and cholinergic drugs imitate the action of acetylcholine. Drugs that oppose the action of epinephrine are called antiadrenergic drugs, and drugs that oppose the action of acetylcholine are called anticholinergic.

CHAPTER 4

1. **d.** *Explanation:* The establishment of an intraosseous line provides a rapid means of vascular access into the bone marrow in patients 5 and younger. Drugs administered by intramuscular injection must be absorbed through muscle tissue and into the capillaries before they enter the circulation. Drugs administered by subcutaneous injection must be absorbed through the subcutaneous tissue and muscle tissue and into the capillaries before entering the circulation. There are fewer capillaries in subcutaneous tissue than in muscle tissue, making drug absorption much slower. Some of the drug will not absorb into the capillaries until it moves through the muscle tissue, because of the scarcity of capillaries in the subcutaneous tissue.

   Drugs administered orally are absorbed from the stomach or small intestines before finding their way into capillaries and into the circulation. Drugs administered orally have a slow and unpredictable rate of absorption, especially if there is food in the stomach, which further slows absorption. Drugs administered intravenously and down the endotracheal tube are absorbed immediately into the circulation.

3. **d.** *Explanation:* The Centers for Disease Control in Atlanta, Georgia has recommends certain universal precautions for protection against contamination and the spread of blood-borne infections, including AIDS. Needles should not be recapped,

bent, broken, or removed from the syringe. Needles and disposable syringes should be disposed of in puncture-resistant containers immediately after use.

CHAPTER 5

Practice Problems

Conversions

1. 110 lb
2. 81.8 or 82 kg
3. 200 μm
4. 3000 mL
5. 300 mg
6. 10 cc
7. 3000 mg
8. 60 mg
9. 90.9 or 91 kg
10. 4000 mg
11. 30 mg
12. 8 g
13. 200 cc
14. 2000 μm
15. 100 mL

Problem Set A

1. a. 80 mg
   b. 4 mL
2. 5 mL
3. a. 2 μg
   b. 60 gtt/min
4. 1600 μm/mL
5. 2 mL
6. a. 400 mg
   b. 8 ml

Problem Set B

1. a. 4 mg/mL
   b. 30 gtt/min

2. a. 0.2 g/mL
   b. 103 gtt/min

3. 111 gtt/min

4. 5 mL

5. a. 4 μg/mL
   b. 15 gtt/min

6. a. 8 μg/mL
   b. 15 gtt/min

CHAPTER 6

1. **a.** *Explanation:* Intracellular fluid is a body fluid contained inside the body's cells; it accounts for approximately 45 percent of total body weight. Extracellular fluid is the body fluid outside the body's cells; it accounts for approximately 15 percent of total body weight. Interstitial fluid is the the extracellular fluid located in the spaces between the body's cells; it accounts for approximately 10.5 percent of total body weight. The remaining extracellular fluid is intravascular fluid, the noncellular fluid portion of the blood; it accounts for approximately 4.5 percent of total body weight.

2. **d.** *Explanation.* Magnesium, a major cation of the body, is required for body temperature regulation, protein and carbohydrate metabolism, and neuromuscular contraction. Potassium is the major intracellular cation, responsible for acid-base regulation, muscle excitability, and nerve impulse conduction. Calcium is the most abundant cation in the body. It is required for bone growth, metabolism, blood clotting, normal cardiac function, and the initiation of neuromuscular contractions. Chloride is the major extracellular anion. Its main function is to maintain fluid balance.

   Sodium is the major extracellular cation and is responsible for fluid balance. Bicarbonate is the major element of the body's buffer system. The main function of this anion is to maintain acid-base balance. Phosphate is the major intracellular anion. It helps maintain acid-base balance.

3. **b.** *Explanation:* An example of an isotonic solution is normal saline solution. A hypotonic solution has a lower osmotic pressure than normal body fluids. If the solution outside a cell membrane is hypotonic, it has a lower osmotic pressure than the solution inside the cell membrane. An example of a hypotonic solution is ½ normal saline solution. A hypertonic solution is that which has an osmotic pressure higher than normal body fluids. If it is hypertonic, the solution outside the cell membrane has a pressure higher than the solution inside the cell membrane. An example of a hypertonic solution is dextrose 50% in water. A colloid is a solution whose molecules are so large that they will not freely diffuse across cell membranes. Colloid solutions remain in the vascular space for longer periods of time, making them the solutions of choice in maintaining vascular volume. Examples of colloid solutions are Dextran and Plasmanate.

4. **a.** *Explanation:* Three mechanisms help the body maintain acid-base balance. The primary mechanism is the buffer system, operating within a fraction of a second. Two components of the buffer system include bicarbonate ion (HCO_3) and carbonic acid (H_2CO_3), which maintain an equilibrium with the hydrogen ion (H^+). The respiratory

system is the second mechanism for acid-base regulation; it takes about 1 to 3 minutes to be effective. The respiratory system works to maintain acid-base balance by altering the carbon dioxide (CO_2) level in the bloodstream. The renal system is the third and slowest mechanism for acid-base regulation, taking from several hours to days to be effective. The kidneys regulate acid-base balance by eliminating excess hydrogen or bicarbonate ions that have accumulated in the body.

CHAPTER 7

Study Questions

1. **b.** *Explanation:* The initial dose of atropine is 0.5–1.0 mg by IV bolus. This dose may be repeated every 3–5 min until an acceptable response is achieved. The maximum total dose of atropine should not exceed 0.04 mg/kg. Doses less than 0.5 mg may cause paradoxical bradycardia. Doses of more than 2 mg may cause tachycardia, delirium, or coma.

2. **a.** *Explanation:* Adverse reactions and side effects of propranolol include the following:
   * *CNS:* Weakness, depression, fatigue
   * *Cardiovascular:* Bradycardia, congestive heart failure, hypotension
   * *Respiratory:* Bronchospasm, wheezing
   * *Endocrine:* Hypoglycemia or hyperglycemia
   * *Gastrointestinal:* Nausea, vomiting, diarrhea.
   Coma has not been noted as an adverse reaction or side effect of propranolol.

3. **d.** *Explanation:* If ventricular fibrillation continues after the initial dose, the dose is increased to 10 mg/kg. This dose can be repeated every 15–30 min, if needed, to a maximum dose of 30 mg/kg.

4. **d.** *Explanation:* The increased cardiovascular effects resulting from the administration of epinephrine include increases in the heart's rate, contractility, and automaticity. Epinephrine also improves blood pressure by increasing systemic vascular resistance. However, these increased cardiovascular effects also cause the heart to require more oxygen. This increased demand is compensated for by epinephrine's bronchodilation effects, which allow more oxygen to enter the system.

5. **b.** *Explanation:* Although bradycardia is not an absolute contraindication for the use of lidocaine, lidocaine should be used with caution in patients who are experiencing bradycardia. Likewise, a history of seizures is not an absolute contraindication for the use of lidocaine, even though a lidocaine overdose can cause seizure activity.

6. **c.** *Explanation:* Digoxin is used to control the heart's ventricular rate in the management of atrial fibrillation, atrial flutter, or paroxysmal supraventricular tachycardia. Digoxin may also be used when treating patients with congestive heart failure.

7. **c.** *Explanation:* Diazoxide causes vasodilation and decreases peripheral vascular resistance. Adverse reactions and side effects include the following:
   * *CNS:* Dizziness, headache, lightheadedness
   * *Cardiovascular:* Tachycardia, hypotension, arrhythmias, chest pain, edema, congestive heart failure

- *Fluid and electrolytes:* Sodium and water retention
- *Endocrine:* Hyperglycemia

Bradycardia is not a side effect of diazoxide.

8. **d.** *Explanation:* Morphine increases the capacity of the venous circulation, which causes the pooling of blood and a decrease in blood return to the heart. The drug also decreases systemic vascular resistance. Therefore, giving morphine to the hypotensive patient is contraindicated.

9. **d.** *Explanation:* Dopamine increases blood pressure and cardiac output and improves blood flow through the kidneys. It causes a minor increase in systemic vascular resistance and preload.

10. **d.** *Explanation:* Isoproterenol is a chronotropic drug, which means it influences the heart's rate. When a chronotropic drug is given too rapidly, ventricular tachycardia or ventricular fibrillation may result.

11. **b.** *Explanation:* Norepinephrine is an adrenergic vasopresser drug; it increases the heart's contractility and arterial and venous vasoconstriction. Administering norepinephrine is very unlikely to result in decreased cardiac output or hypotension.

12. **d.** *Explanation:* Nitroglycerin increases coronary blood flow by relaxing vascular smooth muscle. The result is dilation of coronary blood vessels and decreased peripheral vascular resistance, which decreases the work load of the heart and reduces myocardial oxygen demand.

13. **a.** *Explanation:* Verapamil slows conduction in the sinoatrial and atrioventricular nodes and slows ventricular response. Verapamil is used to stop paroxysmal supraventricular tachycardia and for the temporary control of rapid ventricular response due to atrial fibrillation and atrial flutter.

14. **c.** *Explanation:* Since lidocaine dosage is determined by body weight expressed in in kg, the patient's weight in lb must be converted to kg. One pound equals 2.2 kg. Therefore, 2.2 divided into 180 equals 81.8 kg. This can be rounded to 82 kg. If lidocaine is to be given at the rate of 1 mg/kg, then 1 mg times 82 = 82 mg.

15. **b.** *Explanation:* Adding 4 g to 1000 mL yields a drug concentration of 4 mg/mL. Likewise, adding 2 g to 500 mL also yields 4 mg/mL. Infusing this 4-mg/mL concentration at a rate 2 mg/min requires the IV to run at 30 μgtts/min. The following drip rates apply:
    - 4 mg/min requires 60 μgtts/min.
    - 3 mg/min requires 45 μgtts/min.
    - 2 mg/min requires 30 μgtts/min.
    - 1 mg/min requires 15 μgtts/min

Case Studies

1. **c.** *Explanation:* Lidocaine is the initial drug of choice for treating ventricular ectopy, including premature ventricular complexes (PVCs), ventricular tachycardia, and ventricular fibrillation. The initial dose of lidocaine for stable ventricular tachycardia is 1–1.5 mg/kg by IV bolus.

    Bretylium is used to treat ventricular tachycardia that has not responded to other therapy, including lidocaine. Currently, there is no evidence that bretylium is superior to lidocaine, or vice versa. Therefore, to help in standardizing treatment, bretylium should not be used as a first-line drug for the treatment of ventricular tachycardia.

Verapamil slows conduction in the sinoatrial and atrioventricular nodes and slows ventricular response. It is used to stop paroxysmal supraventricular tachycardia that does not require cardioversion and for the temporary control of rapid ventricular response due to atrial fibrillation and atrial flutter.

Atropine competes with the neurotransmitter acetylcholine for receptor sites, blocking parasympathetic nerve fibers. This blocking action accelerates heart rate in an attempt to improve cardiac output.

2. **a.** *Explanation:* Nitroglycerin decreases the heart's ventricular work load, reduces the heart's oxygen demands, and increases coronary blood flow. These benefits can help to relieve the pain caused by angina or MI.

Lidocaine can be administered to prevent the development of ectopic activity during MI. In such a case, the physician may order lidocaine, but not until the nitroglycerin has been administered and has had a chance to produce any therapeutic benefit.

Bretylium is used to treat ventricular tachycardia and ventricular fibrillation resistant to other therapy including lidocaine. Unlike lidocaine, bretylium is not used to prevent the development of ectopic activity in MI.

Morphine is used to treat pain and anxiety associated with acute MI. However, it is a powerful narcotic analgesic and CNS depressant. Therefore, morphine should not be given until other, more conversative treatment has been tried.

3. **c.** *Explanation:* Adenosine is used to slow conduction through the AV node of the heart. It may also interrupt reentry pathways through the AV node. Adenosine can restore normal sinus rhythm (NSR) in patients experiencing paroxysmal supraventricular tachycardia (PSVT).

Verapamil slows conduction in the sinoatrial and atrioventricular nodes and slows ventricular response. It is the drug of choice to stop paroxysmal supraventricular tachycardia that does not require cardioversion.

Isoproterenol is a pure beta-adrenergic agonist that causes an increase in both heart rate and heart contractility. It is used as an immediate but temporary measure to treat poor cardiac output caused by bradycardia that has not responded to atropine.

Procainamide slows conduction velocity in the bundle of His, decreasing cardiac excitability. It is considered a second-line drug used to suppress ventricular ectopy and arrhythmias and to convert supraventricular arrhythmias.

CHAPTER 8

Study Questions

1. **c.** *Explanation:* Bronchodilators are beta-adrenergic agonists, having their strongest effect on beta$_2$-adrenergic (pulmonary) receptors. This relaxes bronchial smooth muscle, causing increased lung capacity and a decrease in airway resistance.

2. **c.** *Explanation:* The standard dosage of albuterol in patients 12 and older is 2 inha-

lations every 4–6 h. The safe dosage for albuterol for patients under 12 has not been established; therefore, the drug should not be administered to such patients.

3. **a.** *Explanation:* Aminophylline should not be administered to patients who are hypersensitive to the drug or who suffer from uncontrolled cardiac arrhythmias. It should be administered with caution to patients over 60 and to patients with congestive heart failure. For these patients the dose of aminophylline should be less than the adult dose.

4. **b.** *Explanation:* The adult dose of epinephrine for the treatment of bronchial asthma is 0.3–0.5 mg (0.3–0.5 mL) of a 1:1000 solution, SC. The initial dose is usually 0.3 mg. A dose of 0.3–0.5 mg by IV bolus of a 1:10,000 solution is appropriate for severe anaphylaxis (see Chapter 12). The pediatric dose used to treat bronchial asthma is 0.01 mg/kg of a 1:1000 solution, SC. A 3–5 mg SC of a 1:1000 solution is definitely not an appropriate dosage of epinephrine.

5. **d.** *Explanation:* If too much oxygen is given, it may take away the patient's stimulus to breathe **(hypoxic drive).** The oxygen can gradually be increased as needed. If the patient develops respiratory depression, you can assist ventilations. Oxygen should never be withheld from any patient who needs it.

6. **a.** *Explanation:* The adult SC dose of terbutaline is 0.25 mg. This may be repeated in 15–30 min. When terbutaline is administered by inhalation, the adult dose is 2 inhalations every 4–6 h. (200 μm/spray).

7. **d.** *Explanation:* Terbutaline is administered to pediatric patients by inhalation. Patients 12 and older should be given 2 inhalations every 4–6 h (200 μg/spray). It is not recommended to give terbutaline in the prehospital setting to patients under 12.

Case Studies

1. **b.** *Explanation:* Racemic epinephrine causes bronchodilation, increasing tidal volume and vital capacity of the lungs. It is used to treat **laryngotracheobronchitis (croup).** Racemic epinephrine is administered according to body weight. Patients < 20 kg receive 0.25 mg/kg by inhalation; patients > 20 kg receive 0.5 mg/kg by inhalation. This patient should receive 0.25 mg/kg.

   Epinephrine is a bronchodilator indicated for the treatment of bronchial asthma. Isoetharine is a bronchodilator used to treat reversible airway obstruction caused by asthma or COPD. Isoetharine is not to be administered to pediatric patients. Metaproterenol is a bronchodilator used to treat dyspnea caused by asthma or COPD. It is not to be administered to patients under 12.

2. **a.** *Explanation:* In most cases 1:1000 solution of epinephrine is the first drug of choice for an acute asthma attack. The dosage is 0.3–0.5 mg, SC. After the epinephrine administration, the physician may order aminophylline, usually considered the second drug of choice for acute asthma. The dosage of aminophylline is 250–500 mg by IV infusion, given over 20–30 min.

   Epinephrine in 1:10,000 solution is not appropriate for patients experiencing an acute asthma attack. Epinephrine in a 1:10,000 solution is administered to cardiac patients and patients experiencing severe anaphylatic reaction. Racemic epinephrine can be administered to adults, but not usually in the prehospital setting.

Terbutaline is used for asthma, but not with epinephrine in a 1:10,000 solution. The dosage of terbutaline is 2 inhalations every 4–6 h (200 μg/spray). Terbutaline administered parenterally may lose its pulmonary effectiveness.

CHAPTER 9

Study Questions

1. **d.** *Explanation:* $D_{50}W$ is used to increase circulating blood sugar levels to normal. It is also used in cases of coma of unknown cause, in case hypoglycemia is a factor in the coma. Some EMS protocols include $D_{50}W$ in the treatment of selected medical cardiac arrests, if low blood sugar levels are a contributing factor.

2. **c.** *Explanation:* The correct pediatric dosage of $D_{50}W$ is 0.5–1 g/kg by slow IV bolus. Before administration, the $D_{50}W$ should be diluted 1:1 with sterile distilled water to make a 25% solution (0.25 g/mL).

3. **a.** *Explanation:* It is important to draw a blood sample before giving any form of glucose to your patient, so that the receiving emergency facility can record the patient's original glucose level.

4. **b.** *Explanation:* Insulin is administered to the patient experiencing diabetic ketoacidosis. Ketoacidosis is associated with a very high level of glucose in the blood (hyperglycemia).

5. **b.** *Explanation:* The adult dose of glucagon in the prehospital setting is normally 0.5–1 U, IM, SC, or IV. One or two more doses can be administered if the patient does not respond in about 20 min. In emergency situations, $D_{50}W$ is the drug of choice. Generally, glucagon should only be used if an IV cannot be started and glucose cannot be given.

6. **c.** *Explanation:* The brain must have sufficient amounts of glucose for metabolism or it may become permanently damaged. Thiamine is required for the metabolism of carbohydrates. Without enough thiamine, the brain is unable to metabolize glucose effectively.

7. **c.** *Explanation:* The prehospital dosage of thiamine is 100 mg. There are two acceptable ways to administer this dosage: (1) dilute 100 mg of thiamine in 50–100 mL of normal saline solution or D_5W and administer over 15–30 min; (2) administer 50 mg of thiamine by slow IV bolus and 50 mg IM.

8. **d.** *Explanation:* Without insulin, glucose cannot pass into the body's cells and blood glucose levels rise, producing hyperglycemia. Acidosis may develop without adequate insulin, because the body breaks down fat for energy in place of glucose, causing the formation of ketone bodies and other acids.

Case Studies

1. **c.** *Explanation:* This patient is suffering from a coma of unknown cause. However, alcohol is suspected as the cause or at least as a contributing factor. Thiamine is necessary for carbohydrate metabolism. Chronic alcohol intake interferes with the

use of thiamine. Many alcohol-dependent patients are thiamine deficient. If $D_{50}W$ is given to the alcohol-dependent patient who is deficient in thiamine, the glucose may cause the patient to develop Wernicke's encephalopathy or Korsakoff's syndrome. Therefore, it is important to administer thiamine prior to dextrose in the suspected alcohol-dependent patient.

2. **b.** *Explanation:* Signs and symptoms of diabetic ketoacidosis include tachycardia; deep, rapid respirations; warm, dry skin; low blood pressure; and a decreased level of consciousness.

3. **a.** *Explanation:* Warm, dry skin can indicate dehydration, and rapid pulse and low blood pressure can indicate shock. This patient needs IV fluid volume replacement. Diabetic ketoacidosis is associated with excessive amounts of glucose in the body caused from the absence of insulin. Therefore, the patient in diabetic ketoacidosis requires insulin. Insulin therapy is generally administered in the hospital. However, if given prehospital, begin with a loading dose of 2–10 U of regular insulin, IV. Follow with 2–10 U by IV infusion.

CHAPTER 10

Study Questions

1. **b.** *Explanation:* Diazepam should be administered at 5–10 mg by slow IV bolus to the patient in status epilepticus. This can be repeated every 10–15 min, to a maximal dose of 30 mg. The prehospital dosage of diazepam for other seizure activity or as a skeletal muscle relaxant is 2–5 mg by slow IV bolus.

2. **c.** *Explanation:* Diazepam causes CNS depression. If diazepam is given too rapidly or in excess, patients may experience respiratory arrest. Therefore, when giving diazepam, assess the patient's vital signs and respiratory status continuously.

3. **a.** *Explanation:* The three adult dosages for dexamethasone that prehospital emergency care professionals need to know are
   1. *Severe allergic reactions:* 4.0 mg by slow IV bolus.
   2. *Cerebral edema:* 10 mg by slow IV bolus.
   3. *Shock:* 100 mg by slow IV bolus.
   The prehospital use of dexamethasone is not recommended for pediatric patients.

4. **d.** *Explanation:* Mannitol should be administered with caution to patients who show a tendency to develop congestive heart failure, because the drug can cause a sudden expansion of extracellular fluid, which can exacerbate the developing of congestive heart failure. Hypersensitivity, preexisting dehydration, and active intracranial bleeding are all contraindications for the use of mannitol.

5. **c.** *Explanation:* The adult dosage for methylprednisolone is 30 mg/kg by IV bolus. This should be followed by an IV infusion of 5.4 mg/kg/h. To determine the amount needed for the IV bolus:

   180 lb $\div$ 2.2 kg = 81.8 or 82 kg
   30 mg $\times$ 82 kg = 2460 mg

To determine the amount needed for the IV infusion:

82 kg × 5.4 mg = 442.8 or 443 mg.

6. **d.** *Explanation:* Phenobarbital should not be administered to patients who are hypersensitive to barbiturates or patients with CNS or respiratory depression. Phenobarbital should be administered with caution to patients with severe liver or kidney dysfunction. Elderly patients are more prone than adults to experience the side effects of phenobarbital. Therefore, the elderly may require less than adult doses of phenobarbital.

7. **b.** *Explanation:* The pediatric dosage of phenytoin is 10–15 mg/kg by slow IV bolus.

8. **a.** *Explanation:* Phenytoin should not be administered to patients with hypersensitivity to the drug or to patients with bradycardia or heart block, because of its effect on atrioventricular conduction. Phenytoin should be used with caution in elderly patients and in patients with severe cardiac or respiratory problems.

Case Studies

1. **d.** *Explanation:* Cerebrovascular accidents (CVAs) are most often seen in, but not limited to, elderly patients. Predisposing factors of a CVA include heart disease, hypertension, cerebral atherosclerosis, existing thrombi, anticoagulant therapy, and cerebral aneurysm. Signs and symptoms of a cerebrovascular accident include altered level of consciousness, speech impairment, drooling, incontinence, facial drooping, and paralysis affecting one side of the body.

   Treatment in this case is mainly supportive, with rapid transport to the emergency department. Administer oxygen by nasal cannula at about 4–6 L/min. A precautionary IV line should be established in case the administration of drugs becomes necessary.

   Verapamil is indicated in controlling rapid ventricular response seen in atrial fibrillation or atrial flutter. In this case the ventricular rate is 90 beats/min, which is not excessive. Verapamil is not indicated in this case.

2. **b.** *Explanation:* Diazepam causes CNS depression. It is used to control anticonvulsant emergencies. The adult dosage of diazepam is 5–10 mg by slow IV bolus. This may be repeated every 10–15 min to a maximum dose of 30 mg. In this situation, administer diazepam with caution, because the patient may have taken alcohol and/or other drugs. Giving diazepam may cause an additive depressant effect that can compromise respirations. Therefore, you should be prepared to intubate and to assist ventilations.

   Phenytoin is also used to control seizure activity. However, phenytoin is contraindicated in patients with bradycardia or heart block, because of its effect on atrioventricular conduction. This patient has both bradycardia (rate of approximately 50 beats/min) and second-degree heart block.

   Methylprednisolone is indicated in patients who have sustained traumatic spinal cord injury and demonstrate a loss of motor function or sensation. Dexamethasone is used to treat shock, acute cerebral edema, and severe allergic reactions. Therefore, these drugs would not be indicated in this situation.

Other drugs that may be indicated in this situation, after control of the seizure activity, are narcan, in the event the patient has overdosed on narcotic drugs; thiamine, to replace depleted thiamine stores; and $D_{50}W$, to correct possible hypoglycemia.

This patient should be rapidly transported to the nearest appropriate emergency facility.

CHAPTER 11

Study Questions

1. **c.** *Explanation:* Oxytocin is a hormone secreted by the pituitary gland. It stimulates both uterine muscle contraction and uterine blood vessels, which in turn controls postpartum hemorrhage.

2. **a.** *Explanation:* The IV infusion dosage of oxytocin is 10–20 U of the drug added to 100 mL of lactated Ringer's or normal saline and titrated to the severity of the hemorrhage. The IM dosage is 3–10 U. Oxytocin is not given to pediatric patients.

3. **b.** *Explanation:* Magnesium sulfate, by affecting neuromuscular transmissions, depresses the CNS. It is therapeutically beneficial in treating seizures associated with eclampsia. Oxytocin is the drug of choice in controlling postpartum hemorrhage. Both diazepam and labetalol are contraindicated during pregnancy. Diazepam is toxic to the fetus, and labetalol may cause apnea, low Apgar scores, bradycardia, and hypoglycemia in newborns.

4. **d.** *Explanation:* The prehospital dosage of magnesium sulfate is 2–4 of a 10% solution by IV bolus. This should be followed by an IV infusion of 1–2 g/h.

5. **b.** *Explanation:* When a patient is convulsing because of eclampsia, she should be given 5–10 mg of diazepam by slow IV bolus. In most protocols, this is followed by a 10% solution of magnesium sulfate.

Case Studies

1. **d.** *Explanation:* Magnesium sulfate is used as an anticonvulsant in the prevention or control of seizures in preeclampsia or eclampsia. The dosage of magnesium sulfate is 2–4 g of a 10% solution by IV bolus over 3 min. This equates to the following:
   - 2 g = 20 mL
   - 3 g = 30 mL
   - 4 g = 40 mL

   The IV bolus dose of magnesium sulfate should be followed by an IV infusion of 1–2 g/h.

   Diazepam is an anticonvulsant used for the treatment of active seizures or status epilepticus. Oxytocin is used in prehospital medicine to contract uterine blood vessels to control postpartum hemorrhage. Mannitol is an osmotic diuretic used as an adjunct in the treatment of edema.

2. **a.** *Explanation:* In most cases of active seizures in the eclamptic patient, the physician will order diazepam. Diazepam is an anticonvulsant used in the treatment of seizures. In this case, the dosage of diazepam is 5–10 mg by slow IV bolus. Once

the diazepam has been administered, a solution of 10% magnesium sulfate should be given at a dose of 2–4 g by slow IV.

You must remember that both diazepam and magnesium sulfate cause CNS depression, which can depress respirations. If respiratory depression should develop, an antidote for the magnesium sulfate is calcium gluconate. If necessary, administer a 10% solution of calcium gluconate at a dose of 5–10 mEq (10–20 mL) by slow IV.

CHAPTER 12

Study Questions

1. **a.** *Explanation:* During an allergic reaction, histamine stimulates both H_1 and H_2 receptors. Stimulation of H_1 receptors causes bronchoconstriction, and stimulation of both H_1 and H_2 receptors causes peripheral vasodilation. Diphenhydramine competes with histamine for H_1 receptor sites.

2. **c.** *Explanation:* The pediatric dosage for diphenhydramine is 2–5 mg/kg by slow IV bolus or IM. The adult dose of diphenhydramine is 10–50 mg by slow IV bolus or IM. Adult patients may require as much as 100 mg of the drug.

3. **d.** *Explanation:* Epinephrine is the primary prehospital drug in cases of anaphylaxis. It constricts dilated blood vessels, raises the heart rate, improves myocardial contractility, and dilates the bronchioles.

4. **b.** *Explanation:* The adult dose of epinephrine in cases of severe anaphylaxis is 0.3–0.5 mg by slow IV bolus (3–5 mL of a 1:10,000 solution). It may also be necessary to follow this dosage up with an IV epinephrine infusion. Patients experiencing mild to moderate anaphylaxis should initially receive an SC injection of 0.3–0.5 mg of epinephrine (0.3–0.5 mL of a 1:1000 solution of epinephrine).

5. **d.** *Explanation:* Hydrocortisone is a strong anti-inflammatory drug used to replace the naturally occurring hormone in the short-term management of inflammatory and allergic reactions.

6. **a.** *Explanation:* The adult dosage of hydrocortisone is 100–500 mg by IV bolus or IM. IV bolus doses greater than 100 mg should be diluted in 50–100 mL of D_5W or normal saline solution.

7. **b.** *Explanation:* After administration of methylprednisolone, patients should be frequently assessed for signs of peripheral edema, rales, or dyspnea. Other side effects of methylprednisolone include hypertension, hyperglycemia, hypokalemia, and fluid retention.

8. **d.** *Explanation:* Methylprednisolone is not recommended for prehospital use in the pediatric patient.

Case Studies

1. **b.** *Explanation:* Anaphylactic reactions can develop very rapidly after an antigen has invaded the body. Bee stings are common causes. The patient who experiences an anaphylactic reaction may develop any of the following signs and symptoms:

- Difficulty breathing
- Sneezing, wheezing
- Coughing blood-tinged sputum
- Hives
- Itching
- Abdominal cramps
- Facial swelling
- Hypotension
- Rapid pulse
- Diarrhea

Patients who experience severe anaphylaxis may develop cardiopulmonary arrest within seconds or minutes unless immediate treatment is begun.

2. **a.** *Explanation:* Epinephrine is used as the primary drug in treating anaphylaxis. It causes constriction of blood vessels, raises heart rate, improves myocardial contractility, and dilates the bronchioles. After epinephrine, diphenhydramine is usually administered. Diphenhydramine blocks the effects of histamine release. It is used in addition to epinephrine in the treatment of anaphylaxis.

    Methylprednisolone and hydrocortisone should be kept on hand to be used once the patient is stabilized. Methylprednisolone and hydrocortisone suppress the body's inflammatory response and modify the body's normal immune response.

    Dopamine is a vasopressor that increase cardiac output and blood pressure while maintaining good renal perfusion (see Chapter 7).

CHAPTER 13

Study Questions

1. **b.** *Explanation:* Amyl nitrite converts hemoglobin to a substance called methemoglobin, which in turn binds with cyanide, preventing its toxicity. Amyl nitrite is used for the immediate treatment of cyanide poisoning.

2. **c.** *Explanation:* The adult dosage for amyl nitrite is 1–2 ampules crushed and inhaled for 30 sec. This may be repeated until the patient arrives at the emergency department. Each amyl nitrite ampule contains 0.3 mL of the drug.

3. **d.** *Explanation:* Activated charcoal should not be used in patients who have ingested cyanide, mineral acids, strong bases, methanol, and ethanol, because it is ineffective with these substances. Activated charcoal is very effective in binding aspirin, phenytoin, and strychnine.

4. **c.** *Explanation:* The pediatric dosage for activated charcoal is 10–30 g (3–5 tbs) mixed with tap water to make a slurry. The adult dosage for activated charcoal is 30–60 g (5–10 tbs).

5. **b.** *Explanation:* Atropine blocks the action of acetylcholine in the parasympathetic nervous system, aiding in the treatment of cholinesterase poisoning from organophosphate pesticides.

6. **c.** *Explanation:* The initial adult dosage of atropine for organophosphate poisoning is 1 mg by IV bolus. If there is no improvement, repeat at 2–5 mg by IV bolus. Med-

ical control may order additional doses while you are en route to the emergency department.

7. **d.** *Explanation:* Naloxone is a competitive antagonist of opiate receptors in the CNS. This competitive action displaces narcotic analgesics from their receptor sites, blocking their effects.

8. **c.** *Explanation:* The initial adult dose of naloxone is 0.4–2 mg by slow IV bolus. This may be repeated at 2–3 min intervals as needed. If no response is seen after 10 mg has been given, another cause should be considered.

9. **d.** *Explanation:* Atropine is the prehospital drug of choice as an antidote to physostigmine. Atropine has anticholinergic properties that can antagonize the cholinergic effects of physostigmine.

10. **b.** *Explanation:* The pediatric dosage of pralidoxime is 20–40 mg/kg by IV infusion over 30–60 min. The infusion is prepared by adding 1 g of pralidoxime to 500 mL of normal saline solution, making a concentration of 2 mg/mL.

11. **b.** *Explanation:* The recommended dosage of syrup of ipecac for a patient over 1 is 15–25 mL PO followed by warm water. The dosage of ipecac for children under 1 is 5–10 mL PO followed by warm water. The adult dose for syrup ipecac is 15–30 mL PO followed by several glasses of warm water. The adult dose may be repeated once in 20 min, if necessary.

Case Studies

1.
A. **b.** *Explanation:* The signs of organophosphate poisoning include bradycardia, diaphoresis, profuse salivation, and occasionally respiratory distress.

   Organophosphate poisoning can be severe. This type of poisoning is most often seen in rural settings where large amounts of pesticides are used. Prehospital treatment for patients exposed to large amounts of pesticides must be aggressive.

B. **d.** *Explanation:* Two drugs should be used to treat organophosphate poisoning: atropine and pralidoxime. Atropine, a parasympathetic blocker, blocks the release of acetylcholine, which aids in the management of organophosphate poisoning. The initial dose of atropine is 1 mg by IV bolus. If there is no improvement, repeat at 2–5 mg by IV bolus. Medical control may order additional doses while you are transporting the patient to the emergency department.

2. **a.** *Explanation:* Diazepam is usually used to control anticonvulsant and antianxiety emergencies. It has been shown to be effective in controlling advancing CNS stimulation and convulsions caused by cocaine overdose. The dosage for diazepam for advancing CNS stimulation is 2.5–5 mg by slow IV bolus. To control seizure activity, administer 5–10 mg by slow IV bolus. This dosage can be repeated every 10–15 min to a maximum of 30 mg.

   Naloxone is used to treat symptomatic narcotic overdose. However, it may cause seizures and should be used with caution in patients who are experiencing or may develop convulsive disorders.

   Atropine is used to treat organophosphate poisoning and its use is not appropriate in this case. Pralidoxime, used after atropine in severe cases of organophosphate poisoning, is also not called for in this case.

CHAPTER 14

Study Questions

1. **b.** *Explanation:* Antipsychotics are contraindicated in patients with CNS depression, because they cause further depression. Chlorpromazine is indicated in the treatment of mild alcohol withdrawal, and both chlorpromazine and haloperidol can be used *with caution* to treat patients with seizure disorders. The major indication for both chlorpromazine and haloperidol is to treat patients experiencing psychosis.

2. **c.** *Explanation:* The adult dosage of chlorpromazine to treat both psychoses and alcohol withdrawal is 25 mg IM.

3. **d.** *Explanation:* Haloperidol is not recommended for pediatric patients in the prehospital setting.

4. **a.** *Explanation:* The pediatric dosage of hydroxyzine is 1 mg/kg deep IM injection. Your patient weighs 46 lb. Therefore:

   46 lb ÷ 2.2 kg = 20.9 or 21 kg
   21 kg × 1 mg = 21 mg

Case Studies

1. **c or d.** *Explanation:* Of these two drugs, diazepam is probably more often used in prehospital emergency care. Both diazepam and hydroxyzine are antianxiety and sedative agents. They both act as CNS depressants. The prehospital sedative dosage of diazepam is 2–10 mg by slow IV bolus or slow IM injection. The dosage for hydroxyzine is 50–100 mg by deep IM injection.

   Both chlorpromazine and haloperidol are used to treat the signs and symptoms of psychosis.

2. **b.** *Explanation:* The precaution for the use of chlorpromazine is that it may lower the seizure threshold in patients with seizure disorders. Since this patient has a history of seizures, diazepam should be on hand to control any seizure activity that may develop. The dosage of diazepam for controlling seizure activity is 2–5 mg by slow IV bolus. This may be repeated if needed, but not to exceed 10 mg.

   Haloperidol is also used to decrease the signs and symptoms of psychosis. It is highly unlikely that medical control would order haloperidol after chlorpromazine. Hydroxyzine is used in the treatment of anxiety and, therefore, is not indicated for this case. Dextrose 50% in water is given to return blood sugar levels to normal in hypoglycemic patients. Individuals experiencing mental disorders may be hypoglycemic, but that is not the primary concern here.

Bibliography

American Heart Association: Textbook of Advanced Cardiac Life Support. American Heart Association, Dallas, 1988.

Audet, PR: Davis's Physician's Drug Guide. FA Davis, Philadelphia, 1989.

Bledsoe, BE, Bosker, G, and Papa, FJ: Prehospital Emergency Pharmacology, ed 2. Prentice-Hall, Englewood Cliffs, NJ, 1988.

Caroline, NC: Emergency Care in the Streets. Little, Brown & Co, Boston, 1987.

Chameides, L (ed): Textbook of Pediatric Advanced Life Support. American Heart Association, Dallas, 1988.

Clark, JB, Queener, SF, and Karb, VB: Pharmacological Basis of Nursing Practice. CV Mosby, St. Louis, 1982.

Conn, PM and Gebhart, GF: Essentials of Pharmacology. FA Davis, Philadelphia, 1989.

Deglin, JH and Vallerand, AH: Davis's Drug Guide for Nurses, ed 2. FA Davis, Philadelphia, 1991.

Eichelberger, MR, et al: Pediatric Emergencies. Brady (Prentice-Hall Division), Englewood Cliffs, NJ, 1992.

Emergency Cardiac Care Committee and Subcommittees, American Heart Association: Guidelines for Cardiopulmonary Resuscitation and Emergency Cardiac Care, I: Introduction. JAMA 268:2172–2183, 1992.

Finucane, BT and Santora, AH: Principles of Airway Management. FA Davis, Philadelphia, 1988.

Fujisawa Pharmaceutical Company: Adenocard monograph. Deerfield, IL.

Hahn, AB, Oestreich, SJK, and Barkin, RL: Mosby's Pharmacology in Nursing. CV Mosby, St. Louis, 1986.

Jones, SA, et al: Advanced Emergency Care for Paramedic Practice. JB Lippincott Company, Philadelphia, 1992.

Springhouse Drug Reference. Springhouse Corporation, Springhouse, 1988.

Thomas, CL (ed): Taber's Cyclopedic Medical Dictionary, ed 16. FA Davis, Philadelphia, 1989.

Vallerand, AH and Deglin, JH: Drug Guide for Critical Care and Emergency Nursing, ed 2. FA Davis, Philadelphia, 1991.

Glossary

Absorption: passage of a substance through a body surface into body fluids and tissues.

Acetylcholine: naturally occurring body substance necessary for the functioning of the parasympathetic nervous system.

Acid-base balance: a state of equilibrium between acidity and alkalinity of body fluids.

Acidosis: condition resulting from an excess of acid or deficit of alkalines (bicarbonate) in body fluid.

Active transport: mechanism for moving substances across cell membranes from a dilute solution to a concentrated solution.

Adrenergic: term for (sympathetic) nerve fibers that, when stimulated, release epinephrine; also, a class of drugs that produces the effect of epinephrine.

Adrenocorticoid: hormone produced by the adrenal cortex; a class of drugs consisting of such hormones and synthetic versions of them.

Adsorption: Adhesion by a gas or liquid to the surface of a solid.

Affinity: in pharmacology, the attraction between a receptor and a drug.

Afterload: Arterial pressure that the heart must push against to eject blood; tension in the ventricular wall during systole.

Agonist: substance that activates a receptor.

Alkalosis: condition resulting from an excess of alkalines or a deficit of acids in the body fluid.

Ampule: a small glass container that can be sealed and its contents sterilized; a common method of packaging hypodermic solutions.

Analgesic: drug that relieves pain.

Anaphylaxis: allergic hypersensitive reaction to a foreign substance.

Anion: see *ion.*

Antagonist: drug that interferes with the action of an agonist.

Antianginal: drug that relieves the pain of angina pectoris.

Antiarrhythmic: drug that controls or prevents cardiac arrhythmias.

Antibody: a substance produced by the body in response to an *antigen;* each antibody reacts only with its specific antigen.

Antidote: substance that neutralizes a poison or the toxic effects of a drug.

Antigen: foreign particle or substance whose presence in the body causes *antibody* production.

Antihistamine: drug that blocks the effects of histamine.

Antitussive: drug used to prevent or relieve coughing.

Apothecaries' system: a system of weight and measure used mostly by pharmacists.

Arterial oxygen tension (PaO$_2$): partial pressure of oxygen in arterial blood; a measure of how much oxygen is dissolved in the bloodstream after it has left the lungs.

Autonomic nervous system: the component of the peripheral nervous system that controls automatic functions.

Beta-blocker: a beta-adrenergic blocking agent. A substance that blocks the inhibitory effects of sympathetic nervous system agents such as epinephrine.

Biotransformation: changes in chemical makeup resulting from metabolism.

Blood-brain barrier (also called the blood–spinal-fluid barrier): membrane that separates the brain and spinal fluid from circulating blood and prevents certain substances in blood (such as drugs) from reaching brain tissue or spinal fluid.

Bolus: a concentrated mass of a substance; pharmacologically, a rounded preparation for oral ingestion or a single dose, injected all at once.

Bound drug: portion of a drug dose that chemically binds with blood proteins or becomes stored in fatty tissue and is unavailable for therapeutic action; see *free drug.*

Bronchodilator: drug used to relieve airway obstruction caused by constriction of the bronchii.

Cation: see *ion.*

Central nervous system (CNS): the brain and spinal cord.

Chemical name: description, in the specialized language of chemistry, of the structure of a drug; see *generic name, official name, trade name.*

Cholinergic: term for (parasympathetic) nerve fibers that, when stimulated, release acetylcholine; class of drugs that mimic the action of acetylcholine.

Cholinesterase: enzyme essential for the functioning of the nervous system.

Chronic obstructive pulmonary disease (COPD): disease that reduces the lung's ability to perform ventilation; causative diseases include chronic bronchitis, pulmonary emphysema, chronic asthma, and chronic bronchiolitis.

Chronotropic: having an influence on the rate of occurrence of an event, such as a heartbeat.

Colloid: substance that forms a suspension instead of a true solution; the molecules of a colloid do not cross body membrane.

Concentration: the amount of an ingredient relative to the whole compound; in pharmacology, the *strength* of a drug solution.

Contraindication: symptom or circumstance that makes an otherwise desirable action or treatment unadvisable.

Croup: laryngotracheobronchitis.

Crystalloid: crystal-forming substance that can dissolve and cross body membranes in solution.

Cumulative drug effects: effects of repeated doses of a drug that the body does not completely or immediately eliminate; such drugs accumulate in the system, and their effects can be greater than the sum of the effects of individual doses.

Depressant: agent that depresses a body function.

Diffusion: the tendency of particles of substances in solution to move about until the concentration of the substance is the same throughout the solution.

dose-dependent: drug effects that vary with changes in the amount administered.

Drug: substance that, when introduced into the body, causes a change in the way the body functions.

Eclampsia: coma and convulsive seizures between the 20th week of pregnancy and the 1st week after delivery, occurring in 1 out of 200 patients with *preeclampsia.*

Effector organ: muscle or gland that, when stimulated by the nervous system, produces an effect.

Efficacy: power to produce a therapeutic effect.

Electrolyte: a substance that, in solution, separates into *ions* and thus becomes capable of conducting electricity. In body fluid, the electrolytes (sodium, potassium, and calcium, magnesium, and chloride) are necessary for cell function and *acid-base balance.*

Embolus (*plural* emboli): particles of undissolved material (body tissue, air bubble, foreign body) in the bloodstream. A *pulmonary embolus* is an embolus in a pulmonary artery.

Epiglottitis: inflammation of the epiglottis.

Endotracheal (ET): through the throat; also called transtracheal; a method of introducing medication into the airway through a tube down the throat (endotracheal tube).

Excretion: elimination of waste products, including drug metabolites, from the body.

Extract: active ingredient of a substance obtained by distillation: see *fluid extract.*

first-line drug: in a prehospital emergency situation, the first drug called for in local protocols; the drug of choice for any given condition. (See also *second-line drug.*)

Fluid, body: the nonsolid, liquid portion of the body, consisting of:
intracellular fluid—the liquid content of body cells
extracellular fluid—all other body fluid, consisting of:
interstitial fluid—the liquid in the spaces between cells and
intravascular fluid—the nonsolid portion of the blood.

Fluid extract: solution of a drug in a liquid in such a concentration that 1 mL of fluid contains 1 g of drug.

Free drug: portion of a drug dose not bound to blood protein or stored in fatty tissue and thereby available for therapeutic action; see *bound drug.*

Generic name (nonproprietary name): name, usually a shortened form of the chemical name, by which a drug is identified; see *chemical name, official name, trade name.*

Glycogen: starch, the form in which carbohydrates are stored in the body; when needed for metabolism, it is converted to glucose.

Habituation: process of becoming used to a substance or stimulus.

Histamine: a substance, normally present in the body, which, when released from injured cells, causes strong reactions that lead to increased gastric secretion, capillary dilation, and bronchiole smooth muscle constriction.

Hypersensitivity: above-normal susceptibility to a foreign substance, such as pollen.

Hypertonic: having higher osmotic pressure than another solution.

Hypnotic: drug that induces sleep.

Hypotonic: having lower osmotic pressure than another solution.

Hypoxic drive: stimulus for respiration triggered by a deficiency of oxygen.

Immunosuppressant: drug that interferes with the body's natural immune response; the primary use of immunosuppressants is to keep the body from rejecting transplants.

Infusion: a liquid substance introduced into the body through a vein.

Inhalation: act of drawing in air or gas into the lungs; a route of drug administration.

Inotropic: having influence on the contractile force of muscle.

Intralingual (IL): into the tongue; route of drug administration.

Intramuscular (IM): into the muscle; route of drug administration.

Intraosseous (IO): into the bone; route of drug administration.

Intravenous (IV): into the vein; route of drug administration.

Ion: an atom with an excess or shortage of electrons, which gives it a charge of negative *(anion)* or positive *(cation)* electrical energy. See *electrolyte*.

Isotonic: having the same osmotic pressure.

keep-open rate: minimun flow rate necessary to keep vein open. This is usually approximately 20 mL/h.

Ketoacidosis: excess acidity of body fluids due to higher than normal levels of ketone bodies; sometimes caused by inadequate use of carbohydrates due to inadequately controlled diabetes mellitus.

Ketone: compound produced during the oxidation of fatty acids.

Kussmaul respirations: very deep, gasping breaths associated with diabetic acidosis and coma.

Laryngotracheobronchitis: inflammation of the larynx, trachea, and bronchii; *croup.*

loading dose: the initial dose necessary to achieve therapeutic concentration of the drug in the bloodstream.

Mechanism of action: explanation of what a drug does to achieve its therapeutic effect.

Membrane: a thin, pliable sheet or layer of tissue; *permeable membrane* allows molecules of substances to pass through it, while *semipermeable membrane* (such as most cell walls) allows the molecules of some but not all substances to pass through it.

Metabolism: all the physical and chemical changes within an organism resulting in the transformation of ingested substances (food, oxygen, etc.) into cell material or energy.

Metabolite: any substance that results from metabolism.

Methemoglobinemia: condition in which more than 1% of hemoglobin in blood is oxidized to the ferric form; symptoms include cyanosis, vomiting, shock, and coma.

Milliequivalent (mEq): the concentration of electrolytes in a certain volume of solution; measure of the number of ionic charges available in a solution.

Motoneuron: a neuron that stimulates a muscle or gland.

Myocardial infarction (MI): death of heart muscle caused by blockage of blood flow through a coronary artery.

National Formulary: See *U.S. Pharmacopeia.*

Narcotic: a drug that depresses the central nervous system.

Narrow-angle glaucoma: disease in which the pressure inside the eye is higher than normal due to structural abnormality.

Neurotransmitter: substance (e.g., acetylcholine, norepinephrine) that allows the transmission of impulses between synapses in a neural pathway.

Nonproprietary name: generic name of a drug.

Official name: the name of a drug given to it by the U.S. Pharmacopeial Convention; usually it is the generic name, followed by the letters USP. See *chemical name, generic name, trade name.*

Onset of drug action: the time required for a drug preparation to reach a effective concentration at the desired site.

Organophosphate: chemical compound, common in pesticides, that inhibits *cholinesterase.*

Osmosis: the movement of a solvent through a semipermeable membrane (such as a cell wall) into a solution with a higher solute concentration, so as to equalize the concentrations of solute on both sides of the membrane.

Osmotic diuretic: drug or agent that causes increased excretion of water and electrolytes (diuresis) by increasing the *osmotic pressure* of the glomerular filtrate.

Osmotic pressure: the pressure produced by the difference in solute concentration between two solutions separated by a semipermeable membrane.

Overdose: dose of a drug sufficient to cause an acute reaction.

Oxytocic: an agent that stimulates uterine contractions.

Parasympathetic nervous system: a division of the autonomic nervous system.

Parenteral: Describing any route of administration other than the alimentary canal, including intravenous and intramuscular.

Passive transport: the mechanisms for moving substances across cell membrane from a solution with a higher concentration of the substance to a solution with a lower concentration.

Peripheral nervous system (PNS): all nervous tissue found outside the central nervous system.

Permeable membrane: See *membrane.*

pH (potential of hydrogen): a number on a scale of 0 to 14 that expresses the acidity or alkalinity of a substance. A substance with a pH of 7 is neutral, one with a pH of 5 is acidic, and one with a pH of 9 is alkaline.

Pharmacodynamics: the study of the actions of drugs on the body.

Pharmacokinetics: the study of the movement of drugs through the systems of the body.

Pharmacology: the study of drugs, their sources, characteristics, and effects.

Physicians' Desk Reference (PDR): a book, published annually, that describes all currently used drugs.

Poison: any substance taken into the body that interferes with normal physiologic function.

Postpartum hemorrhage: in a woman who has given birth, the loss of more than 500 mL of blood within 24 h of delivery.

Potentiation: the synergistic action of two substances (drugs, hormones, and other body chemicals) in which the total effects are greater than the sum of the independent effects of the two substances.

Preeclampsia: hypertension and other abnormalities resulting from *toxemia of pregnancy* and, in some case, leading to *eclampsia.*

Preload: the degree of stretch of the heart muscle fibers at the beginning of a contraction; the volume or pressure within the ventricle at the end of diastole.

Prophylactic: an agent, device, or process designed to prevent an unhealthy outcome.

Proprietary name: trade name.

Psychosis: mental disorder characterized by loss of contact with reality.

Pulmonary embolus: See *embolus.*

reagent: A substance used to detect the presence of another substance.

Receptor: in pharmacology, a part of a cell that combines with a drug or body substance to alter the cell's functioning.

Reflex arc: the neural pathway of a reflex action.

Reperfusion: resumption of blood flow to a tissue area after it has been blocked, by, for example, a thrombus.

second-line drug: the drug whose administration is called for by local protocols when the maximal dose of first-line drug has not had the desired effect, or when administration of the first-line drug is contraindicated. (See also *first-line drug.*)

Sedative: a drug that has a soothing or tranquilizing effect.

Seizure: a sudden attack of pain or other symptoms. Seizures associated with epilepsy include *tonic-clonic (grand mal)* and *partial* or *absence (petit mal).*

Seizure threshold: level of stimulus intensity sufficient to set off a seizure.

Semipermeable membrane: See *membrane.*

Solubility: the ability to dissolve in a substance.

Solute: see *solution.*

Solution: a mixture of a liquid *(solvent)* and a solid *(solute)* in which the particles of the solid are so well mixed that they cannot be distinguished from the resulting fluid: see *suspension.*

Solvent: see *solution.*

Status epilepticus: epilepsy

Steroid: any of a class of complex compounds important in body chemistry, including sex and other hormones and vitamins.

Subcutaneous (SQ or SC): under the skin; a route of drug administration.

Sublingual (SL): under the tongue; a route of drug administration.

Suppository: a semisolid drug preparation in the form of a cone or cylinder that is inserted into the rectum, vagina, or urethra.

Suspension: a mixture of a solid and a fluid in which the particles of the solid are mixed with, but not dissolved in, the fluid; see *solution.*

Sympathetic nervous system: division of the autonomic nervous system.

Sympathomimetic: drug or agent that produces effects like those produced by stimulating the sympathetic nervous system.

Synapse: the connecting space between two neurons in a neural pathway.

Synergism: the acting together of two substances (drugs, hormones, or other body chemicals) whose combined effect is different from, and perhaps greater than, the individual effect of each substance.

Therapeutic benefit: the desired effect of a drug.

Therapeutic index: a number representing the ratio of the lethal or toxic dose of a drug to its therapeutic dose; an expression of the relative safety of a drug—the higher the number, the wider the margin of safety.

Therapeutics: the study of the effects of remedies, such as drugs, and the treatment of disease.

Thiazide: any of several drugs used as diuretics.

Thrombi: see *thrombus.*

Thrombus (*plural* thrombi): a blood clot that obstructs a blood vessel of heart cavity.

tibial tuberosity: a palpable elevated prominence on the superior-anterior margin of the tibia (just below the knee).

Tincture: a drug preparation consisting of a vegetable or chemical substance dissolved in alcohol.

titrate: Titration is the process of determining the concentration of a chemical solution by adding known amounts of a reagent to the solution until the characteristic change in color or electrical state occurs (see *reagent*). In drug administration, to titrate is to slowly increase the rate of administration until the desired effects are seen.

Tolerance: decreased effectiveness of a drug due to repeated dosage; a person with a tolerance to a drug requires larger doses for the same therapeutic effect.

Toxemia of pregnancy: pathologic condition resulting from metabolic disturbances in pregnant women, manifested in *preeclampsia* and, less often, in *eclampsia.*

Toxicology: the study of poisons.

Trade name: the name of a drug given to it by a manufacturer and registered as a trademark; see *chemical name, generic name, official name.*

Transtracheal: see *endotracheal.*

Troche: lozenge; a drug preparation in the form of a cylinder or disk, intended to be held in the mouth until dissolved or disintegrated.

United States Pharmacopeia (USP): a book, published every 5 years by the U.S. Pharmacopeial Convention, that sets forth the official formulas for all drugs used in the United States and the specifications and standards for preparing and administering them. Since 1975, a similar publication, the *National Formulary,* has been included in the *Pharmacopeia.*

Universal precautions (body substance precautions): uniform procedures of infection control through the use of barrier precautions; *universal* means that the procedures apply to all patients and all work situations, determined by the degree of risk of exposure to body substances and not by the diagnosis of infectious disease.

U.S.P. unit: a standard of measurement determined by the United States Pharmacopeia for a "biologic" (derived from living substance) drug, such as a vaccine, penicillin, and so on; the amount of such a drug that produces a determined therapeutic effect under controlled conditions.

Vagus nerve: one of a pair of cranial nerves, the major sensory and motor nerve of the parasympathetic nervous system.

Vasoconstrictor: a drug used to decrease the diameter of blood vessels.

Vasodilator: a drug used to increase the diameter of blood vessels.

Vasopressor: a drug that causes the muscles of the arteries and capillaries to contract.

Volatile: easily evaporated; volatile drugs are readily excreted through perspiration and respiration.

Volume of distribution: the amount of fluid (body water or plasma) necessary to achieve the desired concentration of a drug in the body.

Withdrawal syndrome: partial collapse resulting from withdrawal of alcohol, stimulants, or some opiates.

Wolff-Parkinson-White syndrome: abnormality of cardiac rhythm characterized by an initial slurring of the R wave (called the delta wave); a shortened P-R interval, and a widened QRS complex.

INDEX

The Drug Index appears on pages 303–307. A "t" following a page number indicates a table; an "f" following a page number indicates a figure.

Abbreviations, pharmacologic, 17, 17t–19t
Absence seizure (petit mal), 290
Absorption, 14–15, 20–23, 26, 285
  administration and, 42–45
  rates of, 23t
Acetylcholine, 13, 32–33, 36, 38–39, 285
Acid-base balance, 76, 78, 84–86, 285
Acidosis, 21, 23, 84–85, 285
Acquired immunodeficiency syndrome
  (AIDS), 57
Activase. See Alteplase
Activated charcoal, 12, 213–214
Active transport, 83, 84f, 285
Adalat. See Nifedepine
Additive effect, 27
Adenocard. See Adenosine
Adenosine, 93–95
Administration of drugs, 15, 20, 26, 40–58,
  61, 86
  alimentary tract routes for, 40–41
  common prehospital techniques for,
  45–57
  dosage calculation and, 58, 61
  pediatric, 260t–263t
  parenteral routes for, 41–45
Adrenalin. See Epinephrine
Adrenergic drugs, 160, 285
Adrenergic nervous system, 36–39, 285
  physiologic actions of, 37t
  receptor sites and functions, 38t
Adrenocorticoid(s), 11, 285
Adsorption, 285
Advanced life support, pediatric, 264t
Adverse reactions, 5, 9, 44. See also
  specific drugs
Aerosol(s), 16
Affinity, 26, 285
Afterload, 285
Agonist(s), 26, 285
AIDS. See Acquired immunodeficiency
  syndrome (AIDS)
Airway obstruction, 13, 22, 42, 160, 168
Albuterol, 13, 160–161

Alcohol/drug abuse, 183
  signs and symptoms of, 184t
Alimentary tract routes, 40–41
Alkalosis, 84–85, 285
Allergen(s), 203
Allergies, 12, 42, 185, 203–204
Alpha-adrenergic receptors, 37–39
  sites and functions of, 38t
Alteplase, 93, 95–96
Alupent. See Metaproteronol
American Heart Association treatment
  algorithms
  adult, 146f–156f
  pediatric, 157f–158f
A-methaPred. See Methylprednisolone
Aminophyllin. See Aminophylline
Aminophylline, 13, 160–162
Ampule(s), 17, 59–60, 60f, 285
  withdrawing medication from, 47f
Amrinone, 14, 96–97
Amyl nitrate, 13, 213–215, 221–222
Analgesic(s), 6, 11, 91, 285
Anaphylactic emergencies, 42, 89, 203–
  211
  drugs for, 204–208. See also specific
  drugs
  therapeutic classification of drugs, 203–
  204
Anaphylaxis, 285
Anectine. See Succinylcholine
Angina pectoris, 11, 38, 41, 121, 124–125,
  134
Animal sources, 6
Animal studies, 9
Anion(s), 77–79, 288
Antagonist(s), 26, 285
Antagonistic, definition of, 28
Antiadrenergic drugs, 36
Antianginal(s), 11, 91, 93, 285
Antianxiety drugs, 11, 183, 195, 228
Antiarrhythmic drugs, 4–5, 11–12, 91–92,
  285
Antibody, 285

293

295

Lidocaine, 4–6, 11–12, 44–45, 256
absorption of, 21–22
cardiovascular emergencies and, 92,
117–119
dosage calculations for, 59, 69–72
Lifeline administration, 49–50
Liniment(s), 15
Liquid drug preparation(s), 16, 60f
Loading dose, 105, 288
Local drug effect(s), 15–16, 41
Lopressor. *See* Metroprolol
Lotion(s), 15
Lozenge(s), 16
Lung congestion, 122
Luminal. *See* Phenobarbital

Macrodrop tubing, 71
Magnesium, 78
Magnesium sulfate, 6, 119–120, 196–199
Mannitol, 184, 187
Masks, 57–58
Mass, 61
Measures. *See* Weights and measures
Mechanisms of action, 5, 20, 25–26, 288.
See also specific drugs
Medicinal gases, 14, 92, 159
Medrol. *See* Methylprednisolone
Membrane, 288
Meperidine. *See* Demerol
mEq. *See* Milliequivalents
Metabolic acidosis, 6, 85, 134–135
Metabolic alkalosis, 85–86
Metabolic emergencies, 175–182
drugs for, 173–179. *See also* specific
drugs
therapeutic classification of drugs, 172–
173
Metabolism, 14, 20, 24–25, 172–173, 288
fluids in, 77–79, 83
Metabolite(s), 24–25, 288
Metaprel. *See* Metaproterenol
Metaproterenol, 13, 165–166
Methemoglobinemia, 24
Methylprednisolone, 12–13, 184, 207–208
Metoprolol, 12, 121–122
Metric system, 63–69
conversions, 67–69
prefixes for, 63t
MI. *See* Myocardial infarction (MI)
Microdrop tubing, 71
MicroNEFRIN. *See* Racemic epinephrine
Milliequivalent(s) (mEq), 60, 79, 289
Minimum therapeutic concentration(s),
27
Morphine, 6, 11, 27–28, 122–123
Motoneurons, 31, 289
Muscle enzymes, 48
Muscle function, 184

Myocardial infarction (MI), 5, 48, 289
treatment algorithm for, 156f
drugs for, 95, 117, 121–122, 135
Myocardial oxygen consumption, 133

Nalbuphine, 11, 123–124
Naloxone, 14, 22, 28, 45, 217–218, 256
Narcan. *See* Naloxone
Narcotic analgesic(s), 27–28, 289
Narcotic antagonist(s), 14, 212
Narrow angle glaucoma, 289
National Formulary (NF), 7, 9, 11
Nervous system, overview of, 30–31, 31f
Neurologic emergencies, 183–194
drugs for, 187–190. *See also* specific
drugs
therapeutic classifications of drugs,
183–184
Neuronal discharge(s), 12
Neurotransmitter(s), 13, 30–33, 36–38,
289
NF. *See National Formulary (NF)*
Nifedipine, 124–125
Nipride. *See* Nitroprusside
Nitro-bid. *See* Nitroglycerin
Nitro-Dur. *See* Nitroglycerin
Nitroglycerin, 11, 13, 21, 41
cardiovascular emergencies and, 93,
125–126
dosage calculations for, 59
Nitrol. *See* Nitroglycerin
Nitrolingual. *See* Nitroglycerin
Nitronox. *See* Nitrous oxide–oxygen
mixture
Nitropress. *See* Nitroprusside
Nitroprusside, 12, 93, 126–127
Nitrostat. *See* Nitroglycerin
Nitrous oxide–oxygen mixture, 11, 14,
127–128
Nomenclature of drugs, 9–11, 10t
Nonelectrolyte(s), 79
Nonproprietary name, 289. *See also*
Generic name
Norepinephrine, 14, 128–129
autonomic nervous system and, 32, 36–
39
Normal values, statistically common
pediatric, 260t
Normodyne. *See* Labetalol
Novolin. *See* Insulin
Nubain. *See* Nalbuphine

Obstetric and gynecologic emergencies,
195–202
drugs for, 196–200. *See also* specific
drugs
therapeutic classification of drugs, 187–
188

298

DRUG INDEX

The General Index appears on pages 293-301.

Activase
in cardiovascular emergencies, 95-96
Activated charcoal
in toxicologic emergencies, 213-214
Adalat
in cardiovascular emergencies, 124-125
Adenocard
in cardiovascular emergencies, 93-95
Adenosine
in cardiovascular emergencies, 93-95
Adrenalin
in anaphylactic emergencies, 205-206
in cardiovascular emergencies, 109-111
in respiratory emergencies, 162-163
Albuterol
in respiratory emergencies, 160-161
Alteplase
in cardiovascular emergencies, 95-96
Alupent
in respiratory emergencies, 165-166
A-methapred
in anaphylactic emergencies, 207-208
in neurologic emergencies, 188
Aminophyllin
in respiratory emergencies, 161-162
Aminophylline
in respiratory emergencies, 161-162
Amrinone
in cardiovascular emergencies, 96-97
Amyl nitrate
in toxicologic emergencies, 214-215
Anectine
intubation and, 258-259
Antilirium
in toxicologic emergencies, 219-220
Apresoline
in cardiovascular emergencies, 113
Arm-a-char
in toxicologic emergencies, 213-214
Arm-a-Med
in respiratory emergencies, 164-165
Atarax
in behavior emergencies, 232

Atropine
in cardiovascular emergencies, 97-99
in toxicologic emergencies, 215-216

Benadryl
in anaphylactic emergencies, 204-205
Benylin
in anaphylactic emergencies, 204-205
Beta-2
in respiratory emergencies, 164-165
Betalin S
in metabolic emergencies, 177-179
Bisorine
in respiratory emergencies, 164-165
Brethaire
in respiratory emergencies, 167-168
Brethine
in respiratory emergencies, 167-168
Bretylium tosylate
in cardiovascular emergencies, 99-100
Bretylol
in cardiovascular emergencies, 99-100
Bricanyl
in respiratory emergencies, 167-168
Bronkosol
in respiratory emergencies, 164-165
Bumetadine
in cardiovascular emergencies, 100-101
Bumex
in cardiovascular emergencies, 100-101
Butorphanol
in cardiovascular emergencies, 101-102

Calan
in cardiovascular emergencies, 136-137
Calcium chloride
in cardiovascular emergencies, 102-103
Calcium gluceptate
in cardiovascular emergencies, 102-103
Calcium gluconate
in cardiovascular emergencies, 102-103

303

Intropin
  in cardiovascular emergencies, 106–107, 107t, 108
Isoetharine
  in respiratory emergencies, 164–165
Isoproterenol
  in cardiovascular emergencies, 114–115
Isoptin
  in cardiovascular emergencies, 136–137
Isuprel
  in cardiovascular emergencies, 114–116

Kabikinase
  in cardiovascular emergencies, 135–136

Labetalol
  in cardiovascular emergencies, 116–117
Lanoxin
  in cardiovascular emergencies, 104–105
Lasix
  in cardiovascular emergencies, 112
Levophed
  in cardiovascular emergencies, 128–129
Lidocaine
  in cardiovascular emergencies, 117–119
Lopressor
  in cardiovascular emergencies, 121–122
Luminal
  in neurologic emergencies, 188–189

Magnesium sulfate
  in cardiovascular emergencies, 119–120
  in obstetric and gynecologic emergencies, 197–198
Mannitol
  in neurologic emergencies, 187
Medrol
  in anaphylactic emergencies, 207–208
  in neurologic emergencies, 188
Meriperidine
  in cardiovascular emergencies, 120–121
Metaprel
  in respiratory emergencies, 165–166
Metaproterenol
  in respiratory emergencies, 165–166
Methylprednisolone
  in anaphylactic emergencies, 207–208
  in neurologic emergencies, 188
Metoprolol
  in cardiovascular emergencies, 121–122
MicroNEFRIN
  in respiratory emergencies, 163–164

Morphine
  in cardiovascular emergencies, 122–123

Nalbuphine
  in cardiovascular emergencies, 123–124
Naloxone
  in toxicologic emergencies, 217–218
Narcan
  in toxicologic emergencies, 217–218
Nifedipine
  in cardiovascular emergencies, 124–125
Nipride
  in cardiovascular emergencies, 126–127
Nitro-bid
  in cardiovascular emergencies, 125–126
Nitro-Dur
  in cardiovascular emergencies, 125–126
Nitroglycerin
  in cardiovascular emergencies, 125–126
Nitrol
  in cardiovascular emergencies, 125–126
Nitrolingual
  in cardiovascular emergencies, 125–126
Nitronox
  in cardiovascular emergencies, 127–128
Nitroprusside
  in cardiovascular emergencies, 126–127
Nitropress
  in cardiovascular emergencies, 126–127
Nitrostat
  in cardiovascular emergencies, 125–126
Nitrous oxide-oxygen mixture
  in cardiovascular emergencies, 127–128
Norepinephrine
  in cardiovascular emergencies, 128–129
Normodyne
  in cardiovascular emergencies, 116–117
Novolin
  in metabolic emergencies, 176–177
Nubain
  in cardiovascular emergencies, 123–124

Osmitrol
  in neurologic emergencies, 187
Oxygen
  in cardiovascular emergencies, 129–130
  in respiratory emergencies, 166–167
Oxytocin
  in obstetric and gynecologic emergencies, 198–199

306

Ventolin
  in respiratory emergencies, 160–161
Verapamil
  in cardiovascular emergencies, 136–137
Vistaril
  in behavior emergencies, 232

Vitamin B1
  in metabolic emergencies, 177–179

Xylocaine
  in cardiovascular emergencies, 117–119